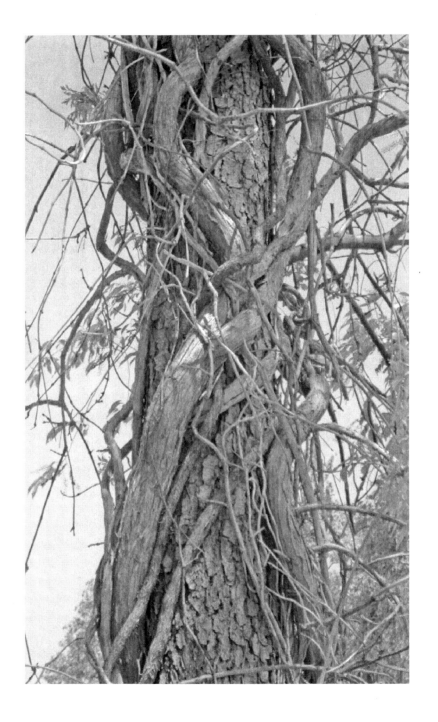

THE KNOWLEDGE OF GOOD & EVIL

THE HISTORICAL COVER-UP OF THE WORD "ABORTION" IN THE BIBLE

שכל

BY

JOSHUA COLLINS

χξς

THE KNOWLEDGE OF GOOD AND EVIL
The Historical Cover-up of the word 'Abortion' in the Bible
Copyright © 2008 by Joshua Collins

Library of Congress Control Number: 2008932725

> Collins, Joshua. 1980
> The Knowledge of Good and Evil
> ISBN 978-0-9801674-9-8
> Subject Codes and Description:
> 1: REL0006060; Religion- Biblical Study- OT
> 2: SOC 041000: Social Science- Abortion
> 3: HS022510: Historical Studies - Jews- Ancient

All rights reserved, including the right to reproduce this book or any part thereof in any form, except for inclusion of brief quotations in a review, without the written permission of the author and GlobalEdAdvance Press.

Printed in the United States of America

Published by
GlobalEdAdvancePress
37321-7635 USA

DEDICATION
HONOR

"... we speak of God's wisdom, secret and hidden, which God decreed before the ages for our glory," (I Corinthians 2:7).

This book is dedicated to serious readers.

Joshua Collins

Please feel free to contact me any time.
(630) 936-9602
JOSHUA.C273@YAHOO.COM

GENESIS
CHAPTER
III

"Every word of God is pure; He is a shield to those who put their trust in Him. Do not add to His words; lest He reprove you, and you be found a liar."
(Proverbs 30:5-6)

"Our sages submit, 'All the verses wherein are written indecent expressions, decent expressions are read in their stead.'"
(*Introduction to the Rabbinic Bible*, Jacob Ben Chajim Ibn Adonijah; p. 51)

"How can you say, 'We are wise, and the law of the Lord is with us,' when, in fact, the false pen of the Scribes has made it into a lie?"
(Jeremiah 8:8)

"For when he saw the captivity was prolonged... and the oral law to be much diminished, – he gathered and scraped up together all the decrees, statutes, and sayings of wise men..."
(*Commentary on the New Testament from the Talmud and Hebraica*, Lightfoot; Vol. 1, p. 161)

"Woe to you, scribes! For you have taken away the keys of knowledge; you did not enter, and those who were entering you hindered."
(Luke 11:52)

TABLE OF CONTENTS

Dedication
Acknowledgement

Structure: 16

Opening Words: 20

Introduction: 72

Disclaimer: 80

Section I: Quest: 96

Section II: The Lock: 152

Section III: A Garden, a Vineyard, or a Paradise?:   282

Conclusion: Drawing Near to the Beginning: 382

Notes:
  Opening words   391
  Section I   393
  Section II   397
  Section III   403

Edited by Rev. Dr. B. Hale, Rev. D. Kasik, & S. Rehanek

ACKNOWLEDGEMENT
PERSONAL DEBT

"Do not be wise in your own eyes; fear the Lord, and turn away from evil. It will be a healing for your flesh and refreshment for your body," (Proverbs 3:7-8).

It is my privilege to make known my debt concerning my small contribution to the pursuit of truth. It is my hope that the glory of Christ will be increased through this book. My first statement of debt is to the Savior, Christ the King. My second statement of debt is recorded in the list below that provides the works utilized for the composition of *The Knowledge of Good & Evil.*

BIBLES:
- The Archaeological Study Bible (NIV)
- The Authorized Version of the 1611 King James Bible
- **Biblia Rabbinica**, by Jacob Ben Chajim
- **The Companion Bible**, by Bullinger (King James, 1611)
- The Ginsburg Edition of The Hebrew Old Testament
- **The Interlinear Bible: Hebrew, Greek, English**, by Green
- J.P.S. Hebrew-English Tanakh
- The New American Standard Version of the Holy Bible
- The New International Version of the Holy Bible
- The New Revised Standard Version of the Holy Bible
- **The Peshitta Version of the Holy Bible**, translated by George M. Lamsa
- The Revised Standard Version of the Holy Bible
- The Septuagint Version of the Holy Bible
- The Stone Edition of the Tanakh

DICTIONARIES/CONCORDANCES:
- **The Analytical Hebrew and Chaldee Lexicon**, Davidson
- **The Analytical Lexicon to the Greek New Testament**, William D. Mounce
- **A Critical Lexicon and Concordance to the English and Greek New Testament**, by Bullinger
- **Dictionary of Biblical Interpretation**, John H. Hayes

- **The Exhaustive Dictionary of Bible Names**, Cornwall & Smith
- **Figures of Speech Used in the Bible**, Bullinger
- **A Greek-English Lexicon of the New Testament and other Early Christian Literature**, (Third Edition; Revised by Danker) based on the work of Bauer
- **The Hatch and Redpath Concordance to the Septuagint** (Second Edition)
- **The Strong's Exhaustive Concordance of the Bible**
- **Vine's Complete Expository Dictionary of Old and New Testament Words**
- **Webster's New World Hebrew Dictionary**
- **Webster's New World English Dictionary**

REFERENCES:

- **Babylonian Talmud**, Schottenstein Edition
- **The Complete Extant Works of Aeschylus**
- **Star Names**, Allen
- **Baal HaTurim Chumash:** (The Davis Edition), Baal HaTurim
- **The Book of Job**, Ball
- **Commentary on the New Testament Use of the Old Testament**, G.K. Beale & D.A. Carson
- **The Book of Job**, Bullinger
- **Commentary on Revelation**, Bullinger
- **The Divine names and Titles**, Bullinger
- **Great Cloud of Witnesses**, Bullinger
- **How to Enjoy the Bible**, Bullinger
- **The Knowledge of God**, Bullinger
- **The Names and the Order of the Books of the Old Testament**, Bullinger
- **Number in Scripture**, Bullinger

- **The Spirits in Prison**, Bullinger
- **The Transfiguration**, Bullinger
- **The Witness of the Stars**, Bullinger
- **Word Studies on the Holy Spirit**, Bullinger
- **The Ten Nequdoth of the Torah**, Butin
- **The Date and Death of Jesus of Nazareth**, Depuydt
- **The Mysteries of Creation**, Errico
- **The Five Millennium Canon of Solar Eclipses (NASA)**, Espenak & Meeus
- **The Complete Extant Works of Euripides**
- **The Illustrated Atlas of the Universe**, Garlick & Tirion
- **Gesenius' Hebrew Grammar**, Edited and Enlarged by E. Kautzsch
- **The Antiquity of the Hebrew Language**, Gill
- **Coheleth**, Ginsburg
- **The Essenes**, by Ginsburg
- **The Kabbalah**, Ginsburg
- **Introduction to the Massoretico-Critical Edition of the Hebrew Bible**, Ginsburg
- **Introduction to the Rabbinic Bible**, Jacob B. Chajim Ibn Adonijah (translated by Ginsburg)
- **Song of Songs**, Ginsburg
- **The Third Book of Moses called Leviticus**, Ginsburg
- **Egypt and the Books of Moses**, Hengstenberg
- **The Expositor's Bible**, Joseph
- **Commentary on the Old Testament**, Keil & Delitzsch
- **Massoreth Ha-Massoreth**, Levita
- **Commentary on the New Testament from the Talmud and Hebraica**, Lightfoot.
- **The Golden Ratio**, Mario Livio
- **Lectures on the Sacred Poetry of the Hebrews**, Robert Lowth

- **The Phoenicians**, Markoe
- **The Astronomy of the Bible**, Maunder
- **Starry Night Companion**, Mosley
- **The Biblical World: An Illustrated Atlas**, National Geographic
- **National Geographic Magazine**, October 2004
- **Classical Mythology**, Harris & Platzner
- **Scripture Parallels in Ancient Classics**, Ramage
- **Ramban (The Torah with Ramban's Commentary)**, Ramban
- **The Vine-Dresser's Manual: An Illustrated Treatise on Vineyards and Wine-Making**, Reemelin
- **Astronomy in the Old Testament**, by Schiaparelli
- **Interlinear Chumash:** (The Schottenstein Edition)
- **The Treasury of David**, by Spurgeon
- **The Revision of the English Version of the New Testament**, by Lightfoot, Trench & Ellicott
- **The Complete Dead Sea Scrolls**, translated by Geza Vermes
- **The Old Testament: Its Formation and Development**, by Weiser
- **The Book of Koheleth**, by Wright

STRUCTURE
THE DESIGN OF THIS BOOK

All of the literature that precedes Section III (page 282) is arranged as a preparatory tutorial system designed to provide the reader with the information necessary to understand the assertions of Section III regarding abortion in the Bible. The design of this book was devised so that the reader is not allotted the burden of making connections for this book, but that the book makes the connections for the reader. Section III utilizes its entirety to display the development and consequences of history's

first abortion as recorded in Scripture.

The Knowledge of Good & Evil is organized into rubrics. The rubric-style in which the text forwards its assertions is provided for the reader in an effort to aid reference and absorption. For instance, Section 1 Rubric 8 is indicated in this way: [1.8]. The rubric style is also provided so that the reader may ponder a particular point in isolation as easily as the reader may consider a collection of connected assertions. The reader may comfortably cease reading at the termination of a given rubric as easily as one would otherwise cease reading at the end of a given chapter.

The message of this book you are reading is told by way of a simple narrative, a story formed by a historical mystery whose figuration became ensconced in the dusty halls of erosive memory and oral tradition. The reader of *The Knowledge of Good & Evil* needs no knowledge of any language besides English. Non-English examples found within this text are merely supplements accompanied by *Strong's Exhaustive Concordance* reference numbers, and these examples are provided for the English reader in case the reader wishes to check against any assertion forwarded in this text. *Strong's Exhaustive Concordance* reference numbers will appear in this way: (ref. 888) and (ref. *888*). The first example (ref. 888) is not italicized and signifies Hebrew and Chaldee references. The second example (ref. *888*) is italicized and signifies Greek references. All references to non-English words are strictly products of dictionary and concordance definitions; the author takes no liberties with any of these references, though thematic connections are given in brackets so that the reader is aware of an inclusion by the author. The part of speech concerning each non-English word in this text will be apparent by the dictionary definitions provided. Dictionary definitions are used in this text to describe the CONCEPT and ESSENCE of each word so as not to burden the reader by repeatedly writing, "verb," "noun," etc.

In some cases, the diction definitions of *E.W. Bullinger's Critical Lexicon and Concordance to the English and Greek New Testament*, *Vine's Complete Expository Dictionary of Old and New Testament Words*, *The Davidson Analytical Hebrew and Chaldee Dictionary*, *The Analytical Lexicon to the Greek New Testament*, and *The Brown-Driver-Briggs Hebrew and English Lexicon* are used in conjunction with *Strong's Exhaustive Concordance* definitions. *Strong's Exhaustive Concordance* definitions are used almost exclusively in this text because *Strong's* reference numbers allow the reader with no experience in Hebrew, Chaldee, or Greek to locate the definitions of the non-English words quickly if the reader chooses to check against the assertions of this text. Furthermore, all literary references will be provided within this text so that the reader will never be forced into the position of merely accepting the author's assertions without being equipped personally with the ability to validate this body of information.

On account of the many Bible translations utilized within *The Knowledge of Good & Evil*, the reader will notice that one passage of Scripture may be quoted more than once, and in these multiple quotations, the English quotations may differ slightly. *The Knowledge of Good &*

Evil attempts to maneuver around the discrepancies of English by providing more than one translation to facilitate its assertions. However, the original Biblical languages are relied upon because of the fact that various English translations supply extra words, that do not occur in the Bible, in an attempt to give the sense of difficult passages. In conjunction with the many English translations used within this book, there are no alterations in any of the quotations (Biblical or otherwise) used within this text beyond what can be effected by a change in the character of the type (bold letters, italics, all capital letters, etc.). End-notes, indicated within this text in this way: [#], are found following the conclusion of this book.

Let us now exhume the great Aposiopesis.

OPENING WORDS
PREFACE

"Behold, I stand at the door and knock: if any man hear My voice, and open the door, I will come in to him, and will sup with him, and he with Me," (Revelation 3:20).

[i. 1]   The goal of this text is to examine only one chapter of the Bible: Genesis Chapter III, the story of lost innocence. In this book, Genesis Chapter III will be studied by utilizing many corresponding Scriptures from both the Old Testament and the New Testament in order to show parallel themes, words, and concepts. Though it may seem that this text jumps rapidly through the Bible, each Scriptural and historical example is set in the sequence of the theme under discussion in order to examine Genesis Chapter III. Of the many corresponding Scripture passages and historical quotations utilized within this book, only one definite conclusion is drawn, and this determination is summarized and restated in the "Conclusion" section at the end of this book where all of this book's contents are explained plainly in one paragraph.

As a multitude of references in Scripture point to Genesis Chapter III, it is useful to examine those related accounts also in order to grasp a more complete picture of the speedily stated events of Adam and Eve. In short, the manner of investigation used in this book is similar to studying a tree from the lowest point of its root-system to its tallest branch, and then returning to that root-system in order to draw a conclusion; the Bible's internal design is more than adequate for such a task, and as such, a host of historical explanations are viewed alongside the Biblical narrative in an effort to provide the reader with an array of support regarding this Biblical investigation. The reader can be assured that even when seemingly remote Biblical passages are quoted, the perspective of this book never shifts away from Eden's garden, its inhabitants, and the lessons provided therein.

This text attempts to loosen the knots of forgotten history and to help unriddle the dark intricacies that have separated those fractions of people who would otherwise join hands in camaraderie. This book is written to inspire you to advance beyond what research is provided here so that, in a collective effort of faithful camaraderie and peaceful unity, we may separate fact from fable and lucidity from legend. The story of Eden is the first point in history where error passed into humanity, and it is this point (connected with its historically consequential ramifications) that Christ came to rectify. This text is but a beginning mark meant to invigorate you with passion past what has been inexplicably assumed by hazy traditions of which few attempt to sift but of which many attempt to mandate as fact. For instance, it has been stated that the Holy Bible never discusses the topic of abortion, though the very word "abortion" is used more than once, in both the Old Testament and the New Testament, with explicit applications, as we will soon investigate.

> "It is the glory of Elohim to conceal a thing: but the honor of kings is to search out a matter," (Proverbs 25:2).

[i.2]   The New Testament accounts are mirrors of the Old Testament accounts. We can understand that any tear in a garment's collar is not sewn up on the garment's sleeve, but on the tear itself from where the tear ends to where it begins (compare Luke 1:17 to Malachi 4:6). The Greek New Testament is not a mere continuation of the Hebrew Old Testament. The Greek New Testament is the grand fulfillment of the Hebrew Old Testament that shines as face-to-face with its Hebrew origin. The Greek

New Testament serves as the textual elucidation of the meaning of the Hebrew Old Testament beyond the oral law and the traditional rendering(s) of the Old Testament. Both Testaments are exquisitely terse, yet incisively precise, as they both are united by a wellspring that flows from a common source of antiquity still present today and in the same strength as yesteryear.

[i.3] The narrative of the Bible is a braid of joy and sorrow, a weaving of which the extremities of its Canon begin and end tied to joy. The entire Torah extends from Genesis 1-3, the Prophets and the Writings extend from the Torah, and the New Testament clutches every branch of the Old Testament and allows the reader to peer backward into the mysterious root of the Scriptural accounts so that the end of one's blooming pursuits for truth lead to the beginning of one's eternally fruitful bliss. Wading through the words of Eden is a tearful deluge of shock, horror, and devastation, but it is beneficial to remember that salty water does not proceed from the same surge as fresh water. Eden's wellspring is a sublime outpouring of surprise and elation that became overwhelmed with stinging tears.

[i.4] Through the prophet Isaiah we learn that Satan's fall from perfection came about because he desired to be "like the Most High," (Isaiah 14:14); how hair-splitting this desire was! The Most High God is entirely righteous, and the desire to be righteous should certainly be our desire as well: "...You shall be holy, for I the Lord your God am holy," (Leviticus 19:2); "Be perfect, therefore, as your heavenly Father is perfect," (Matthew 5:48). However,

Satan lusted to be "like the Most High" in power as well – a dire mistake that expelled him from the splendors of the heavenly Paradise (as we may read of in Ezekiel 28:11-19).

Satan forsook the free gift of God's love and attempted to steal God's throne, and as such, there was no longer a place for Satan, the "Dragon," found in Heaven (Revelation 12:8). We cannot help but notice some peculiarities in the description of this "Dragon" who was cast down, as it is written, "The great dragon was thrown down, that ancient serpent, who is called the Devil and Satan, the deceiver of the whole world – he was thrown down to the earth, and his angels were thrown down with him," (Revelation 12:9); it does not say that Satan, the "dragon" (or serpent) was cast down to hell, but that he was cast down to the earth; it does not say that he became recognized as a "dragon" (or serpent) after he fell, but that he was recognized as such before he fell to the earth. "How you have fallen from heaven, O morning star, son of the dawn! You have been cast down to the earth..." (Isaiah 14:12). The first story we have of Satan, in the order of the Sacred Canon, calls Satan a "serpent" in Genesis 3:1. As to the chronology of Satan's description in Revelation 12, we might consider that Joshua's death is described in Joshua 24:29 and Judges 1:1, but that he is recounted again, alive, in Judges 2:6-7, and his death is stated again in Judges 2:8; we might also reflect on the flash-back of Mark 6 regarding John the Baptist, etc. Biblical pattern often differs from what we call "chronological." Considering the "serpent" called "Satan," the "dragon" of Revelation 12, perhaps we might better understand the concept of a "serpent" or "dragon" by considering the angels of Isaiah 6, the famous "Seraphs."

The word "Seraph" means "fiery serpent," but the Seraphs in Isaiah 6 are righteous, not wicked. These "fiery serpents," the angelic Seraphs, are described as having six wings (Isaiah 6:2); our common English term for a winged, fiery serpent is "dragon," and so it is clear that the concept of a "dragon" or a "serpent" cannot automatically indicate evil: "...therefore be wise as serpents and pure as doves," (Matthew 10:16) – notice the combination of *serpents* and *wings* (wings being signified by the "*doves*"). Whatever the truest signification of a "dragon" may be as intended by the Scriptures, particularly for the sake of righteousness, is mysterious. However, the conceptual imagery of a "dragon," with respect to *death*, is preserved in part by the celestial mappings of the *autumnal* equinox near 2,700 B.C. (as we will discover in Rubric 2.35). Interestingly enough, the Egyptians called guardian griffins "Serref," (*Brown-Driver-Briggs Hebrew and English Lexicon*, p. 976). We might also take notice of Isaiah 14:29, "Do not rejoice, all you Philistines, that the rod that struck you is broken, from the root of the snake will come forth an adder, and its fruit will be a flying fiery serpent": here we have a description of a "root," a "snake," an "adder," "fruit," and a "flying fiery serpent." When we consider the imagery of a "root," a "snake" and "fruit," it is difficult to avoid Ezekiel 15: "The word of Jehovah was to me, saying, 'Son of man, how is the vine-tree more than any other tree, or than a branch that is among the trees of the forest? Shall wood be taken from it to do work? Or will men take from it to do work? Or will men take from it for a peg to hang every vessel on it? Behold, it is put in the fire for fuel. Both its ends the fire devours, and its middle is charred. Will it prosper for work? Behold, when it was whole it was not made for work. How much less when the fire has devoured it, and it is charred! Shall it yet be made to work? Therefore, so says the Lord Jehovah: As the vine-tree among the trees of the forest, which I have given it to the fire for fuel, so I will give the dwellers of Jerusalem. And I will set my face against them. They shall go out from the fire, and the fire shall devour them. And you shall know that I am Jehovah when I set My face against them. And I will give the land to be desolate, because they have done a treacherous act, declares the Lord Jehovah.'"

D. Kimchi paraphrased the sense of Ezekiel 15 concerning the "vine-tree" to mean, "I do not ask thee concerning the vine that bears fruit (for so it ought to be accounted), but concerning the branch which is amongst the trees of the wood, unfruitful, even as the trees themselves are," (*Commentary on the New Testament from the Talmud and Hebraica,* Lightfoot, Vol. 3; p. 403)

Ezekiel 15 refers to a wild vine as a "tree," and if we consider this terminology along with Isaiah 14:29 ("the rod that struck you is broken, from the root of the snake will come forth an adder, and its fruit will be a flying fiery serpent") perhaps we understand more of the account of Paul in Acts 28:3-5: "Paul had gathered a bundle of brushwood and was putting it on the fire, when a viper, driven out by the heat, fastened itself on his hand... He, however, shook off the creature into the fire and suffered no harm." Consider again Deuteronomy 32:32-33:

"Their vine comes from the vinestock of *Sodom* [*Flaming; Burning*], from the vineyards of *Gomorrah* [*Rebellious People*]; their grapes are grapes of poison, their clusters are bitter; their wine is the poison of Serpents, the cruel venom of asps." In a similar way, II Kings 4:32-37 tells us this story: "When Elisha returned to Gilgal, there was a famine in the land. As the company of prophets was sitting before him, he said to his servant, 'Put the large pot on, and make some stew for the company of prophets.' One of them went out into the field to gather herbs; he found a wild vine and gathered from it a lapful of wild gourds, and came and cut them up into the pot of stew, not knowing what they were. They served some for the men to eat. But while they were eating the stew, they cried out, 'O man of God, there is death in the pot!'" (II Kings 4:38-40).

Wild vines, which grow onto trees, are to be distinguished from vines used for wine-grapes; however, the Essenes used related imagery when discussing people and their actions: "The serpents are the kings of the peoples and their wine is their ways," (*The Complete Dead Sea Scrolls: Damascus Document*, Vermes; p. 136). When we think of the "serpent" of Genesis 3:1 in Eden, it is beneficial to note that the Hebrew word for this "serpent" is "נחש" (ref. 5175) which is, essentially, the same name as "Nachash" the Ammonite of I Samuel 11:1 who said, "...I will make a treaty with you, namely that I gouge out everyone's right eye, and thus put disgrace upon all Israel"; the "serpent" of Genesis 3 promised the woman, "...your eyes will be opened..." (Genesis 3:5). Obviously, Nachash the Ammonite was not in the garden of Eden with Adam, but, equally as obvious, the Scriptures contain no futile words, as each account of the Torah stems from Genesis 1-3, the Prophets and the Writings extend from the Torah, and the New Testament clutches every branch of the Old Testament and allows the reader to peer backward into the mysterious root of the Scriptures.

[i.5] Righteousness is mightier than wickedness; yet, good and evil can focus on the same subject. A given subject can have both positive and negative applications. For instance, steroids can be administered to an accident victim in order to help restore a damaged limb to promote the recovery process, or steroids can be taken recreationally to the point of one's own demise. A chemist can help heal someone, or a chemist can aid in a person's destruction. A solider can defend the weak with his superior strength, or a soldier can oppress the weak with his superior strength. Jesus described Himself as a serpent in John 3:14; Satan is referred to as a "serpent" in Genesis 3:1. Jesus described Himself as, "the bright Morning Star" in Revelation 22:1; Satan is referred to as "morning star" in Isaiah 14:12. Jesus said, "Behold, I come like a thief..." in Revelation 16:15; Jesus said of Satan, "The thief comes only to steal and kill and destroy" in John 10:10. Jesus is described as a "lion" in Revelation 5:5; Satan is described as a "lion" in I Peter 5:8.

"And the Lord sent fiery serpents [*nacheshim seraphim*] among the People, and they bit the People; and many people of Israel died. Therefore the People came to Moses, and said, 'We have sinned, for we have spoken against the Lord, and against thee; pray unto the Lord, that He take away the serpents from us.' And Moses prayed for the People. And the Lord said to Moses, 'Make thee a *fiery serpent* [*seraph*], and set it upon a pole: and it shall come to pass, that every one that is bitten, when he looketh upon it, shall live.' And Moses made a *serpent* [*nachash*] of brass, and put it upon a pole, and it came to pass, that if a serpent had bitten any man, when he beheld the serpent of brass, he lived," (Numbers 21:6-9). "And just as Moses lifted up the serpent in the wilderness, so must the Son of Man be lifted up, that whoever believes in Him may not perish but may have eternal life. For God so loved the world that He gave His only Son, so that everyone who believes in Him may not perish but may have eternal life," (John 3:14-16). Before the Dragon was cast from Heaven, he was called the "signet of perfection," (Ezekiel 28:11), but he became a "profane thing," (Ezekiel 28:16). The serpent on the pole that Moses constructed was used for righteous purposes initially, but after Moses' death, it became used for idolatrous purposes and had to be destroyed (II Kings 18:4); this brazen serpent was called "*Nehushtan*" that some define as "A Brass Thing," (*Companion Bible*, Bullinger; p. 516), and that others define as "Brazen; Enchanted" (*The Exhaustive Dictionary of Bible Names*, Cornwall & Smith; p 183); in either case, this brazen work became thought of as being "enchanted" and was therefore destroyed accordingly.

[i.6]   Satan's fatal desire was to be like God in power, and since he could not be like God in the manner he desired, he attempts to fool us today into thinking that he is like God, through confusion based on our own desires: "You will not surely die; for God knows that when you eat of it your eyes will be opened, and you will be like God, knowing good and evil," (Genesis 3:4-5). Satan is a counterfeiter, which is why the greatest sins can appear initially in the guise of righteousness. God is all righteous, but Satan is all evil. "God is light," (I John 1:5), but "...Satan disguises himself as an angel of light," (II Corinthians 11:13-14). The Psalmist asked in righteousness, "Open my eyes, so that I may behold wondrous things out of Your Law," (Psalm 119:18); Satan promised the woman, "...your eyes will be opened..." to her own demise.

In a disturbing way, descriptions of Satan are close to descriptions of God at times, though Satan is exactly opposite of God, and Satan is far weaker than God. There is a Christ, and there is an antichrist. In order for there to be an "anti" anything, there must first be a thing. Goodness is the standard, but evil is a parasite. In Genesis 2:9, the Tree of Life is named before the "Tree" of the Knowledge of Good and Evil is named. Jesus said, "I am the TRUE vine..." (John 15:1) – we may consider the opposite of this statement. "So we are ambassadors for Christ, since God is making His appeal through us; we entreat you on behalf of Christ, be reconciled to God. For our sake He made Him to be sin Who knew no sin, so that in Him we might become the righteousness of God," (II Corinthians 5:20-21).

[i.7]   The words of the Greek New Testament have been sharply debated as somehow being at variance with teachings of the Hebrew Scriptures – a false claim that has split those whose union would otherwise prove more than fruitful. Let us take account of Revelation 19:13, as it says that Jesus' Name is called "The Word of God," that is, "The *Logos* of God." When we recall the creation account in Genesis 1&2, we remember that is was by the Word that creation was brought into existence, and as such, we cannot ignore the inspired writer who wrote:

"In the beginning was the *Word* [*Logos*], and the *Word* [*Logos*] was with God, and the *Word* [*Logos*] was God. He was in the beginning with God. All things came into being through Him, and without Him not one thing came into being," (John 1:1-3).

Jesus, connected to the plural Name "Elohim" (the Creator), is identified as the "Word" [*Logos*] in John 1:1-3, and the specific term used for "Word" here serves a peculiar function in sifting through the shadows of Eden. We must distinguish between the Greek terms "*logos*" = "word," and "*rhema*" = "word." "There is a difference between the two: λογος (logos), generally speaking, is taken as meaning a word as made up of letters; and ρημα (rhema), a saying as made up of words," (*How to Enjoy the Bible, Bullinger,* p. 183). The word "logos" is sometimes used in the sense of a "formula" {1} or "computation" {2}.

[i.8] The ancients used tablets covered in dust for purposes of calculation that allowed for quick writing and erasing. God made trees "out of the ground," (Genesis 2:9), and God made every beast of the field and every fowl of the air "out of the ground," (Genesis 2:19). However, according to Genesis 2:7, Jehovah Elohim made Adam

32   The Knowledge of Good and Evil

"from the dust of the ground," and we see the connection to God as the great artificer of creation, calculating the substance and function of all things by specific designs to function in particular, yet connected ways, as He makes clear in Job 38 (Job being the oldest Book of Scripture). God created by the Word (Who is God), through meticulous computation, and there was a special emphasis placed on the creation of humanity.

[i.9]   The notion of "computation" regarding the words of the Bible can often prove to be a foreign concept to many Bible-readers as they pour through the Text with the aid of the useful chapter and verse divisions. However, the Hebrew Bible, in which the story of Adam and Eve is found, was not stamped with chapter or verse divisions originally, but only became so marked after time. "The Hebrew Scriptures in manuscript have no division into chapters at all. The text is divided into sections, of which there are no less than 669 in the Pentateuch [*Torah*]. The book of Leviticus has ninety-eight of these sections while in our Authorized Version it has only twenty-seven chapters. The divisions into chapters, now to be found in the Hebrew Bibles, were adopted in the fourteenth century by the Jews from the Christians for polemical purposes, and the figures attached to each verse are of a still later period," (*Leviticus*, Ginsburg; p. 35).

The divisions of the Hebrew Bible have a curious number with respect to the Torah that is far from random. The ancient Scribes were called the "Sopherim," that is, "The Numberers." "Indeed, the first original word סופרים [*Sopherim*] did more peculiarly signify the numberers... [so called] because they numbered all the letters of the law: for they said ו (vau) was the middle letter in the whole book of the law," (*Commentary on the New Testament from the Talmud and Hebraica,* Lightfoot, Volume 3; p. 98). The concept of Biblical number has been long-lost in much current Christian Biblical study with the exception of a very few obscure works that, I must personally admit, have the tendency to become inadvertently fanciful, though they are well-intentioned, honest attempts aimed towards understanding a complex topic. There are some extant works on the subject of Biblical number that are more admirable and scientific than others and that wield a very respectable amount of true scholarship {3}. However, when considering the 669 divisions of the Torah, one cannot escape the fact that Hebrew letters are also numbers, and that it is for this reason that the Hebrew Bible was divided as such as is seen in the design sealed by the Scribes. That is, the letter-as-number system of Scripture is not by any means "Numerology," but rather a linguistic formula of a precision beyond the structure of, say, English.

Language is, essentially, mathematical as grammarians will attest to this fact, for there is a strict formula necessary for one language to be distinguished from another. The mathematical components of languages are not codes, but these components are standards that define language systems as independently functioning programs of communication. To a much higher extent, the Bible is written in a system where each letter of a given word is also a number, and the addition of the letter/numbers of a word (or words) computes to a total number that defines a word (or words) and connects words thematically so that individual accounts are revealed to be bound by a common thread – for Scriptural accounts are not a development of individual experiences, but Scriptural accounts are components of a cohesive whole illustrated cyclically throughout time: "What has been is what will be, and what has been done is what will be done; there is nothing new under the sun," (Ecclesiastes 1:9). The ancient Scribes were certainly numberers. The letter-number formula of the Bible is called "gematria," and the gematriaos of the Bible led the ancient Scribes to divide the Torah into its 669 divisions.

Again, *The Knowledge of Good & Evil* requires only a command of English so as not to impose any burdens on the reader. This text has also sought to never leave the reader in the unwanted position of merely accepting an assertion without personally scrutinizing it first; therefore the number-system called "Gematria" is provided. Simply put, each letter of the Hebrew alphabet corresponds with a number so that it may be understood that the words of Scripture are made up of numbers:

Hebrew

(א) = 1	(י) = 10	(ק) = 100
(ב) = 2	(כ) = 20	(ר) = 200
(ג) = 3	(ל) = 30	(ש) = 300
(ד) = 4	(מ) = 40	(ת) = 400
(ה) = 5	(נ) = 50	(ך) = 500 or 20
(ו) = 6	(ס) = 60	(ם) = 600 or 40
(ז) = 7	(ע) = 70	(ן) = 700 or 50
(ח) = 8	(פ) = 80	(ף) = 800 or 80
(ט) = 9	(צ) = 90	(ץ) = 900 or 90

Again, the letter-number formula of the Bible is called "gematria," and this formula was significant to the ancient Scribes when they divided the Torah into its 669 divisions. That is, "gematriaos" = "גמטריאות" = "ת+ו+א+י+ר+ט+מ+ג" = 400+6+1+10+200+9+40+3 = **669**. The Bible was written by a specific formula, and recognized as such, the Bible was divided accordingly by the Scribes (the Numberers) who preserved the sacred Text. Unfortunately, Gematria has often been mistaken as Numerology, and such a mistake has led to the abandonment of Gematria as a main-stream discipline of study for many. Gematria has been obscured even further by auxiliary and inflated "rules" imposed upon the study of number that allow for a more than liberal manipulation of Biblical number in an attempt to justify various assertions.

[i.10] The author of this book is staunchly opposed to Numerology, for Numerology is but the parasite of Gematria in the same way that Astrology is the parasite of Astronomy. Unfortunately, Christians largely abandoned both Gematria and Astronomy because of these respective disciplines' promiscuous misuses that fell into occult pursuits; because of the degeneration to which these closely related disciplines became subject, even the greatest Church fathers were often denied such knowledge. Gematria is sometimes regarded as Numerology, though what is meant by such a regard is that Numerology sometimes utilizes the rules of Gematria: "One special version of numerology is the Jewish Gematria (possibly based on 'geometrical number' in Greek), or its Muslim and Greek analogues, known as Khisab al Jumal ('calculating the total'), and Isopsephy (from Greek 'isos,' equal, and 'psephizein,' to count), respectively. In these systems, numbers are assigned to each letter of the alphabet... By adding together the values of the constituent letters, numbers are then associated with words or even entire phrases. Gematria was especially popular in the system of Jewish mysticism practiced mainly from the thirteenth to the eighteenth century know as cabala. Hebrew scholars sometimes used to amaze listeners by calling out a series of apparently random numbers for some ten minutes and then repeating the series without an error. This feat was accomplished simply by translating some passage of the Hebrew scriptures into the language of Gematria," (*The Golden Ratio*, Livio; p. 22). The "gematria" discussed above is numerology, a parasitic system that employed the rules of Gematria for purposes outside of its design. Gematria, as it was intended to be recognized, is not a component of mysticism, nor was its design intended to be imposed artificially. Gematria is not numerology, but numerology can employ the rules of gematria. The host is pure, but the parasite is impure. Livio did not make an errant statement, but rather, Livio defined the abuses of Gematria, as we should all avoid such abuses. On account of the gross misapplications of the parasite, the host was widely rejected. (As far as the word "gematria" being based on "'geometrical number' in Greek," *The Ginsburg Edition of the Hebrew Bible* notes that "γεωμετρια" = "גמטריא" = "gematria" on p. 26.)

[i.11] The struggle of Good vs. Evil is often fueled by a single question: "What did God say?" – as this struggle often concerns how God's Word is observed, perceived, and obeyed, and thus compels one to make judgments (errant or accurate) regarding what is permissible. The very first temptation began not with a lie, but with a simple question: "Did God say, 'You shall not eat from any tree in the garden?'" (Genesis 3:1), and this question brought rise to an attempt to rationalize that which is irrational, as (regardless of English) Satan mentioned nothing of the "fruit" that the woman was contemplating in Genesis 3:2, and neither did God mention anything of "fruit" in His command to Adam in Genesis 2:17, for this "fruit" was the subject of the woman's desire (Genesis 3:16 in connection with Genesis 1:28-29): "But one is tempted by one's own desire, being lured and enticed by it; then, when that desire has conceived, it gives birth to sin, and that sin, when it is fully grown, gives birth to death," (James 1:14). "Desire" is often the most expedient vehicle of sin. The woman (named "Eve" after her sin and the subsequent judgments of God), was punished in this way: "...I will greatly increase your pangs in childbearing: in pain you shall bring forth children, yet your desire shall be for your husband, and he shall rule over you," (Genesis 3:16).

The human mistakes of Eden began with the premise that humanity possessed the capability of determining the utmost rationale beyond the framework of the Word of God, and the first human error came by humanity's knack for inflating the Holy Word of God as yeast makes dough rise. "...*Bread* is very frequently used in the Jewish writers for *doctrine*," (*Commentary on the New Testament from the Talmud and Hebraica*, Lightfoot, Vol. 3; p. 307-308). Jesus called Himself the "Bread of Life" (John 6:35). As "knowledge" is defined by acquisition (whereas "wisdom" is defined by application) the first humans wanted a knowledge of which the acquisition thereof proved to be an unwise possession. Ironically, for having eaten of the Tree of the Knowledge [not "wisdom"] of Good and Evil, God punished Adam in this way: "...Because you have listened to the voice of your wife, and have eaten of the tree about which I commanded you, 'You shall not eat of it,' cursed is the ground because of you; in toil you shall eat of it all the days of your life; thorns and thistles it shall bring forth for you; and you shall eat the plants of the field. By the sweat of your face you shall eat *bread* until you return to the ground, for out of it you were taken; you are dust, and to dust you shall return," (Genesis 3:17-19).

Adam was to eat bread by the sweat of his face until he returned to the ground. Interestingly enough, consider the words of Job regarding the pursuit of wisdom: "Miners put an end to darkness, and search out to the farthest bound the ore in gloom and deep darkness. They open shafts in a valley away from human habitation; they are forgotten by travelers, they sway suspended, remote from people. As for the earth out of it comes *bread*; but underneath it is turned up as by fire. Its stones are the place of sapphires, and its dust contains gold. The path no bird of prey knows, and the falcon's eye has not seen it. The proud wild animals have not trodden it; the lion has not passed over it. They put their hand to the flinty rock, *and overturn mountains by the roots.* They cut channels in the rocks, and their eyes see every precious thing. The sources of the rivers they probe; hidden things they bring to light. But where shall *wisdom* be found? And where is the place of understanding?" (Job 28:3-12).

The common expression of "uprooting mountains" or "overturning mountains" was used to describe the removal of difficulties, as a great teacher was called a "rooter up of mountains," hence our Savior's words: "Truly I tell you, if you have faith and do not doubt, not only will you do what has been done to the fig tree, but even if you say to this mountain, 'Be lifted up and thrown into the sea,' it will be done," (Matthew 21:21). Accordingly, Proverbs 3:5-6 states, "Trust in the Lord with all your heart; and lean not unto your own understanding. In all your ways acknowledge Him, and He shall direct your paths." Love for God entwined with faith in God allows wisdom to take root in a person, and such wisdom can uproot mountains that are immovable by one's own understanding apart from God. "And though I have the gift of prophecy, and *understand all mysteries and all knowledge*, and though I have all faith, so that I could *remove mountains*, and have not love, I am nothing," (I Corinthians 13:2).

Proverbs 3:13-18 calls "Wisdom" a "tree of life": "Happy are those who find wisdom, and those who get understanding, for her income is better than silver, and her revenue better than gold. She is more precious than jewels, and nothing you desire can compare with her. Long life is in her right hand; in her left hand are riches and honor. Her ways are the ways of pleasantness, and all her paths are peace. She is a tree of life to those who lay hold of her; those who hold her fast are called happy,"

If "Wisdom" is "a tree of life," how then, regarding the forbidden tree, could it have been that when the woman looked at "the tree," she saw that it was "to be desired to make one wise," when eating of it was the most foolish mistake in human history? Furthermore, why does she not specifically qualify which tree was under discussion in her conversation with Satan (Genesis 3:3) when she said, "the tree that is in the middle of the garden"? – for Genesis 2:9 informs us that both principle "trees" were in the garden's middle. Why also does she inflate God's word, like yeast in dough, by discussing "fruit," and the act of "touching" the tree?

Consider the Torah, the Law, the Books of "Moses" in light of the word "dough":

"Moses" = "משה" (ref. 4872) = "ה+ש+מ" = 5+300+40 = **345**

"dough" = "עריסה" (ref. 6182) = "ה+ס+י+ר+ע" = 5+60+10+200+70 = **345**

In Luke 12:1-2, Jesus said, "Be on your guard against the yeast of the Pharisees, which is hypocrisy. Nothing is covered up that will not be uncovered, and nothing is secret that will not become known." As the religious elites of Christ's earthly days inflated the laws of Moses similar to yeast in dough, Christ's identification of Phariseeism's follies is piercingly apparent.

[i.12] Knowledge is defined by acquisition, but wisdom is defined by application. Humanity sought the heights of wisdom from a source of knowledge that led to folly. "Does a spring pour forth from the same opening both fresh and brackish water? Can a fig tree, my brothers and sisters, yield olives, or a grape-vine figs? No more can salt water yield fresh," (James 3:11-12). As such, we cannot ignore this enigmatic Scripture:

"How can you say, 'We are wise, and the law of the Lord is with us,' when, in fact, the false pen of the Scribes has made it into a lie?"(Jeremiah 8:8).

Where can we find evidence of this false pen? Where in the law of the Lord did the Scribes transmit lies? This text does not mean to imply that the true story of Scripture is somehow altogether different from what we know, or that it is even altogether metaphorical. This text does not contend that the Scriptures are flawed – by no means! What this text does affirm is that each portion of Scripture is connected within a multi-layered system similar to an onion. No matter how many layers of an onion one peels away, whatever layer is underneath is still just as much a part of that onion; the onion never "changes," but rather provokes more tears as one digs deeper into it. This text also affirms that the Old Testament contains numerous places that the Scribes deliberately altered and that this information is not secret to Jews as the Scribes themselves catalogued most of their "emendations" to be read by successive Scribes. The New Testament specifically addresses these alterations and exposes the motivations behind the choices of the Scribes so that our Bibles today serve as both a lock and a key connected to the mystery of time itself. By the New Testament's respective addresses regarding the Scriptural manipulations of the Scribes, we can begin to understand the immense threat that Christ innocently posed to the Sanhedrin by His adherence to the Torah – which is the reason that the Sanhedrin wanted to remove Him from a position of influence over the commoners, lest their own misconduct be openly exposed.

[i.13] The computation of Biblical words is apparent when one reads through a Biblical Lexicon, as these lexicons often begin indicating a given letter of the alphabet by listing the letter's numeric equivalent before relating all of the following words that begin with that given letter. The numbers of the Bible and their computations are not esoteric, for they are merely overlooked and forgotten. The numbers are no secret to those prone to use a dictionary. The information you are about to read may seem altogether new, but it is actually ancient.

[i.14] The Hebrew language originally lacked vowels, and the current system affixed to it, for the purposes of specificity, is an extremely helpful teaching tool. At the same time, we cannot help but notice a relationship between words of differing parts of speech that carry differing definitions when these differing words, even those of differing parts of speech, are composed of the exact same consonants (particularly in the exact same order); this facet of the Hebrew language was preserved by its numeric system. In other words, terms composed of the same consonantal spelling, but that have different vowels, compute to the same number to show parallel ideas and concepts. "Many of these roots represent theological, moral, and ceremonial concepts that have been obscured by the passage of time..." (*Vine's Expository Dictionary of Old and New Testament Words*, Forward – Introduction).

Opening Words 43

As we read the New Testament along with the Old Testament, we also cannot help but notice an unyielding congruence of the respective accounts between the two Testaments. The terminology of the New Testament, specifically as it applies to the attributes of a given entity, can seem arcane and cryptic, but they are not random, and the system by which they are employed is beyond beautiful. Gematria illustrates terse thematic relation. Let us examine a few Hebrew words and their definitions:

"*naw-khash*" = "נחש" (ref. 5172) = "to hiss, whisper a (magic) spell, to prognosticate, enchanter, diligently observe, learn by experience"

"*nakh-ash*" = "נחש" (ref. 5173) = "an incantation, augury, enchantment"

"*naw-khawsh*" (from ref. 5172) = "נחש" (ref. 5175) = "a serpent"

These three words have distinct pronunciations that determine the meanings of the spelling "נחש" to communicate the definitions above. In other words, each term is its own word, but all three of these terms are spelled with the exact same consonants in the exact same order. The number-system (Gematria) that the Scriptures contain shows us that, regardless of how each respective word above is pronounced, all three words indicate the same number of 358.

"*naw-khash*" = "נחש" (ref. 5172) = "נ+ח+ש" = 300+8+50 = **358**

"*nakh-ash*" = "נחש" (ref. 5173) = "נ+ח+ש" = 300+8+50 = **358**

"*naw-khawsh*" (from ref. 5172) = "נחש" (ref. 5175) = "ש+ח+נ" = 300+8+50 = **358**

In more explanatory terms:
"naw-khash" = "נחש" (ref. 5172) = "to hiss, whisper a (magic) spell, to prognosticate, enchanter, diligently observe, learn by experience" = "ש+ח+נ" = 300+8+50 = **358**
"nakh-ash" = "נחש" (ref. 5173) = "an incantation, augury, enchantment" = "ש+ח+נ" = 300+8+50 = **358**
"naw-khawsh" (from ref. 5172) = "נחש" (ref. 5175) = "a serpent" = "ש+ח+נ" = 300+8+50 = **358**

What is the relationship between the three words above? Let us consider the Sanhedrin, the high court of the Jews during the earthly days of Jesus. "Members of the Sanhedrin had to be 'masters of sorcery'..." as the term, "...'masters of sorcery'... referred to Torah scholars who had studied the black arts..." (Baal Ha Turim, Gold; p. 2009). The Sanhedrin's excuse concerning their knowledge of the black was "Members of the Sanhedrin had to be 'masters of sorcery' in order to be able to carry out the death sentence against sorcerers who might otherwise have been able to use their sorcery to protect themselves from capital punishment," (Baal Ha Turim, Gold; p. 2009). The Torah scholars who were masters of sorcery understood that the Torah forbids the practice of black arts, but they claimed that the Torah did not forbid the knowledge of the black arts, and therefore such knowledge was a necessary acquisition. It is quite unbelievable to assume that none of the Sanhedrin would ever resort to using such knowledge for personal (and wicked) purposes. As the hypocrisy becomes more apparent concerning the Sanhedrin, we notice that John the Baptist called the Pharisees and Sadducees a "brood of vipers," in Matthew 3:7. That is, the words "to hiss," "whisper," "sorcery (or magic)," and "serpent," serpent are all "נחש" = "ש+ח+נ" = 300+8+50 = 358 despite their respective pronunciations and definitions. The Greek New Testament was written to explain the Hebrew Old Testament and to show how it was fulfilled. Gematria shows the relationship between words despite the vowels written around them, as the current system of vowels used in Hebrew did not exist as such when the Scriptures were written. The Greek New Testament accounts for all of the definitions of the Hebrew words presently discussed by calling the practitioners of magic "vipers" so that the reader may understand the fulfillment of the Hebrew Scriptures by way of the Greek New Testament.

[i.15] Gematria is but one system of deduction: its correct applications can never somehow alter the content of Scripture that is read in the light of the simple meaning of a passage. Gematria is not the mere recognition of mathematically symmetrical words – which is why the illustration of this symmetry is explained by Biblical STORIES, not merely other Biblical words. Though there have been many systems of numerology that have perverted the uses of the gematria, particularly those that attempt to alter Scripture, gematria is actually an illustration that runs parallel to the content of Scripture; gematria is not some tool provided to manipulate Scripture. Our study does not rely on gematria, but rather, this book shows how gematria runs parallel to the accounts of Scripture that we might better understand the marriage of the Old and New Testaments as it was intended despite the fact that many have (for whatever strange reasons) attempted to divorce the two Testaments from each other. Again, the reader needs only knowledge of English, and the reader is never expected to use any mathematical skill. Gematria is merely displayed herein to show how the ancients viewed Scripture, and to exhibit more of the intricate design of Scripture.

[i.16] When considering the Sadducees and Pharisees and Scribes during the earthly days of Christ, it proves quite strange that the most learned Torah scholars were also Jesus' most adamant critics. Who better to identify the Savior than the Torah scholars? The Sadducees, Pharisees, and Scribes were not renegade upstarts, but they ruled the religious and social order of the people in both official and lay capacities from both official and lay positions. The "laws" that these sects claimed Jesus' routinely broke are not laws found in the Hebrew Scriptures, but these broken laws were their "laws," i.e. their additional interpretations above the words of the Torah called the "oral law"; notice how the "...Pharisees and Scribes came to Jesus from Jerusalem and said, 'Why do you break the tradition of the elders?" – for they did not speak of the tradition of the Torah (Written Law), but of the tradition of the elders (oral law – their own traditional and official laws that they claimed extended from the Torah, but those laws that were not actually found written in the Torah). Jesus said to the Pharisees and Scribes, "... for the sake of your tradition, you make void the word of God," (Matthew 15:6). It was and is a common opinion that the Torah is an insufficient to guide the entirety of human life, and as a result of this so-called deficiency, the oral traditions of the elders must be adhered to in order for the Written Law to be upheld; as such, the traditions of the elders became a written law unto itself, and these traditions are viewed as necessary to understand the Word of God. In other words, it is a common opinion that human reasoning is to be relied upon in order to understand God's reasoning, and that the practical applications of His Word are insufficient without human traditions regarding those applications; by reasoning as such, the adherence to the words of the elders often overrides personal Scripture reading. The Pharisees and Scribes asked Jesus, "Why do your disciples disregard the tradition of the elders..." (Matthew 15:2), and Jesus asked the Pharisees and the Scribes, "...why do you break the commandment of God for the sake of your tradition?" (Matthew 15:3).

Jesus never broke any of the 613 laws of the Torah, but He did deliberately break the traditional and human (oral) laws to show how such human traditions themselves actually breached the confines of the Torah. Jesus kept the Written Law perfectly, and He showed how such a holy adherence breaks the bonds that humanity has forged. Keep in mind that the "serpent's" first temptation involved a question and an emendation of the Law that God *spoke* to Adam. It would make little sense to assume that Christ somehow broke the very laws He was willing to die on account of for our sakes, as He was entirely innocent because He kept all 613 of those very same laws of the Torah. The fact that the rulers of the people claimed one thing or another does not make such claims true. For instance, the Pharisees said, "Search, and look: for out of Galilee ariseth no prophet," (John 7:50) – an odd comment considering that Jonah had come from Galilee; Jesus said in another place, "This generation is an evil generation; it asks for a sign, but no sign will be given to it except the sign of Jonah," (Luke 11:29). The "brood of vipers" did not tell the truth, and their magic and manipulations profited them little in the end, despite their venomous words that often gave the appearance of sweetness.

[i.17] When we consider the discourse between Adam's wife and the "serpent" in Eden, it is quite strange to assume that the Tree of the Knowledge of Good and Evil somehow held a wisdom within its fruit when the action of eating of it was, again, the most foolish mistake in human history. The Pharisees affirmed that nowhere in Scripture had a prophet arisen from Galilee, and their accusatory sight was errant. We may also consider the fact "...the woman saw that the tree was good for food..." (Genesis 3:6), but it is also odd to consider the food of the forbidden tree "good" when it not only brought about suffering for the woman, Adam, and all of his posterity; Job 20:12-16 also vividly describes Adam vomiting this food that contained "the poison of serpents" (Job 20:14). A helpful tip the New Testament provides for us is that Hebrew was a dead language in the earthly days of Christ, for it was not the common tongue of the people, but was instead confined largely to the Scripture reading in the Synagogues – from the elites to the common people. The elites would elaborate to the non-Hebrew-speaking Jews of Jesus' earthly days concerning what the reading apparently meant, and this elaboration became defined as the tradition(s) of the elders, the oral law. In other words, what the religious leaders said was God's Law was the official law of the elders over the people, often despite God's Law.

Terms like "oral law" may seem foreign to the reader of this book. One way to think of it is that, though there are disagreements concerning the applications of the Hebrew Scriptures, there must have been a specific way that Moses read the Torah aloud to the people despite the expansiveness of Hebrew diction, and along with the Torah there must also have been extensions to this specific reading that applied to particular circumstances that *appeared* to be not specifically mentioned in Scripture so that Moses was given other instruction that he did not write down but that was instead transmitted orally from generation to generation along side what was written at Sinai. In a similar way, Ezra must have delivered a specific reading, aloud, to the people, and this specific reading must have been extended beyond what was spoken initially so that it was applicable to situations that *seem* to have no apparent ruling inside the Torah. The religious regulations outside of the Torah (but viewed equally with the Torah) are called the "oral law." Even the way Hebrew is pronounced is subject to question, for no one alive today knows how the language sounded exactly when it was recorded in the Torah, and how a word is pronounced determines what the word means. For the reasons now named, we can better understand why Hebrew Bibles do not all agree, for the various Hebrew Bibles are little different from the many English translations (in a manner of speaking). English Old Testaments are often influenced by the traditions of the elders (the rulers of the oral law) as English Old Testaments record many of the editing choices of the Scribes that differ from the Sacred Text that the Scribes received prior to their redaction of God's Word. The Scribes edited the Scriptures because they viewed the Sacred Text as being sometimes "indelicate." Again, this may be new news to Christians, but it is old news to Jews, and Christians received the Sacred Text from the Jews – in its edited format that reflected the traditions of the elders.

Many of the Scribes, along with various members of the Sanhedrin, deemed it unfit to disseminate their more intricate knowledge of the Written Law to the common people, and as such, they but expounded upon the oral law, and they often swelled these words of "interpretation" into teachings that were not found on pages of Scripture – teachings that were even antithetical to Scripture. When Jesus began explaining the Written Law and then proving His claims with miracles, He was perceived as a direct threat to the conspiracies of the Sanhedrin. He said, "The Scribes and the Pharisees sit on Moses' seat; therefore, do whatever they teach you and follow it; but do not do as they do, for they do not practice what they teach… They do all their deeds to be seen by others…" (Matthew 23:2-5); for, "…a person is tested by being praised," (Proverbs 27:21), and "…the Lord tests the heart," (Proverbs 17:3). When Jesus refused to cease from exposing the errors of the rulers' traditions by following the Written Law flawlessly to their shame, they conspired against Him falsely so that He would be put to death (as it is written in the *Hebrew* Scriptures as we will soon examine). Satan challenged what God had *said,* in Genesis 3:1, and the woman "interpreted" the true Oral Law incorrectly with her own oral law whereby human reasoning led to human sin that ushered death into human history; for the Written Law was already marked out above the two humans before they were created, as it was pointed out to them (Genesis 3:15) after they breached the confines of what God had said so that the "law of liberty" discussed in James 1:25 might show itself in the fulfillment of time.

[i.18] The Torah, essentially, gives all the meanings of the Prophets, the Writings, and the New Testament as these Canonical divisions tie to the 613 laws of the Torah that had sprung from the sins of Eden. No one knows all of everything found within the Scriptures, yet the Scriptures were written to be understood. The Written Law is often examined by systems that are categorized as belonging to the "realm of allusion," which simply means passages, words, numbers, etc. that allude to and elucidate other passages, words, numbers, etc. Unfortunately, various exegetical systems employed to interpret the Scriptures have often been used to assert that there are "alternate" readings of Scripture. The various allusions, of which gematria is but one, should at no time whatsoever offer Scriptural alternatives against the simple meaning of a verse; rather, allusions were intended to serve to explain the simple meaning of a verse in more detail and to a greater extent through concise means. In order to "affirm" allusions, commentators (with masterful minds, I must admit) have imposed foreign systems on top of the various systems of allusion, which is a mistake that further separates respective "interpretations." As we make many allusions in our daily speech through figures and such, the word "allusion" should not evoke any negative feelings, though Biblical allusions have been viewed through negative lenses because of their sore abuses that have transformed allusions into illusions. An allusion is but an indirect reference, so, technically speaking, when one refers to an account, scenario, or quotation, yet one does not cite his or her source directly (assuming/requiring the reader to have prior knowledge in order to comprehend the reference), that could be considered an "allusion," a tendency that occurs consistently in the New Testament relative to the Old Testament as the New Testament accounts reflect Old Testament accounts. However, what may be considered allusions today may not have been considered as such in ancient times, for the Scriptures are very specific in providing dating systems by the names of the various mapped regions of the sky, though these provisions are given according to the names they were known by when the Scriptures were written; current society has also changed many of these names similar to how the Scribes "edited" the Scriptures.

[i.19] Both the Hebrew and Greek alphabets are numeric. An example of the numeric qualities of the Hebrew and Greek alphabets can be observed in the case of the Corban Chamber where the 13 trumpet-shaped receptacles in the Temple stood: "There was also a chamber in which whatsoever money was collected in these chests, of which we have spoken, was emptied out into three other chests; which is called by the Talmudists, emphatically as... the chamber. 'There were three chests, each containing three seahs, into which they empty the

Corban, and on them were written ג ב א. And why, saith R. Jose was Aleph, Beth, Gimel written upon them? namely, that it might be known which of them was filled first, that it might first be emptied. R. Ishmael saith, The inscription was in Greek, Alpha, Beta, Gamma,'" (*Commentary on the New Testament from the Talmud and Hebraica*, Lightfoot; Vol. 1, p. 224).

It may also prove useful to remember that, though the New Testament is written in Greek, the speech of the people within the New Testament was often not Greek. Instead, the speeches recorded in the New Testament are often but recorded in Greek, a fact that allows a reader a clearer conception of the confusion over the word "yeast/leaven" in Matthew 16:7: the Greek word was perfectly placed there for a specific reason, but Jesus charged His listeners with error when thinking in terms of edible "bread," an indication as to why He then illustrated His point by discussing edible bread in order to explain His original point as the Greek definition of "yeast" was a word that, when spoken in the Hebrew tongue, sounds similar to a Hebrew word indicating a bond : "maw-so-reth" = "מסרת" (ref. 4562) = "band, bond"; "mish-eh-reth" = "משארת" (ref. 4863) = "a kneading-trough (in which dough rises); from ref. 7604 in the original sense of swelling." "I will give you the keys of the kingdom of Heaven, and whatever you bind on earth will be bound in Heaven, and whatever you loose on earth will be loosed in Heaven," (Matthew 16:19). Remember:

"Moses" = "משה" (ref. 4872) = "מ+ש+ה" = 5+300+40 = **345**

"dough" = "עריסה" (ref. 6182) = "ע+ר+י+ס+ה" = 5+60+10+200+70 = **345**

In Matthew 4:3, Satan tempted Jesus first by stating his temptation without specifically identifying anything that was "written"; Jesus responded by saying "It is written..." to which Satan then exacted his next temptation by also stating, "It is written..." once he realized that Jesus was no easy target.

"...say Shibboleth..." (Judges 12:6).

It may further be considered that no language on earth preserves its original pronunciation over vast quantities of time, for to assume so would be similar to saying that current American English-speakers pronounce every English word the exact same way that Shakespeare pronounced English (which is a much shorter time-period than from Moses until today). No one today knows how the Hebrew spoken at Sinai specifically sounded. However, we do still possess what was written at Sinai. We also have the New Testament, written in Greek, whose letters are also numbers that perfectly correspond to the Hebrew given to Moses. "Jesus," connected to "Elohim" is called "The Word" = "The Logos" = The Computation in John 1. The Greek New Testament (written by the Hebrews and according to the idioms and style of Hebrew) was also constructed in accordance with the rules of Gematria:

Greek

(α) = 1	(ι) = 10	(ρ) = 100
(β) = 2	(κ) = 20	(σ) = 200 or 6
(γ) = 3	(λ) = 30	(τ) = 300
(δ) = 4	(μ) = 40	(υ) = 400
(ε) = 5	(ν) = 50	(φ) = 500
(ς) = 6	(ξ) = 60	(χ) = 600
(ζ) = 7	(ο) = 70	(ψ) = 700
(η) = 8	(π) = 80	(ω) = 800
(θ) = 9	Koppa = 90	(϶) = 900

The New Testament mirrors the Old Testament. The New Testament is the fulfillment of the Old Testament. The accounts of the New Testament reflect the assertions of the Old Testament. "In the beginning was the Word, and the Word was with God, and the Word was God. He was in the beginning with God. All things came into being through Him, and without Him not one thing came into being," (John 1:1-3).

"Jesus" = "Ιησους" = "Ι+η+σ+ο+υ+ς" = 10+8+200+70+400+200 = **888**; Genesis 2:4: "Jehovah Elohim made" = "עשות יהוה אלהים" = "ע+ש+ו+ת+י+ה+ו+ה+א+ל+ה+י+ם" = 40+10+5+30+1+5+6+5+10+400+6+300+70 = **888**.

As can be seen by the computation of 888 above, the New Testament words of John 1:1-3 are related to the Old Testament words of Genesis 2:4. As John 1:1-3 describes Christ as the Creator, we can also understand these two New Testament passages:

1) "He has rescued us from the power of darkness and transferred us into the kingdom of His beloved Son, in Whom we have redemption, the forgiveness of sins. He is the image of the invisible God, the firstborn of all creation; for in Him all things in heaven and on earth were created, things visible and invisible, whether thrones or dominions or rulers or powers – all things have been created through Him and for Him," (Colossians 1:13-16).

2) "From of old God spoke to our fathers by the prophets in every manner and in all ways; and in these latter days he has spoken to us by His Son, Whom He has appointed Heir of all things, and by Whom also He made the ages; for He is the brightness of His Glory and the express image of His being, upholding all things by the power of His Word; and when He had through His Person cleansed our sins, then He sat down on the right hand of the Majesty on high, (Hebrews 1:1-3).

[i.20] When we consider what Jehovah Elohim made, we can hardly avoid the first story of humanity in Eden. "Eden" is often called "Paradise" even though the word "Paradise" does not appear in the Genesis story. The word "Paradise" was recorded from the mouth of Christ as He hung on the cross in Luke 23:43. When the word "paradise" is uttered, it has the tendency to be tethered to ethereal conceptions in connection with Eden, yet this word "paradise" has more applications than only those of but one place. Regarding the word "paradise," its peculiarity of definition, the culture from which the word originated, and it's link to Eden is quite weighted. A "paradise" was the term used to describe a type of walled or hedged geography; though, as time passed, those walls became used for purposes against their original design.

[i.21]   It should be noted that Genesis 2:8 says that the Lord God planted a garden "*in* Eden"; it does not say that the Lord God planted the Garden *of* Eden. However, it is written that, "The Lord God took the man and placed him in the Garden of Eden…" in Genesis 2:15 and "…the Lord God sent him forth from the Garden of Eden…" in Genesis 3:23; the order is "in Eden," (Genesis 2:8), "in the garden of Eden," (Genesis 2:15), and "Garden of Eden," (Genesis 3:23). By the design of the distinctions observed above, a purpose is intended to be unfolded for us below.

[i.22]   We cannot overlook the importance of vineyards when we consider the fact that Jesus referred to himself as the "True Vine" in John 15:1, and that the word "vine" used here is "αμπελος" (ref. *288*) which means "a vine (as coiling about a support)." The word "vineyard" = "כרם" (ref. 3754) is also considered a "garden," as the prominent scholars Keil and Delitzsch render this word as "vine-garden" (*Commentary on the Old Testament: Song of Songs*, Keil & Delitzsch; p. 518). Hence, we see a connection between "vineyard" and "garden." Anyone who has visited a vineyard has also noticed the caution vinedressers take regarding who comes within the grounds, for vines require much care and are extremely valuable. As such, the preciousness of life within the famous garden in Eden is similarly described in the Bible.

[i.23]   Jehovah Elohim planted a garden "*in* Eden," for Eden was a place in which a smaller section, a hedged district that was the home of Adam, was planted within a larger fortification. The word "garden" used to describe Adam's home describes something hedged about or fortified against intrusion. The fortification of the garden in Eden was to be guarded by Adam (Genesis 2:15), for outside of Adam's garden abode lurked an enemy, a hunter bent on the destruction of humanity. Humanity was, initially, the only animate life mentioned within the garden in Eden, a fact that made humanity most exotic, most prized, and most sought after.

[i.24] Gardens and paradises have an intimate connection with respect to the ancient world's reckoning of these two entities. The gardens and paradises discussed in the Scriptures were linked in two main ways: 1) both were hedged or walled in, and 2) both encompassed thriving life found within their hedges. The main distinction between a garden and a paradise was that a paradise was stocked with animate life amongst vegetable life, whereas a garden was stocked with vegetable life only. Animate life, besides the necessary caretaker(s) of a garden who cultivate and care for the grounds, is not altogether welcome within a properly cultivated and well-preserved garden. It is written: "Jehovah Elohim took the man and put him in the Garden of Eden to cultivate it and to *guard* [or *preserve*] it," (Genesis 2:15). The garden in Eden was the home of Adam, whereas the paradise around it was the home of the animal life created before him in Genesis 1.

[i.25] "Paradise" = "Παραδεισος" (ref. *3857*), "is an Oriental word, first used by the historian Xenophon, denoting 'the parks of Persian kings and nobles.' It is of Persian origin (Old Pers. pairidaeza, akin to Gk. peri, 'around,' and teichos, 'a wall') whence it passed into Greek," (*Vine's Expository Dictionary*, p. 457). The word "paradise" is an "old Persian word," (*Commentary: Song of Songs*, Keil & Delitzsch, p. 559) that denoted an enclosing, a manner of fortification by walls (similar to those erected by a military), a circumvallation, and something defended – though the notion of this word being originally Persian is debated: "The Hebrews, who had gardens at so early a period, would surely not borrow names for them from other nations. [The word "paradise"]... is a compound of... [the word] *to divide*, and [the word] *to separate, to enclose*; hence *a protected, an enclosed place, a garden*," (*Song of Songs*, Ginsburg; p. 161). It is safe to say that the concept of a "paradise" eventually became used in the Persian sense to describe the exotic, lush geography that contained animal life, but animal life placed there for the purposes of hunting for sport, as the walls surrounding paradises were so designed (eventually) that animals could not escape the hunter, but those animals were instead compelled to face the hunter. The predatory sense of the word "paradise" became more related to the sense of Luke 19:43: "Indeed, the days will come upon you, when your enemies will set up ramparts around you and surround you, and hem you in on every side." However, it should be understood, as we will later discover in more detail, that the *original* design of a "paradise" was to preserve animate life... animate life that was supplied with sweet water, abundant food, and serene protection. The word "paradise" later became used as the sporty mingling of stalked blood with pruned nature's voluptuously sublime inhabitants against its original design and original definition. When Christ promised the dying criminal to His side that he would be with Him in "Paradise" (Luke 23:43), it can hardly be thought that this criminal was ensured by the Savior to be hunted down as Adam was hunted down by Satan (the Enemy Adam was specifically commissioned to guard against in Genesis 2:15 so that such hunting would not occur), nor that this criminal would engage in predatory acts, for the reign of the Messiah is one where, "The wolf shall live with the lamb, the leopard shall lie down with the kid, the calf and the lion and the fatling together, and a little child shall lead them. The cow and the bear shall graze, their young shall lie down together; and the lion shall eat straw like the ox. The nursing child shall play over the hole of the asp, and the weaned child shall put its hand on the adder's den. They will not hurt or destroy on all My holy mountain; for the earth will be full of the knowledge of the Lord as the waters cover the sea," (Isaiah 11:6-9). However, later in history, the concept of "hunting" became connected to the word "paradise." King Solomon burned for the Shulamite, as the Shulamite is compared to a "paradise" (rendered "orchard" in English) in Song of Songs 4:13; we make take notice of another passage in light of this "paradise": "...for love is strong as death; jealously is cruel as the grave: the coals thereof are coals of fire, which hath a most vehement flame," (Song of Songs 8:6).

[i.26] Since the sense of the word "paradise" is most commonly remembered in light of the Persians, it is beneficial to contemplate some of the most famous and mysterious Persians – the Magi – particularly with respect to their "sorcery" from which we derive the word "magic."

Again "Members of the Sanhedrin had to be 'masters of sorcery'..." as the term, "...'masters of sorcery'... referred to Torah scholars who had studied the black arts..." (*Baal Ha Turim*, Gold; p. 2009). Like the word "paradise," the word "Magi" also came to have more than one application: originally, it denoted the royal Persian priesthood of whom the Hebrew prophet Daniel was affiliated, and whose descendents found the Christ Child (Matthew 2:1) with the aid of Daniel's work; later, it also became connected with various practitioners of the dark arts who were not necessarily connected with any particular (let alone royal) priesthood (Acts 8:9-13). The most dangerous of the sorcerers during Christ's earthly days were those of the Sanhedrin, the Torah scholars, who routinely revised the oral law by questioning what God had said in His Written Law. In a similar way, the "serpent's" first question to Eve was, "Did God say...?" The main doctrine of the Pharisees was that the oral law (what is said by human authority concerning God's Word) completed the Written Law (God's Word).

[i.27] "From Heaven He caused you to hear His voice in order to teach you, and on earth He showed you His great fire, and you heard His words from the midst of the fire," (Deuteronomy 4:36).

Ancient "magicians" like the Magi were scientists and fire worshippers, astronomers and astrologers, wise men and sorcerers, chemists who were masters of medicine and also masters of poison; of these sorcerers, it proves difficult to decipher how far the originally regal Magi leaned to one side or the other of the "sorcerer's" spectrum, but it is known that the Magi were responsible for educating the king, and it is also known that they possessed a distinct respect for the religious uses of fire. It is remarkable to note that the Hebrew word "gall" = "ראש" (ref. 7219) is also rendered "poisonous plant," "venom," and "poison (even of serpents)." The word "Magi," like the word "paradise," became entangled with a definition that did not exist originally, a parasite that fed off of the success of its host, an illusion that had the appearance of an allusion; Gematria, in its exactitude, is little different. Consider that the first time the number "13" appears overtly in Scripture is in Genesis 14:4: "Twelve years they had served Chedorlaomer, but in the thirteenth year they rebelled"; however, "love" = "אהבה" (ref. 160) = "ה+ב+ה+א" = 5+2+5+1 = **13**. The number 13 is applied to both "love" and "rebellion," for there are both positive and negative applications to various entities. In a similar way, the term "sorcerer" could indicate merely a perception about one who possessed superior and apparently esoteric knowledge or one such person who applied such knowledge in a Satanic fashion. As we can see, "אהד" (ref. 258) = "to unify, i.e. (figuratively) collect (one's thoughts):- go one way or other" = "ד+ה+א" = 4+8+1 = **13**. In a similar way, "one (or as an ordinal first)" = "ד+ה+א" = 4+8+1 = **13**.

[i.28] The manner of personal devotion that can be credited to the sciences (as opposed to the black arts) that defined the Magi as a whole throughout history is nearly anybody's guess, but it can be reasonably assumed that what began with scientific discovery eroded into less noble pursuits – what began in devout forms of curiosity, ended in unwholesome forms of manipulation. The Magi were also interpreters of dreams, priests of the Medes and Babylonians who claimed that God spoke out from flames, wise men who had knowledge of substances aimed to remedy sickness, but that, if handled improperly, could be employed to administer sickness. Ancient "knowing ones," "wise men," or "sorcerers" were usually masters of producing physical effects by artificial means, for mixed purposes. The Magi were a peculiar and nebulous order, and they were regal and famous originally; however, their shining reputations became infected by the ill-inclined renegades among them to the point that their title became one of wonderment and fear as much as it had originally been one of wonderment and admiration. As the Scriptures provide descriptions of North Celestial Polar positions, the North Ecliptic Pole, and various constellations according to the identifications that they were known by when the Scriptures were written, it is understandable as to why the Magi followed celestial lights to the Christ Child. Partially through Bible scholarship's rejection of astronomy, and partially because of the current official standardization of the names and boundaries of celestial maps, many Scriptural accounts are now, unfortunately, viewed as unexplainable by Christians and as nearly mythological by skeptics. However, because of the errant liberties taken by astrologers who mapped the heavens in whatever manner that pleased them personally, standardization was necessary – though the standardization of the celestial maps does not reflect the reckonings of antiquity completely.

The story of Eden, the fortified enclosure that housed

animate life in both prosperity and peace, is also the story of a master sorcerer, an expert hunter, who sought to transform the abode of Adam into a place of poverty in the guise of prosperity, and a place of bloodshed in the guise of freedom. The words "paradise" and "Magi" reside within a shady realm of initial grandeur and eventual erosion. Adam was the first human and our oldest human descendent. The "serpent" was the first sorcerer or "knowing one," though he "... disguises himself as an angel of light," (II Corinthians 11:13-14). Like the Magi, the strictest Pharisees wore white as a symbol of purity. The Sanhedrin claimed that the knowledge of the black arts was necessary should one attempt to identify those who practice the black arts. The Sanhedrin was comprised of the Jewish elites. The High Priest was called "The Priest Messiah" = "The Anointed Priest" (Leviticus 4:3,5,16; 6:22). The Priest Messiah of Jesus' earthly days once challenged Jesus by asking, "Are You the Messiah, the Son of the Blessed?" (Mark 14:61). Jesus referred to Himself as a "serpent," (John 3:14). Before Satan fell, he was called "the signet of perfection," (Ezekiel 28:12). Hebrews 4:14 calls Jesus the "Great High Priest." The enemy, Satan, seeks to cause confusion, and what appears like a remedy is often his poison.

[i.29] The word "garden" is used in the Eden account of Genesis 2 & 3 for very specific reasons. God's creation illustrates God's Word. Biblical principles are accompanied by examples of the very same principles found in nature that are bound to scientific laws. No claim of the Holy Scriptures is unreasonable, and those claims of the Holy Scriptures that are thought to be unreasonable are only misunderstood. "For since the creation of the world God's invisible qualities – His eternal power and divine nature – have been clearly seen, being understood from what has been made, so that men are without excuse," (Romans 1:20).

[i.30] When we consider the fact the Bible was written without punctuation, it can become confusing to understand a Biblical assertion tethered to the punctuation choice of an editor, for the placement of a mere comma alone can alter the perception of an entire passage. The Scriptures are precisely worded for explicit detail, and so the diction employed must be recognized as possessing an absolute value prior to its placement within the body of the sacred Text. In other words, there is a strict reason as to why one word is used instead of another, and the reason must have existed prior to its placement within the Scriptures in order for it to be used to describe something particular. At the same time, the specific usages of words also allude to concepts of unutterable beauty. It is beneficial to examine the methods in which the ancients read the Bible as opposed to placing a modern mindset on top of these famous, ever-fruitful Words of antiquity. There can be several Hebrew words constructed by the same letters in the same order, more words constructed by the same letters in a different order, and even more words that all compute to the same number; the ancients understood an intimate relationship between every word composed of the same letters and every word that computed to the same number, and by a system of deduction, they inductively gained insight.

The Knowledge of Good & Evil strives to use the lens of the ancients to facilitate the discovery of those who live on earth today. Any system can be but vaguely discovered by rules that it did not contain originally. Furthermore, *The Knowledge of Good & Evil* utilizes the Greek New Testament, particularly the Words of Christ, to unlock the mysteries of the Old Testament, as it is apparent that the accounts of the New Testament are parallel stories to those of the Old Testament despite the fact that they occurred at a different time in history. "Is there a thing of which it is said, 'See, this is new?' – it has already been in the ages before us," (Ecclesiastes 1:10). The entirety of this book concerns but one chapter in the entire Bible: Genesis Chapter III.

[i.31]   How can a serpent speak?

"There exists... the so-called "deficient" spelling (also known as the 'pointed' or 'dotted' one). This format uses different combinations of dots for different vowels, and is thus not difficult to read. For technical and traditional reasons, however, 'pointed' writing and printing is reserved only for Holy Scriptures, prayer books and poetry. It is also used in textbooks for children and beginners as well as in literature for children in their first 3-4 years of reading. Thereafter, everyone switches to the 'plene' (also known as 'unpointed' or 'undotted') spelling where vowels are nearly nonexistent and therefore replaced by mere intelligent guessing," (*Webster's New World Hebrew Dictionary*, p. xv).

Our English Old Testaments are translated from a system

of Hebrew meant for children in their first 3-4 years of reading – a system in which the Scriptures were not written originally, and a system that became copied by the ancient Scribes. In essence, we are reading the children's version of the Old Testament; we have not been reading the full story.

"Whom shall He teach knowledge? And whom shall He make to understand doctrine? Them that are weaned from the milk, and drawn from the breasts," (Isaiah 28:9).

"I tell you the truth, unless you change and become like little children, you will never enter the kingdom of heaven. Therefore, whoever humbles himself like this child is the greatest in the kingdom of heaven," (Matthew 18:3-4).

"Brothers and sisters, do not be children in your thinking. In regard to evil be infants, but in your thinking be adults," (I Corinthians 14:20).

"For in the first place the Jews were entrusted with the oracles of God. What if some were unfaithful? Will their faithlessness nullify the faithfulness of God?" (Romans 3:2-3 NRSV)

"How can you say, 'We are wise, and the law of the Lord is with us,' when, in fact, the false pen of the Scribes has made it into a lie?" (Jeremiah 8:8).

"Since, then, we have such a hope, we use great plainness of speech, not like Moses who put a veil over his face to keep the people of Israel from gazing at the end of the glory that was being set aside. But their minds were hardened. Indeed, to this very day, when they hear the reading of the old covenant, that same veil is still there, since only in Christ is it set aside. Indeed, to this very day whenever Moses is read, a veil lies over their minds," (II Corinthians 3:12-15).

[i.32] Let us consider the manifold concept of "fruit":

1) "And the fruit of righteousness is sown in peace of them that make peace," (James 3:18).

2) "If you will only obey the Lord your God, by diligently observing all His commandments that I am commanding you today, the Lord your God will set you high above all nations of the earth; all these blessings shall come upon you and overtake you, if you obey the Lord your God… Blessed shall be the fruit of your womb, the fruit of your ground, and the fruit of your livestock…" (Deuteronomy 28:1-4).

3) "Then you shall again obey the Lord, observing all His commandments that I am commanding you today, and the Lord your God will make you abundantly prosperous in all your undertakings, in the fruit of your body, in the fruit of your livestock, and in the fruit of your soil…" (Deuteronomy 30:8-9).

4) "Reuben, you are my firstborn, my might and the first fruits of my vigor…" (Genesis 49:3).

5) "Shall I give my firstborn for my transgression, the fruit of my body for the sin of my soul?" (Micah 6:7).

[i.33] No description of Scripture is arbitrary. Metaphors

are often employed within Scripture, but they are not so esoteric or conceptual that they are only applicable to topics outside of observable nature or even diction reference. Scriptural illustrations serve to aid our comprehension of the subjects the Bible discusses, for we must (at all times) keep in the forefront of our minds that the Scriptures are meant to be understood for our sustenance and edification. Let us consider the concept of a "needle" and of a "camel":

NEEDLE:
"Did You not pour me out like milk and curdle me like cheese? You clothed me with skin and flesh, and *knit* me together with bones and sinews. You have granted me life and steadfast love, and Your care has preserved my spirit," (Job 10:10-12).

"I will praise Thee; for I am fearfully and wonderfully made: marvelous are Thy works; and that my soul knoweth right well. My substance was not hid from thee, when I was made in secret, and curiously *wrought with a needle* in the lowest parts of the earth. Thine eyes did see my substance, yet being unperfect; and in thy book all my members were written, which in continuance were fashioned, when as yet there was none of them," (Psalm 139:15).

CAMEL:
"בכר" (ref. 1070) = "(in the sense of youth); a young camel:- dromedary"; from "בכר" (ref. 1069) = "to burst the womb, i.e. (caus.) bear or make early fruit (of woman or tree); also to give the birthright:- make firstborn, be firstling, bring forth first child (new fruit)."

"Truly I say to you, whoever does not receive the kingdom of God as a child may in no way enter into it... Children, how hard it is to enter the kingdom of God! It is easier for a *camel* to go through the eye of a *needle* than for someone who is rich to enter the kingdom of God," (Mark 10:15... 24-25). The word "eye" of a *needle* used here is "orifice" = "τρυμαλια" (ref. *5168*). It is easier for one to be birthed through an orifice the size of a needle's eye than for a rich man to enter the Kingdom of God. "Jesus answered him, 'Very truly, I tell you, no one can see the kingdom of God without being born from above.' Nicodemus said to Him, 'How can anyone be born after growing old? Can one enter a second time into the mother's womb and be born?' Jesus answered, 'Very truly, I tell you, no one can enter the kingdom of God without being born of water and Spirit... The *wind [same word as "Spirit"]* blows where it chooses, and you hear the sound of it, but you do not know where it comes from or where it goes. So it is with everyone who is born of the Spirit,'" (John 3:3-8). It is impossible for flesh to pass through the eye of a needle. It is quite easy for wind to pass through the eye of a needle. "For mortals it is impossible, but not for God; for God all things are possible," (Mark 10:27).

"But someone will ask, 'How are the dead raised?' With what kind of body do they come?' Fool! What you sow does not come to life unless it dies. And as for what you sow, you do not sow the body that is to be, but a bare seed... So it is with the resurrection of the dead. What is sown is perishable, what is raised is imperishable. It is sown in dishonor, it is raised in glory. It is sown in weakness, it is raised in power. It is sown in a physical body, it is raised a spiritual body. If there is a physical body, there is also a spiritual body. Thus it is written, 'The first man, Adam, became a living soul'; the last Adam became a life-giving spirit... flesh and blood cannot inherit the kingdom of God... Listen, I will tell you a mystery! We will not all die, but we will all be changed, in the twinkling of an eye ['οφθαλμος' (ref. *3788*)], at the last trumpet. For the trumpet will sound, and the dead will be raised imperishable, and we will be changed." (I Corinthians 15-52).

Again, "I will praise Thee; for I am fearfully and wonderfully made: marvelous are Thy works; and that my soul knoweth right well. My substance was not hid from thee, when I was made in secret, and curiously *wrought with a needle* in the lowest parts of the earth. Thine eyes did see my substance, yet being unperfect; and in thy book all my members were written, which in continuance were fashioned, when as yet there was none of them." (Psalm 139:15): "Whoever observes this... may, indeed, feel the beauty and gracefulness of this well-adapted metaphor, but will miss much of its force and sublimity, unless he be apprised that the art of designing in needlework was wholly dedicated to the use of the sanctuary, and, by a direct precept of the divine law, chiefly employed in furnishing a part of the sacerdotal habit, and the veils for the entrance of the Tabernacle," (*Lectures on the Sacred Poetry of the Hebrews*, Lowth; p. 85).

INTRODUCTION
QUESTIONS

"You do not have, because you do not ask," (James 4:2).

[ii.1]   What a sublime pleasure it is to expound upon the love of the Savior! How exhilarating it is to explain what we believe and the hope that is within us! However, even the best among us often trip into humiliation and stinging defeat when the skeptic asks "Why?" – and how woeful it is when fellow believers contend with each other as to the what of the matter without ever asking why?

As we know, it is quite easy to hold firmly to whatever we choose, at least for a while. It is another matter altogether to explain why we believe what we believe in a practical manner, especially when we must articulate precisely how our beliefs work in any congruence with consistent, rational, immovable factuality carried out to an end of unquestionable truth – for to deny any of these qualities opens us to scorn from every direction, and rightfully so. An all-too-common concession is that the Words of Holy Scripture function as a related but loosely-connected collection of moral principles that developed over the course of history. As such, many seemingly devout arguments lack the force to defend the hope that is within us when an account is demanded from us by the opposition – an account that we are held responsible for giving the opposition.

[ii.2]   How is it that a common conception of Christianity has claimed the Greek New Testament to be merely a continuation of the Hebrew Old Testament when the same claim adamantly denounces the additions forwarded by other "continuations" held by major belief systems outside of Christianity that recognize the Books of Scripture as well? – when pondering this question, an all too common answer claims that "You just have to believe..." which is one of the weakest arguments that any human can present to another concerning any assertion about any topic. For instance, try "just believing" that you have one million dollars in your bank account, and after defending that belief staunchly, observe how well your monthly bank statement accords with your unshakable belief in the million dollars you claim to have.

How often do groups who claim to be "Christian" wrangle over topics like abortion only to present nothing but personal feelings, experiences, and philosophies in conjunction with disconnected and poorly-quoted portions of Scripture? – just as often as we meet people who can quote more movie-lines and song-lyrics than passages of Scripture (and it is certain that we have all met these types on various occasions). If the Holy Bible is the standard by which we are supposed to live, how can the Holy Bible be subject to what we think of it? If the Holy Bible is subject to our thoughts and desires, then it is we who are the standard and not the Holy Bible. For instance, one may claim that a tree in his/her backyard is 6,000 feet tall, speaks Portuguese, and is home to the world's largest 7-legged elephant; no matter how firmly one believes about the qualities of this magnificent tree, none of those beliefs add to or detract from the nature of the tree itself. One's beliefs can only, at best, add to or detract from the validity of one's own understanding.

Certainly, 100% accuracy is unquestionably impossible for any human mind to achieve. The only Book in existence without flaw is the Holy Bible, for there is no book produced out of a human mind that is perfect in its construction. Sadly, it is because of human shortcomings that Holy Scripture is assumed to have its faults, and this assumption has lead to countless errors in copies of Scripture beyond mere scribal slips, as is evinced when attempting to find perfect uniformity (even if only spelling is concerned) between various manuscripts of Scripture. A personal lack of reason concerning an entity does not make the entity itself unreasonable; that is, it was eventually found to be unreasonable to assume the earth to be flat, but the discovery of the round earth did not make the earth before it unreasonable, it only made the conceptions of the earth before this discovery unreasonable.

[ii.3] Because the Holy Scriptures' sophistication is unmatched, it can sometimes appear daunting to discern even the basic mechanics of how the Truth is revealed on the pages of Scripture. However, it is an errant assertion to claim that God Almighty's Holy Word, designed specifically for our sustenance, liberation, and perpetuity is so esoteric and recondite that it is beyond our grasp to experience what it was designed specifically to offer us on a daily basis; such a claim implies that God is somehow incapable of communicating with us adequately, and such a claim shows, with immediacy, that it is we who render ourselves incapable of receiving what we are actually capable of comprehending. When we prove unable to articulate the Truth logically and instead only possess an intuitive "understanding" of the Truth, how is it that two people's claims of the exact same "truth" do not align with each other when both people claim the common source of the Holy Scriptures?

[ii.4]   God is flawless, and so are the fruitful Words He gave us to guide us and to guard us from what we cannot overcome ourselves. God can empower us to overcome what we ourselves have let consume us. The power of God is not limited to the power of our minds. I now ask some questions: If God Almighty is perfectly just, why did He curse the ground for Adam's sin? If God Almighty is perfectly ordered, why did He punish the womb for Eve's sin? If God Almighty is perfectly loving, why then did He require bloodshed to forgive sins?

"For, first, when all the books of the New Testament were written by Jews, and among Jews, and unto them; and when all the discourses made there, were made in like manner by Jews, and to Jews, and among them; I was always fully persuaded, as of a thing past all doubting, that that Testament could not but everywhere taste of and retain the Jew's style, idiom, form, and rule of speaking," (*Commentary on the New Testament from the Talmud and Hebraica*, Lightfoot; Vol. 2, p. 3).

Let us consider the language in which Matthew wrote his Gospel. Matthew 1:23 states, "'Look, the virgin shall conceive and bear a son, and they shall name Him Emmanuel,' which being interpreted, means 'God with us.'"   Why would Matthew have to "interpret" the very words that he himself scribed? Concerning the common language in the days of Matthew, Dr. Lightfoot noted the following:

"...that the Hebrew was not at all understood by the common people may especially appear from two things:

1) "That, in the synagogues, when the law and the prophets were read in the original Hebrew, an interpreter was always present to the reader, who rendered into the mother-tongue that which was read, that it might be understood by the common people. Hence those rules of the office of an interpreter, and of some places which were not to be rendered into the mother-tongue.
2) "That Jonathan the son of Uzziel, a scholar of Hillel, about the time of Christ's birth, rendered all the prophets... into the Chaldee language; that is, into a language much more known to the people than the Hebrew, and more acceptable than the mother-tongue," (*Commentary on the New Testament from the Talmud and Hebraica*, Lightfoot; Vol. 2, p. 19-20).

"... the Hebrew was altogether unknown to the common people: no wonder, therefore, if the evangelists and apostles wrote not in Hebrew when there were none who understood things so written, but learned men only," (*Commentary on the New Testament from the Talmud and Hebraica*, Lightfoot; Vol. 2, p. 22). "Rabban Simeon Ben Gamaliel saith, 'Even concerning the holy books, the wise men permitted not that they should be written in any other language than Greek.'" (*Commentary on the New Testament from the Talmud and Hebraica*, Lightfoot; Vol. 2, p. 23). Again, "Rabban Simeon Ben Gamaliel saith, '... They searched seriously, and found... that the law could not be translated according to what was needful for it, but in Greek,'" (*Commentary on the New Testament from the Talmud and Hebraica*, Lightfoot; Vol. 2, p. 24).

Accordingly, we can understand more of why the New Testament was written in Greek, though there are more reasons than those listed above. However, due to the respect that the Jews had for the Greek Language, and due to their acceptance of the works of Plato (particularly of the dialogue format of which Plato was a master), it can be observed how extensive a link was made possible through the Greek language to the Gentile world for the purposes of Christ. At the same time, it proves difficult not to experience some manner of dejection to think that the very language of the people whose ancestors walked through parted water, parted themselves from their own mother-tongue – little different than how many people today of all walks sever themselves from the Bible on a daily basis.

DISCLAIMER
WHAT LIES HIDDEN

"But where shall wisdom be found? And where is the place of understanding?"
(Job 28:12).

(The words of this book were written independently of the views of the publisher. The author holds no ecclesiastical office.)

[iii.1]   Some of the methods of interpretation (if you will) found within this book may seem obscure if not altogether foreign to the reader. This book takes many avenues in its investigation, but every avenue taken arrives at the same end. If there are various disciplines concerning Biblical interpretation that all point to the same facts from "different" perspectives, then the various disciplines must be only fragments of an original whole. As the reader will see, each discipline employed within these pages arrives at a common conclusion by its own uniqueness. For instance, scholars may use the study of diction and the exploration of syntax in conjunction with more seemingly esoteric methods in order to draw conclusions about the absolute. However, because supposedly differing disciplines are seemingly varying tunnels dug towards the same Truth, it is apparent that, at one point in time (or perhaps before time), all of the so-called "differing" disciplines were one. The height of our blunders is most quickly achieved by the denunciation of an absolute. The apex of our apostasy is most notable in the assumption that our own minds can be the absolute, and that anything that exists outside the small box of our own personal recognition is somehow errant because it does not accord with our presuppositions that have been cultivated by our cultures and traditions.

[iii.2]   Small, brief, and elementary examples concerning the science of astronomy are used within this work.

Views concerning astronomy have suffered degradation regarding the various disciplines within Biblical interpretive spheres because of astronomy's gross perversion called astrology that wars against any sound reason whatsoever. Astrology is Satanic, foolish, and unprofitable, for it is only a cheap counterfeit based on astronomy. The few, brief, and elementary examples of astronomy are used within this text for the purposes of dating history. The Church has often abandoned astronomy because of the lamentable abuse of astrology. The Father has given us an inheritance that is superior to any inheritance the world has to offer us, for He offers what is far above any corruption the world attempts to infect us with in the guise of edification. It is only to our own injury that we discard portions of our inheritance because the world has squandered its inheritance. I urge the reader not to be bound by the deceit of the enemy so that the reader may not be kept from his/her own inheritance. There is no astrology and no numerology found within any portion of this text. Let us be reunited with what has been robbed from us by the Enemy.

[iii.3]   Before we advance in our studies, let us note a few observations:

"*Chodesh* and *yareach* are masculine words... But nowhere throughout the Old Testament is the moon personified*, and in only one instance is it used figuratively to represent a person... Jacob understands that the moon (*yareach*) stands for a woman, his wife," (*Astronomy of the Bible*, Maunder; p. 86-87).
*(Possibly compare to Habakkuk 3:10-11)

The reference to the moon made by Dr. Maunder concerns the gender of words and their applications and is found in Genesis 37:9-11. It is apparent that the gender of words cannot fully indicate the entire concept and essence of words despite the rules of diction that individual words are bound to out of context. Consider that Israel was a man, but that the nation named after him is referred to as a woman (Jeremiah 3). Consider the fact that the human author of Ecclesiastes was a man, but his title is a feminine name.

[iii.4] That rules of diction need not be abandoned, but such rules cannot yield final determinations regarding the entire concept and essence of a word, though the rules of diction are a precise science of high value, especially in the case of Jepthah in Judges 11:29 -37; "*Jepthah* means "*He will open, i.e. He will set free and liberate; He sets free; God opens; the breaker through*":

"The Spirit of the Lord came upon Jepthah, and he passed through *Gilead* [*Perpetual Fountain; A Heap of Testimony; A Witness; Mass of Testimony; Strong*] and *Manasseh* [*One Who Causes to Forget; Forgetfulness*]. He passed on to *Mizpah* [*A Watch Tower*] of Gilead, and from Mizpah of Gilead he passed on to the *Ammonites* [*People of Strength*]. And Jepthah made a vow to the Lord, and said, 'If You will give the Ammonites into my hand, then whatsoever comes out of the doors of my house to meet me, when I return victorious from the Ammonites, shall be the Lord's, to be offered up by me as a burnt offering.' So Jepthah crossed over to the Ammonites to fight against them; and the Lord gave them into his hand. He inflicted a massive defeat on them from *Aroer* [*Childless*] to the neighborhood of *Minnith* [*Small; Allotment; From Her*], 20 towns, and as far as *Abelkeramim* [*Mourning of the Vineyards*]. So the Ammonites were subdued before the people of Israel. Then Jepthah came to his home at *Mizpah* [*A Watch Tower*]; and there was his daughter coming out to meet him with timberels and with dancing. She was his only child; he had no other son or daughter except her. When he saw her, he tore his clothes, and said, 'Alas, my daughter! You have brought me very low; you have become the cause of great trouble to me. For I have opened my mouth to the Lord, and I cannot take back my vow.' She said to him, 'My father, if you have opened your mouth to the Lord, do to me according to what has gone out of your mouth, now that the Lord has given you vengeance against your enemies, the Ammonites.' And she said to her father, 'Let this thing be done for me: Grant me two months, so that I may go and wander the mountains, and bewail my VIRGINITY...'"

The story of Jepthah has been sadly tainted far too often by a claim that asserts that Jepthah conducted the human sacrifice of his own daughter, and that he was somehow lauded for his devotion to God (Hebrews 11:32) Who Himself despises human sacrifice, and Who would not have accepted Jepthah's offer if Jepthah had actually communicated that he would even kill a human as a sacrifice – a sacrifice against the guidelines of the Torah:

"... Jepthah's vow consisted of two parts; one alternative to the other. He would either dedicate it to Jehovah (according to Lev. xxvii.); or, if unsuitable for this, he would offer it as a burnt offering. It should be noted also that, when he said, 'Whatsoever cometh forth of the doors of my house to meet me,' the word 'whatsoever' is Masculine. But the issuer from his house was Feminine..." (*Great Cloud of Witnesses*, Bullinger; p. 328).

Leviticus 27 explains the vow of Jepthah:

(1st Condition: concerning humans; Leviticus 27:2-8) – "If anyone makes a special [or singular] vow to dedicate persons to the Lord by giving equivalent values, set the value of a male between the ages of twenty and sixty at fifty shekels of silver, according to the sanctuary shekel, and if it is a female, set her value at thirty shekels. If it is a person between the ages of five and twenty, set the value of a male at twenty shekels and of a female at ten shekels. If it is a person between one month and five years, set the value of a male at five shekels of silver and that of a female at three shekels of silver. If it is a person sixty years old or more, set the value of a male at fifteen shekels and of a female at ten shekels. If anyone making the vow is too poor to pay the specified amount, he is to present the person to the priest, who will set the value for him according to what the man making the vow can afford."

(2nd Condition: concerning animals; Leviticus 27:9-13) – If what he vowed is an animal that is acceptable as an offering to the Lord, such an animal given to the Lord becomes holy. He must not exchange it or substitute a good one for a bad one or a bad one for a good one; if he should substitute one animal for another, both it and the substitute become holy. If what he vowed is a ceremonially unclean animal – one that is not acceptable as an offering to the Lord – the animal must be presented to the priest, who will judge its quality as good or bad. Whatever value the priest then sets, that is what it will be. If the owner wishes to redeem the animal, he must add a fifth to its value."

Concerning Leviticus 27:2 ("... shall make a singular vow..."), Dr. Ginsburg commented, "According to the interpretation of this phrase which obtained during the second Temple it denotes *shall pronounce a vow*. Hence the ancient Chaldee Versions render it, "shall distinctly pronounce a vow." Accordingly, no vow mentally made or conceived was deemed binding. It had to be distinctly pronounced in words. The form of the vow is nowhere given in the Bible. Like many other points of detail, the wording of it was left to the administrators of the law. They divided vows into classes: (1) Positive vows, by which a man bound himself to **consecrate for religious purposes** his own person, **those members of his family over whom he had control**, or any portion of his property, and for this kind of vow the formula was, 'Behold I consecrate this to the Lord'; and (2) Negative vows, by which he promised to abstain from enjoying a certain thing, for which the formula was, 'Such and such a thing be unlawful to me for so many days, weeks, or for ever,'" (*Leviticus*, by Ginsburg; p. 286).

Jepthah dedicated his daughter to a celibate devotion to Jehovah (similar to a nun), for she lamented her permanent virginity, not her certain loss of life. Who would lament a denial of copulation when faced with the certainty of physical doom? There is never a point in the Scriptures that accepts human sacrifice to God, a point that is made quite clear concerning the life of Abraham as the Lord tested Abraham's cultural misunderstandings only to overrule such despicable cultural misunderstandings by the fulfillment of the His divine command of substitution; concerning the pagan culture of Abraham prior to his knowledge of God, what greater sacrifice above child sacrifice was there to such lost people? Jepthah, having only one child, certainly lamented the stunting of his family line (*"Mourning of the Vineyards"* & *"Childless"*), specifically in that he had no son. Consider the augmentation of Jepthah's sorrow in light of the fact that he himself was the product of prostitution weighed against his own apparent sense of familial belonging.

Since it is evident that God honored the vow of Jepthah by giving Jepthah victory over the Ammonites, it would be more than contradictory for God to have entered into an agreement against His Own holy will concerning human sacrifice... for certainly had Jepthah vowed to slaughter even his own daughter, Jepthah would not have been mentioned in the Hall of Faith (Hebrews 11:32) for blatantly opposing the will of God, nor would Jepthah have made a vow according to the guidelines of the Torah if his intention was to attempt to keep the Torah by breaking the specific guidelines of his vow that he devotedly kept. Confusion concerning the account of Jepthah has led various Bible translations to employ the word "whosever" instead of "whatsoever" concerning the conditional victim of sacrifice versus the conditional subordinate dedicated for religious purposes. The victim of righteous sacrifice cannot be a human sacrificed by another human. According to Scripture, the only acceptable human "sacrifice" is not one who kills another, but only one who lays down his or her life (at the hands of others) for the sake of others who cannot possibly repay them for their "sacrifice," hence our Savior's words: "No one has greater love than this, to lay down one's life for one's friends," (John 15:13). Christ was the final sacrifice that paid all debt (of which none was His own) so that others might live, not die. According to John 15:13, it can hardly be deduced that one can "love" another so strongly as to kill another, otherwise, by such perverted logic, God then could have certainly "loved" us so much that He would have killed us instead of dying for us in order to save us from what perils might otherwise come. The battle between good and evil concerns God's Word.

[iii.5] "In the beginning was the Word, and the Word was with God, and the Word was God. He was in the beginning with God. All things came into being through Him, and without Him not one thing came into being. What has come into being in Him was life, and the life was the light of all people. The light shines in the darkness, and the darkness did not overcome it," (John 1:1-5). "And the Word became flesh and tabernacled among us, and we have seen His glory, the glory as of a father's only son, full of grace and truth," (John 1:14). Satan intended to diminish and ultimately extinguish God's Holy word on earth, and as a result of this ill attempt, God's Holy Word came down and *tabernacled* among us (being *born* of a *Virgin*) that we might live forever with Him, as He is ever-living. We will investigate the italicized words in due time.

[iii.6]   No system of deduction or induction found within *The Knowledge of Good & Evil* will be left unexplained. Every system of deduction is provided and explained to the reader so that the reader can discover the same truths for him/herself and not be left to depend upon *The Knowledge of Good & Evil* for an attempt at a greater measure of correctness. We have names for our letters in English: "A" is called "Ay"; "B" is called "Bee"; "C" is called "See," etc., though the only concepts attached to such names are, for the most part, the sounds of the letters themselves (or at least the sounds they are capable of when pronounced in conjunction with other letters: "H" = "Aych" as it can produce this sound with the letter "C" in front of it). However, Hebrew letters have names that describe various concepts symbolized by a given letter. For instance, the first Hebrew letter "א" signifies "an ox." The "א" is considered to be the "revealed part" of the concept of "an ox" signified by this letter, but "an ox" is "אלף" and the remaining two letters "לף" are called the "secret parts." Here are what are commonly called the "revealed parts" (letters) and the "secret parts" (the remaining letters of the full letter-names) of the Hebrew alphabet separated by the "=" sign; (this list is generously provided in the *Introduction to the Ginsburg Edition of the Hebrew Old Testament: Vol. I*, by Rev. Alfred S. Geden, M.A., D.D. & Rev. R. Kilgour, D.D.; p. 18-19):

א	=	אָלֶף
ב	=	בֵּית
ג	=	גִּימֵל
ד	=	דָּלֶת
ה	=	הֵא
ו	=	וָיו
ז	=	זַיִן
ח	=	חֵית
ט	=	טֵית
י	=	יוֹד
כ	=	כַּף
ל	=	לָמֶד
מ	=	מֵים
נ	=	נוּן
ס	=	סָמֶךְ
ע	=	עַיִן
פ	=	פֵּא
צ	=	צָדִי
ק	=	קוֹף
ר	=	רֵישׁ
שׁ	=	שִׁין
שׂ	=	סִין
ת	=	תָּו

Satan's first words in Genesis are "Yea, hath," or "Is it so," as in "Is it so that God said, 'You shall not eat from any tree in the garden?'" (Genesis 3:1). These letters and their names will be explained later. As for now, let us consider that the battle between good and evil is over the word of God. The first letter-name of the Hebrew alphabet is "aleph" = "אֶלְף" = "א+ל+ף" = 80+30+1 = **111**. Like the first letter-name of the first letter of the Hebrew alphabet, the first letter that Satan spoke in Eden was "א" = "אֶלְף" = "א+ל+ף" = 80+30+1 = **111**, and Satan's first words in Genesis are "אַף כִּי" = "א+ף+כ+י" = 10+20+80+1 = **111**. As this first Hebrew letter (**111**) signifies "an ox," we can see a connection to this first letter when God said, "...thou art cursed above all cattle, and above every beast of the field..." (Genesis 3:14).

■■■

The reader will notice in the Gematria examples of this book that mostly *single words* from the lexicon are displayed out of context numerically in relation to the themes of the Bible (in context). The reason for this book's usage of single words from the lexicon is that these words cannot be manipulated numerically to assert a point that suits the author of this book himself. The author of this book is not a numerologist, and he has no desire to manipulate numbers to assert a particular doctrine. Instead, this book's display of Gematria (NOT Numerology) merely shows how the words of the lexicon compute to a congruence that mirrors **the related themes of the Bible** so that the reader might understand that the Bible's internal design is far above mere mortal cognition. In other words, one could merely compute the gematria values of the lexicon and state a case for word-parallels based on such a computation (and to no worthwhile effect); however, this book illustrates how the word-parallels in the lexicon (through gematria) also parallel Biblical accounts (in context) – it is the congruence of the Bible's parallel stories to the Biblical lexicon's parallel gematria values that is elucidated by this book's deliberate usage of single words. Various Biblical accounts mirror other Biblical accounts, and the themes of such parallel accounts are mirrored also by the gematria values of numerically congruent words in the Biblical lexicon. For example, let us consider these words:

"עור" (ref. 5782) = "(through the idea of *opening* the eyes) to *wake* (literally or figuratively)" = "ע+ו+ר" = 200+6+70 = **276**

"עור" (ref. 5783) = "to (be) bare:- be made naked" = "ע+ו+ר" = 200+6+70 = **276**

"עור" (ref. 5785) = "skin (as naked); hide, leather" = "ע+ו+ר" = 200+6+70 = **276**

"עור" (ref. 5786) = "to blind" = "ע+ו+ר" = 200+6+70 = **276**

When we observe that the number "**276**" links the ideas of **opening the eyes, nudity, hides/leather,** and **blindness**, we might also observe that Genesis Chapter III states that the serpent intimated Eve's **blindness** and stated that her **eyes would be opened** (Genesis 3:5), for both Adam and Eve's **eyes were opened** and they were aware of their **nakedness** upon realizing their sins (Genesis 3:7), and Jehovah Elohim made them garments of **leather** (Genesis 3:21) to cover their **nudity**. Thus, by knowing that the accounts of the Bible mirror each other, we can see that these parallel Biblical accounts also mirror the Gematria of *the single words of the Biblical lexicon that mirror each other numerically*.

Without accounting for the single words of the Biblical lexicon, the uses of Gematria can draw near to the abuses of Numerology, for Numerology is not Biblical and Numerology is against the numeric uniformity of Scripture. The divine design of the Bible shows how the concept and essence of each Biblical word as found in the lexicon agrees with the concept and essence of other Biblical words in the lexicon that compute to the same number, and this agreement is reflected intimately by the themes of the Bible's accounts that also parallel each other thematically.

Regardless of the lexicon, when the specific themes of Scripture reflect each other overtly, the gematria of words in context also reflect each other (see Rubrics i.19 & 2.54) – and this point is asserted because the computation of Gematria is unnecessary in order to discover overt Biblical parallel; rather, this book merely shows an example as such to reemphasize an allusion already provided by the simple meaning of a Biblical passage. The computation of Gematria regarding Biblical passages that parallel each other is but a reduced version of the parallel themes already obvious to the reader. Simply put, one does not need an intricate knowledge of mechanics to drive a car, but should one desire to learn more of how, specifically, a car operates, one might study auto-mechanics.

The Author of the Bible must have fully understood the

concept and essence of each of the 8,674 Hebrew words and 5,624 Greek words used in the Bible in conjunction with all of these words' individual and related mathematical computations in order to mirror His Book's parallel accounts to these computations, as Biblical accounts are validated even by celestial pattern. The Holy Bible cannot be but a masterful book in which its stories are written around the Gematria parallels of the Biblical lexicon, for history itself attests to the Holy Bible; therefore, history has unfolded along the lines of the Holy Bible, and the lines of the Holy Bible are written in congruence to the Gematria values of the Biblical lexicon – thus proving that, "In the beginning was the Word, and the Word was with God, and the Word was God," (John 1:1). The design of the Bible is far above human invention and imagination, as **the concept, essence, and computation of each Biblical word reflects the themes of history itself** explained in the Bible. Gematria and Numerology may appear similar, but they are not the same: Gematria is the host, but Numerology is the parasite.

SECTION I

א
QUEST

"Always be ready to make a defense to anyone who demands from you an accounting for the hope that is in you," (I Peter 3:15).

[1.1] How often do those who believe the Scriptures worship what they cannot explain, and how often do those who do not believe the Scriptures worship what they can explain? Far too often, fanciful stories are concocted concerning the history of the Scriptures' development and safeguarding. Far too often tradition persuades us to read stories into the Scriptures that are not truly there. The Holy Bible we read commonly is both a lock and a key. The Old Testament, as we know it, displays a lock; the New Testament displays the key. The Bible is wrapped in a giant mystery with a labyrinth inscribed around its borders that hedges in secrets beyond the capacities of our imaginations.

[1.2] It can become easy to read and re-read the New Testament in rapt joy while pondering the seemingly incomprehensible love of our Savior. It can also become easy to neglect the Old Testament because the Law was fulfilled by our Savior long ago. By neglecting the Old Testament in favor of the New Testament, we render ourselves utterly helpless in understanding why Christ did anything in the manner that He did anything, other than for the obvious fact that He loves us. Yet, did you ever slaughter an animal and sprinkle its blood all over your friend's living room because you cared for your friend? When you became tired of slaughtering animals for your friend, did you spill your own blood on your friend? If you have never done such things for someone else out of "love," it might be beneficial to consider why Jesus did similar things for you out of "love."

[1.3] We are much acquainted with the story of the

talking snake that tempted Eve and Adam to eat from a forbidden tree, an action that resulted in every crime and pain imaginable. We are also much acquainted with the fact that Christ died for our sins, and through His blood, we are saved. As far as Christ dying for our sins, we are certain of His love for us. As far as a talking snake and a piece of sinful fruit, I have yet to hear any solid, definite, clearly connected answer as to how Christ's blood fixes such a legendary story, or even how such a mythic account is possible in reality. Let us peer into an almost lost history whose skeleton has been buried in a garden since before Christ began His earthly ministry. The resounding questions of this book are: WHAT is the Eden story about and WHY did Christ do and say the things He did and in the manner that He did and said them? Far too often we are told, "It's just a mystery; now accept it!" Then why not believe in the mysteries of Cabala or Astrology? – why not just accept them? Are we to accept unanswerable mysteries over other accounts, legends, myths, and philosophies? Furthermore, are we supposed to tell others to just accept such things as well – an acceptance of certain things over those things that can appear to be defined and grasped as concrete? How can we accept such a strange premise that discusses talking snakes and seemingly magic fruit when the Scriptures say, "Now faith is the substance of things hoped for, the evidence of things not seen," (Hebrews 11:1). "Just accept it?" What happens when someone asks you why? How convincing will your answer be when it is limited to the all too common response: "Because." Furthermore, since when do the feelings of the heart rightfully outweigh reason? – for if the feelings of the heart could rightfully outweigh reason, then all of our unreasonable feelings would outweigh the reason God commands our obedience to Him for our own good.

"Because sentence against an evil deed is not executed speedily, the human heart is fully set to do evil," (Ecclesiastes 8:11).

There must be some reason as to why we have feelings and as to why our feelings can be unreasonable as often, or even more often, than they are reasonable. Often, feelings and physical sight are linked, for visual art is passionately appreciated by many. Often, a lack of feeling exists in conjunction with a lack of physical sight. We can believe that we can stand on a particular surface because our physical sight communicates to us that the surface is solid, and yet people perish each year by falling through thin surfaces of frozen bodies of water. Often, people claim not to put trust in that which they cannot see, and yet those same people dive headlong into water floating above an unseen and shallow bottom – whether for summer recreation or in personal pursuits – and often to the result of an injured and ignoble crown. The lack of physical sight cannot possibly indicate a lack of reality, despite what human feeling claims about either, for claiming ultimate reality based solely on physical sight could never prove the existence of wind beyond the reality of its effects. The same words rendered "spirit" in the Holy Scriptures are also rendered "wind."

How can one explain that the story of Salvation works apart from how the story of Salvation works? Often, the only defense that is personally articulated regarding the story of Salvation is that one personally believes one thing or another, and often the only apparent assuredness of such beliefs is intuitive and without qualifiable (let alone quantifiable) reason. God's reason knows everything: "Come now, let us reason together, says the Lord: though your sins are like scarlet, they shall be like snow; though they are red like crimson, they shall become like wool; If you are willing and obedient, you shall eat the good of the land; but if you refuse and rebel, you shall be devoured by the sword; for the mouth of the Lord has spoken," (Isaiah 1: 18-19).

[1.4]   The Scriptures say that, "... without the shedding of blood, there is no forgiveness of sins," (Hebrews 9:22). How can such a gruesome declaration be reconciled with a belief system that demands that, "... whatever is just, whatever is pure, whatever is pleasing, whatever is commendable, if there is any excellence and if there is anything worthy of praise, take account of these things," (Philippians 4: 8), and at the same time require that there must be a horrific, unjust slaying of a completely innocent Man? How is it that, if "God is love," (I John 4: 16), that blood must be shed at all? What must be remembered is that there is a consistent formula in the Holy Bible that threads every story together and binds them unwaveringly to Genesis 1-3:

The punishment for sin perfectly fits the crime of sin, and God's grace perfectly fits the punishment.

This book does not intend to argue the notion of divine

"punishment" in our lives today, but this book does intend to demonstrate how our Savior accepted the punishment that should have been entirely ours under the Law.

[1.5]   The entire unified progression of Scripture stems from Genesis 1-3. The Garden of Eden story in Genesis 2 & 3 is among the most famous on earth. Concerning the Scriptures, the believer and non-believer alike have heard the famous story of the talking snake that tempted the first woman into eating from a forbidden tree that somehow ruined all humanity. The believer often holds firm to such a tale as the origin of humanity's plight, whereas the non-believer often holds firm to such a tale as the origin of the believer's mistake. If the Holy Scriptures actually claimed that there was a talking snake that tempted the first woman to eat from a forbidden tree that somehow resulted in all of humanity's pain, suffering, and trouble, the non-believer would be correct. However, the Holy Scriptures never claim such an incredible tale, and both the believer and non-believer often share the same tradition as pointed from the parallax of traditional assertion and opposition. Such a claim about a talking snake is as outrageous as a claim that a world-wide flood occurred over the ludicrously brief time period of 40 days. There is no story of a 40-day flood in the Holy Bible, nor is there any story of a talking snake. Errant tradition, not Holy Scripture, is the sole reason for such mythical tales of obscured truth. Visual depictions of such mythical accounts frame honest mistakes that have left lamentably longer impressions than the Literary Truth of accurate historical record. Before you discard this book indignantly, let us briefly examine the story of the flood of Noah's time in order to make a point about the fabled talking snake.

[1.6]   According to tradition, many people claim that the Holy Scriptures clearly state that 40 days of rain flooded the entire earth. Where does Holy Scripture ever say that 40 days of rain flooded the entire earth? In the Book of Genesis, Jehovah said "... I will cause it to rain on the earth 40 days and 40 nights..." (Gen. 7:4); "Noah was 600 years old when the flood waters came on the earth," (Genesis 7:6); "In the 600th year of Noah's life, in the second month, on the 17th day of the month, on that day all the fountains of the great deep burst forth, AND the windows of the heavens were opened," (Gen. 7:11). The Holy Bible clearly states that the rain fell on the earth 40 days and 40 nights. Where does it say that the rain was the only water that constituted the great flood?   The Scriptures specifically state that all the fountains of the great deep burst forth. So we see that the waters came both from the bottom-up, and from the top-down to meet in one great flood with Noah's ark between the two waters; notice how this description is the exact opposite of "Day Second" in Genesis 1:6 where Elohim commanded, "Let an expanse be in the midst of the waters, and let it divide between the waters AND the waters," hence, the sky waters (in the imagery of those above the firmament) and the sea waters (in the imagery of those below the firmament). Noah was the human root of the regeneration of the earth, so when both of the waters of the flood of Noah's time finally abated, the waters of the sky and sea both separated themselves from the ground, just as they did on "Day Second" and "Day Third" before Noah walked the earth. The pattern is as a giant blink: the sky waters were separated from the sea waters (Genesis 1:6), the sky waters were joined again to the sea waters (Genesis 7:11), and the sky waters were again separated from the sea waters (Genesis 8:2) before the sea waters were eventually separated from the ground (Genesis 8:3). Genesis 1:2 says that the "Ruach," that is "Wind" or "Spirit" of God blew over the waters, just as it did in the flood of Noah's time (Genesis 8:1). Essentially, the literary formula employed in the Noah story is a reflection of the creation story of Genesis 1.

The Scriptures never say anything about a flood lasting 40 days and 40 nights, only that it rained 40 days and 40 nights, for all the fountains of the great deep burst forth. "In the 600th year of Noah's life, in the second month, on the 17th day of the month, on that day all the fountains of the great deep burst forth, AND the windows of the heavens were opened," (Gen. 7:11). "In the 601st year, in the first month, on the first day of the month, the waters were dried up from off the earth," (Genesis 8: 13). "The waters flooded the earth for 150 days," (Genesis 7:24). That is, the actual flooding process itself was 150 days. Once the 150-day flooding stopped, the waters had to abate – which, obviously, took quite some time; thus the entire duration of the great deluge until it abated was one year, not 40 days. Now we see why the flood began when Noah was 600 years old and finally abated when he was 601 years old. The Astronomer G. Shiaparelli wrote that, "The flood would therefore have lasted for twelve moons and eleven extra days. It is hard not to recognize here the intention of making the flood last for an exact solar year; for if 354 days be assumed for the duration of twelve moons... the total duration of the flood comes to 365 days," (*Astronomy in the Old Testament*, Schiaparelli; p. 127). We note that, "The waters increased and bore up the ark," (Genesis 7:17), that is, the great springs of the deep rose also as opposed to water having only fallen down upon the ark in the form of rain.

What then of the talking snake and the famous fruit?

[1.7]   We must always keep in the forefront of our minds that Christ fulfilled every part of the Law to forgive every sin so that existence could be realigned with how it was intended to be originally prior to human error. The entire Holy Bible is as a mirror, and each story is reflected by some other story within the Text, which is only one reason that the New Testament is not merely some continuation of the Old Testament, but rather a reflection of the Old Testament. The Old Testament cannot be comprehended to the intended extent without the New Testament, and neither can the New Testament be comprehended to the intended extent without the Old Testament. "But you, O Bethlehem of Ephrathah, who are one of the little clans of Judah, from you shall come forth for me one who is to rule in Israel, whose origin is from of old, from ancient days," (Micah 5:2 & Matthew 2:6).   Christ's innocent death ended sin's dominion, just as a former innocent death began sin's dominion.

Genesis 3:6 says, "So when the woman saw that the tree was good for food, and that it was a delight to the eyes, and that the tree was to be desired to make one wise, she took of its fruit and ate..." The English words, "to make wise" are only one Hebrew word: להשכיל from שכל ; these three letters in this order have more than one meaning as their identical gematria values display part of the link, though only one meaning can be rendered in context while reading. Why then is only one meaning put down in our English Bibles? Acknowledging the fact that only one word can be selected while reading (as it is impossible to articulate related meanings/allusions all at once while reading), it is also well known that the ancient Scribes endeavored their utmost to euphemize various portions of difficult Scripture so as not to utter displeasing words when reading the tradition aloud. Consider the words "to make wise": how could the forbidden tree have been good "to make wise" when this description of wisdom is linked to the Tree of Life that is described in Proverbs 3:18?

When reading the Hebrew dictionary, one finds multiple words composed of the exact same letters in the exact same order. The difference between two words with identical letters can be seen in the dots and dashes that surround these letters. The "dots and dashes" are vowels and articulation aids, and they display the system that distinguishes one word from another despite two words being constituted by the exact same consonant letters in the exact same order. However, the vowels, as we know them, did not fully exist in Hebrew when the Scriptures were written originally, but the full set of the vowels was a later invention instead. The Hebrew Bible was not originally written with the dots and dashes, that is, with the vowels and articulation aids we now read today. What we read today is our introduction to what was written originally. The invention of vowel points helped to provide a standard reading of the Text, but the invention limited the differentiated messages that work in unison within the written Text. Simply put, the insertion of the vowels facilitated reading so that the reader would not be allotted the onus of trying to pronounce almost every word one way or another to fit a tradition. The vowels themselves fixed the tradition(s), in a manner of speaking.

Some Bibles (both Jewish and Christian) render Genesis 1:1-2 to say, "In the beginning, *when* God created the heavens and the earth, the earth was formless and void and darkness covered the face of the deep..."; this rendering ignores two major points: 1) it conflicts with Isaiah 45:18, and 2) it ignores the fact that the Jewish calendar is based on the cycles of the moon.

1) Isaiah 45:18 states that, "For thus says the Lord, Who created the heavens (He is God!), who formed the earth and made it (He established it; He did not create it a chaos, He formed it to be inhabited!)." In other words, Genesis 1:2 states that, "...the earth was [/became] *without form* [*tohu*]..." and Isaiah 45:18 states that, "He created it not *tohu*..."

2) Considering the importance of the seven-day week (as marked by the Sabbath), one month (based on the round reckoning of four weeks) equates to four portions of seven, that is 28 days (reckoning only whole numbers when averaging the sidereal month of 27.32166 days and the synodic month of 29.53059 days); the sidereal month is not regarded in Jewish law. The set of four sevens is the first and most ancient form of a week. The Jewish months are composed of either 29 days (a "deficient" month, which is slightly less than a synodic month) or 30 days (a "pregnant" month, which is slightly more than a synodic month). The official declaration of a new moon

was (apparently) determined by the sighting of the first sliver of the moon – which is after the true conjunction – and the Jewish month only reckons whole days and does not include fractions of days. The numbers 28, 29, and 30 are fitted together in Ecclesiastes 3:1-8 that lists the famous 28 "times" and these times are introduced by the figuration of Synonymous Parallel regarding "season" and "time" (3:1) so that, technically speaking, 28 days (four periods of seven), 29, and 30 days are all recognized in unison and in relation to the reckoning of a month – which is the first Law of the Torah addressed to the Jews as a nation (Exodus 12:2) – a law that reflects the first statement of the Torah written in seven words and 28 letters. The calculation of the month is of extreme importance to Jews, as this calculation regulates the festivals commanded in the Torah.

The week is of great significance in the Scriptures, for the eventual 27-letter alphabets of both Hebrew and Greek are also numeric, and their first letter is both the number 1 and the number 1,000 (considering the beginning – 1 – and the end – 1000 – of a circuit) whereby 28 components are reckoned (cyclically speaking) so that the alphabets can be divided into four equal portions of seven based on the week of seven days (though being constituted of only 27 letters, a constitution that recognizes final letter-forms). Genesis 1:1 should read, "In the beginning, God created the heavens and the earth" (as some versions still render it), for this original rendering shows Genesis 1:1 to be, again, seven words long constructed by 28 letters in accordance with the week, no different than how we have observed the flood of Noah's time to be in congruence with the solar year.

[1.8] Technically speaking, there is no way to account for all the meanings of the Hebrew Scriptures in any language all at one time – the Scriptures are too expansive as the same message is relayed over and over through increasing levels of specificity and potency, like the layers of an onion. The Hebrew Scriptures were written originally in a language system that lacked the vowel-markings that we know today, and due to this complexity, the ancient Scribes invented a system of vowels that were placed into the Scriptures and solidified there some time considerably after the final Hebrew Scripture was written. The history of the Hebrew vowel insertion and its official Scribes is contested as it is more than clouded by the lack of record concerning who these Scribes actually were. The chronology and specificity of the Scribal history of the Scriptures is often shaded into the tinctures of legend. However, the Scribes' work is documented, as it has served to define the exactitude of some of the most devoutly held traditions.

The two most famous groups of Scribes were called the "Sopherim" and the "Massorites": "The labors of the Massorites may be regarded as a later development and continuation of the early work which was carried on by the *Sopherim* (סופרים, γραμματεις) = the doctors and authorized interpreters of the Law soon after the return of the Jews from the Babylonish captivity (comp. Ezra VII 6; Neh. VIII 1&c.). And though it is now impossible to describe the chronological order the precise work which these custodians of Holy Writ undertook in the new Commonwealth, it may safely be stated that the gradual substitution of the square characters for the so-called

Phoenician or archaic Hebrew alphabet was one of the first tasks," (*Introduction to the Massaretico-Critical Edition of the Hebrew Bible*, Ginsburg; p. 287).

The Scribes gradually introduced letters that serve also as vowels to help pronounce the Hebrew Scriptures that were yet without the famous vowel-points; however, as to this vowelization of the Scriptures, such sharp contention came about that two major divisions arose in opposition to each other: the Pharisees and the Sadducees. The Sopherim introduced the written changes in order to aid laity in the study of Scripture (*Introduction to the Massaretico-Critical Edition of the Hebrew Bible*, Ginsburg; p. 299), and the Pharisees were, "an essentially lay group formed from one of the branches of the Hasidim of the Maccabaean age," (*The Complete Dead Sea Scrolls*, Vermes; p. 53). "After the ephemeral rule of the successor to Herod the Great, Herod Archelaus (4 BCE-6 CE), who was deposed by Augustus for his misgovernment of Jews and Samaritans alike, Galilee continued in semi-autonomy under the Herodian princes Antipas (4 BCE- 39 CE) and Agrippa (39-41 CE), but Judaea was placed under the direct administration of Roman authority. In 6 CE, Coponius, the first Roman prefect of Judaea, arrived to take up his duties there. This prefectorial regime, whose most notorious representative was Pontius Pilate (26-36 CE), lasted for thirty-five years until 41, when the emperor Claudius appointed Agrippa I as king. He died, however, three years later, and in 44 CE the government of the province once more reverted to Roman officials, this time with the title of procurator. Their corrupt and unwise handling of Jewish affairs was one of the chief causes of the war of 66 which led to the destruction of Jerusalem in 70 CE, and to the subsequent decline of the Sadducees, the extinction of the Zealots in Masada in 74, the disappearance of the Essenes, and the survival and uncontested domination of the Pharisees and their rabbinic successors," (*The Complete Dead Sea Scrolls*, Vermes; p. 53). However, regarding the Massorah (the work of the Sopherim and Massorites), as it eventually came to be, it "refers to everything transmitted with the biblical text except its consonants. It includes: vowel signs, accent signs, arrangements of poetry, marginal notes and endnotes, as well as separate treatises on the copying and use of manuscripts. Massorah exists independently of halakhah (rabbinic law). The early medieval masters of the biblical text who developed this documentation are known in English as 'masoretes' [*Massorites*]. Many masoretic annotations seem designed to reduce loss or distortion in transmission of the text," (*J.P.S. Tanakh*, p. ix). The officers and the learned laity had the Sopherim to guide their learning; however, when the Massorites later received the Sacred Text, their work existed independently of rabbinic law (though the Massorites came to have divisions amongst themselves). We can see the battle over the Holy Word of God and its preservation. The main difference between the Sopherim and the Massorites is that the Sopherim were the authorized revisers of the Scriptures, whereas the Massorites were the authorized custodians of the Scriptures. The Sopherim set the Text in order, and the Massorites preserved and guarded it.

"Most Hebrew words are built upon verbal roots consisting of three consonants called radicals. There are approximately 1,850 such roots in the Old Testament, from which various nouns and other parts of speech have been derived. Many of these roots represent theological, moral, and ceremonial concepts that have been obscured by the passage of time... Hebrew language and literature hold a unique place in the course of Western civilization. It emerged sometime after 1,500 B.C. in the area of Palestine, along the eastern shore of the Mediterranean... The Hebrew language probably came into existence during the patriarchal period, about 2,000 B.C. The language was reduced to writing about 1,250 B.C., and the earliest extant Hebrew inscription dates from about 1,000 B.C.... Greek tradition claims that the Phoenicians invented the alphabet. Actually, this is only partly true, since the Phoenician writing system was not an alphabet as we know it today. It was a simplified syllabary system – in other words, its various symbols represent syllables rather than separate vocal components. The Hebrew writing system grew out of the Phoenician system. The Hebrew writing system gradually changed over the centuries. From 1,000 to 200 B.C., a rounded script (Old Phoenician style) was used. This script was last used for copying the biblical text and may be seen in the *Dead Sea Scrolls*. But after the Jews returned from their Babylonian Captivity, they began to use the square script of the Aramaic language, which was the official language of the Persian Empire [*the empire to whom the Magi and the word 'paradise' is principally linked*]. Jewish scribes adopted the Aramaic book hand, a more precise form of the script. When Jesus mentioned the "jot" and "tittle" of the Mosaic Law, He was referring to the manuscripts in the square script. The book hand is used in all printed editions of the Hebrew Bible... From A.D. 200 to nearly A.D. 900, groups of scholars attempted to devise systems of vowel markings (later called points) to aid Jewish readers who no longer spoke Hebrew. The scholars who did this work are called Masoretes [*Massorites*], and their markings are called the Masora [*Massorah*]. The Masoretic text that they produced represents the consonants that had been preserved from about 100 B.C. (as proven by the *Dead Sea Scrolls*); **but the vowel markings reflect the understanding of the Hebrew language in about A.D. 300**. The Masoretic text dominated Old Testament studies in the Middle Ages, and it has served as the basis for virtually all printed versions of the Hebrew Bible," (*Vine's Expository Dictionary of Old and New Testament Words*; Forward – Introduction).

Adam was placed in the garden in Eden to "cultivate it and to guard it," (Genesis 2:15); "Now the serpent was subtle above every beast of the field which the Lord God had Made," (Genesis 3:1); "...only a place that is cultivated is called a 'field,'" (*Ramban: Genesis, Vol. 1*, Ramban; p. 93). The ancient Scribes treated the Scriptures as a "garden," = "גן" (ref. 1588) = "garden (as fenced)"; from "גנן" (ref. 1598) = "to hedge about; protect; defend." Similarly, a "paradise" is also something "hedged" in, and a "vineyard" = "כרם" (ref. 3754) is also considered a "garden," as Keil and Delitzsch render this word as "vine-garden" (*Commentary on the Old Testament: Song of Songs*, Keil & Delitzsch; p. 518). The Massorah is called a hedge, or a "Fence to the Scriptures," (*Companion Bible*, Bullinger; Appendix 30) because, as it was written on the actual pages of Scripture (around the holy words), it served to lock every letter of every word in place safely protected against intrusion. However, the work of the Massorites was only completed (A.D.), after the Scriptures were handed to them from the Sopherim (who began B.C.), to be guarded or "hedged in." Consider the title "Sopherim" in light of these words:

"סֹפֵר" (ref. 5608) = "to score with a mark as a tally or record, to inscribe, to enumerate" = "ס+פ+ר" = 200+80+60 = **340**

"סֵפֶר" (ref. 5609) = "a book, roll" = "ס+פ+ר" = 200+80+60 = **340**

"סֹפֵר" (ref. 5610) = "a census:- numbering" = "ס+פ+ר" = 200+80+60 = **340**

"סֹפֵר" (ref. 5612) = "writing (the art or a document); by implication, a book, bill, evidence, register" = "ס+פ+ר" = 200+80+60 = **340**

The guarded, garden-like approach to hedging in the Scriptures conducted by the Scribes probably had something to do with the fact that consonants "נצר" can be rendered these ways:

"נצר" (ref. 5341) = "to guard (in a good sense; to protect, maintain) or in a bad sense (to conceal), subtle" = "נ+צ+ר" = 200+90+50 = **340**

"נצר" (ref. 5342) = "in the sense of *greenness* as a striking color; *a shoot* (figuratively) a descendant, *branch*" = "נ+צ+ר" = 200+90+50 = **340**

Christ is called the "Righteous Branch" in Jeremiah 23:5 and the "Word" or "Computation" ["λογος" (ref. *3056*)] in John 1:1, for "...He opened their minds to understand the Scriptures," (Luke 24:45).

Unfortunately, the work of the Sopherim eventually hid critical elements of the Scriptures (probably after Ezra and Nehemiah died) to the point that the mysterious Sopherim decided to make many "emendations"; some of the most famous of these are called "The 18 Emendations of the Sopherim." These emendations were devised partially to eliminate, "indelicate expressions and anthropomorphisms," (*Introduction to the Massaretico-Critical Edition of the Hebrew Bible*, Ginsburg; p. 347).

[1.9] "You must neither add anything to what I command you nor take away anything from it," (Deuteronomy 4:2); "You must diligently observe everything that I command you; do not add to it or take anything from it," (Deuteronomy 12:33). Regarding the garden in Eden, consider that in Genesis 3:2-3, the woman (later named "Eve" after her punishment) subtracted the Holy Name "Jehovah" from Jehovah Elohim's command and only referred to Him as "Elohim," added the word "fruit" to Jehovah Elohim's command, subtracted one of the two trees from the "midst" of the garden in her accounting, added a clause about touching the ambiguous "tree," and turned Jehovah Elohim's certain declaration into a condition – all in only one statement! "Every word of God is pure; He is a shield to those who put their trust in Him. Do not add to His words; lest He reprove you, and you be found a liar," (Provebs 30:5-6).

We might feel an in initial uneasiness, if not resentment, towards the choices of some of the unknown Scribes, though we can hardly blame every one of those Scribes for what became of originally honest work. However, we all, at one time or another, have committed recitative blunders regarding the word of God similar to Eve's blunder. Though it does not necessarily excuse the matter of Scriptural alteration, it is difficult to believe that deliberately alternative editing choices existed in Ezra's Great Synagogue while he lived, though such degenerative choices certainly occurred later in history. Good intentions are never enough. Satan desired to be like the Most High (Isaiah 14:14), and he tempted the woman with the promise of being like God herself (Genesis 3:3-5). Without defining a capacity, being like God appears to be nothing but good as He Himself is entirely good, hence the power of the Tempter's terse allusions and nebulous illusions. Though there is no acceptable excuse for error concerning God's Word, there is no group of people who are all entirely good; so let us keep this in mind as we unearth the ancient labors exerted upon the Scriptures, and let us view these labors from a historical viewpoint.

Many have vehemently asserted that the earth broke apart because of the contents of some magic apple that humanity chose to eat, but where does it say "apple," and how does such a fruit destroy the entire earth? How are God's judgments in Genesis Chapter 3 connected to the presumed magic fruit? We cannot ignore the fact that the *Introduction to the Rabbinic Bible*, p. 51) states the common fact that "Our sages submit, 'All the verses wherein are written indecent expressions, decent expressions are read in their stead,'" as this introduction provides list after list of assumed Biblical discrepancies, alterations, etc.

[1.10] There was a vast array of conflicting assertions

made by the ancient Rabbis regarding what the Scriptures actually communicated, how they should be read, and how they should be copied. Various Rabbis asserted that their particular traditions amend what other Rabbis considered anomalies or even mistakes concerning printing (copying/transmission) of the Holy Scriptures. Some ancient Scribes and Rabbis actually believed that the inspired Word of God lacked adequate grammar, was speckled with poor spelling, and that it was only by their superior command of Hebrew that they could fix what the prophets wrote! The ancient Scribes made a list of 56 known instances where the letter י was inserted in the middle of a word articulated by the official reading that did not occur in the actual Text of the Scriptures. The Scribes made another list of 18 words that omitted the letter ו at the end of a word.

The Sopherim made the famous "18" emendations to the Bible. The number 18 is put in quotes because the various lists of the "18" emendations the Sopherim differ from each other, thereby producing more than 18 in number: Genesis 18:22; Numbers 11:15, 12:12; I Samuel 3:13; II Samuel 12:14, 16:12; I Kings 12:16, 21:10, 21:13; II Chronicles 10:16; Job 1:5, 1:11, 2:5, 2:9, 7:20, 32:3; Psalms 10:3, 106:20; Ecclesiastes 3:21; Jeremiah 2:11; Lamentations 3:20; Ezekiel 8:17; Hosea 4:7; Habakkuk 1:12; Zechariah 2:8; Malachi 1:13, 3:9. Why would the sages of numbers miscount a number as small as 18? – perhaps because "חוד" (ref. 2330) = "to tie a knot, i.e. (figuratively) to propound a riddle" = "ד+ו+ח" = 4+6+8 = **18**, though this is only a suggestion and not an assertion. The religious elites were aware of the alterations to the copies of Scripture as such alterations led to the eventual theological divisions, even amongst themselves; but after enough time had elapsed, the people who heard the Scriptures in the Synagogue were unaware as to the intricacies of the Scriptures that the Scribes' alterations covered.

"Whom shall He teach knowledge? And whom shall He make to understand doctrine? Them that are weaned from the milk, and drawn from the breasts," (Isaiah 28:9). "I tell you the truth, unless you change and become like little children, you will never enter the kingdom of heaven. Therefore, whoever *humbles* himself like this child is the greatest in the kingdom of heaven," (Matthew 18:3-4) – as an attitude, not a knowledge-base, is being discussed, for it is written, "Brothers and sisters, do not be children in your *thinking*. In regard to evil be infants, but in your thinking be adults," (I Corinthians 14:20).

Unfortunately, the edited copies of Scripture became translated into English, and our edited copies were translated again into simpler and simpler English. Such a regression is similar to taking the most monumental of epics, converting it into an amended children's book, and then making dozens of successive copies of which each is even simpler and farther removed from the source than the one that immediately preceded it... and once the simplest version of a children's book is accepted by a multitude, this children's book becomes doctrine; after this doctrine is established, more than half of the simplest copy of the children's book becomes neglected under the slander of being considered out-dated. As to the number of deaths that have resulted over the reduced and simplified copies of Scripture, we can see childish reasoning spurring childish actions. Some who discard the Old Testament as being too violent might be quick to argue that the New Testament negates such violence because Christ commanded, "...You shall love your neighbor as yourself," (Matthew 19:19); "You shall not take vengeance or bear a grudge against any of your people, but you shall love your neighbor as yourself; I am the Lord," (Leviticus 19:18).

[1.11] The Scribes disliked any anthropomorphic descriptions of God, and they considered such anthropomorphic descriptions to be displeasing to the ear. For instance, Genesis 18:22 says, "... God still stood before Abraham"; the Scribes changed this to "...Abraham still stood before God" – as is found in English Bibles today. The Scribes also did their best to rewrite the Scriptures in a manner that could, in no way, be interpreted that God is somehow evil; so in Numbers 11:15, it is said, "Kill me, I pray ... that I may not see THY evil"; the Scribes changed this to say, "... that I may not see MY evil" – as is found in English Bibles today. The original sense given in Numbers 11:15 does not indicate that God is evil, but that He can and will bring about various disciplinary calamities, like pruning, in order to produce a righteous end for His people. "No such difference of opinion, however, can possibly be entertained about the statement made by the redactors of the text with regard to the principles by which they were guided in the work of redaction. The classical passage which sets forth these principles is as follows: 'In every passage where the text has indelicate expression a euphemism is to be substituted for it, as for instance for... *ravish, violate, outrage* [Deut. XXVIII 30; Isa. XIII 16; Jerem. III 2; Zech. XIV 2]... *to lie with,* is to be substituted; ...*urine* [2 Kings XVIII 27; Isa. XXXVI 12] read... *water of the feet...*'" etc. (*Introduction to the Massoretico-Critical Edition of the Hebrew Bible*, Ginsburg; p. 346).

Among the most noticeable alterations/euphemizations of Scripture, for our purposes, is that the Scribes changed Numbers 12:12 to say, "Let her not be as one dead born, which when it proceeds from the womb of ITS mother has half of ITS flesh consumed," (as this sense is also found in English Bibles today); but Numbers 12:12 originally said, "Let her not be as one dead, who proceeded from the womb of OUR mother, and half of OUR flesh be consumed," (*Introduction to the Rabbinic Bible*, Chajim; p. 68), and this alteration of Numbers 12:12 is also documented in the *Introduction to the Massoretico-Critical Edition of the Hebrew Bible*, Ginsburg; p. 348). The "OUR mother" referred to here is Adam's wife, which is why after she sinned and her WOMB was punished, then "...Adam called his wife's name *Eve* [*Life*] because she *became* the mother of all the living," (Genesis 3:20).

As applied to infants, *Webster's New World Dictionary* defines the word "abortion" in these ways:

"1:a) any spontaneous expulsion of an embryo or a fetus before it is sufficiently developed to survive; miscarriage;

1:b) any deliberate procedure that removes, or induces the expulsion of a living or dead embryo or fetus; 2) an aborted embryo or fetus; 3) anything immature and incomplete or unsuccessful, as a deformed creature."

The emendations of the Scribes were devised to eliminate, "indelicate expressions," (*Introduction to the Massaretico-Critical Edition of the Hebrew Bible*, Ginsburg; p. 347). Among the most notable emendations occurred at Numbers 12:12, for this graphic and "indelicate" description is not arbitrary or random. No part of Scripture is arbitrary or random. Concerning Jewish practice, "Seven relatives of the deceased are required to mourn (father, mother, brother, sister, son, daughter, and spouse). The mourning period, called *aveilus*, begins with the sealing of the grave. Until that time, the mourners are in a state of *aninus*... there is no *aninus* for a *neifel* ["נפל" (ref. 5309) = "something fallen, i.e. an *abortion:- untimely birth*"]... a nonviable infant, and an infant that died within thirty days of its birth is considered a *neifel*," (*Baal Ha Turim*, Gold; p. 978); according to ancient custom, such person was not provided a coffin, but the person who suffered such a dark birth was planted in the ground like a seed and the memory of the grim event was hushed as Ecclesiastes 6:3-4 indicates: "...I say that a stillborn child is better off than he. For it comes into vanity and goes into darkness, and in darkness its name is covered."

Here is the oldest secret of human history, the reason why the earth was rent into a tear of despair: the firstborn of all humanity was born dead, at the ignorant, but sinning, hands of both of *his* parents who consumed forbidden food that stunted God's first command to "be fruitful and multiply" (Genesis 3:28) – and this is why Jesus, the "Firstborn of the Dead" (Colossians 1:18; Revelation 1:5) died on a tree in His innocence at the ignorant, but sinning, hands of the religious and political elites:

"...Father, forgive them; for they do not know what they are doing," (Luke 23:43). As the "serpent" commented negatively on the sight of Adam's wife for evil purposes (Genesis 3:5), so Christ commented negatively on the Pharisees' sight for righteous purposes (John 9:39-41), for the Pharisees were considered serpents (Matthew 23:33). The Scribes themselves admitted to altering Numbers 12:12, among many other places in Scripture, in order to avoid the unpleasantries of reading such statements aloud. However, such an emendation also served to obscure this statement: "I will greatly increase your pangs in CHILDBEARING; **in pain you shall bring forth children**..." (Genesis 1:16), for the punishment fit the crime, and the grace fit the punishment through the Savior, the "Firstborn of the Dead" (Colossians 1:18; Revelation 1:5). "Some of the Pharisees near Him heard this and said to Him, 'Surely we are not blind, are we?' Jesus said to them, 'If you were blind, you would not have sin. But now that you say, 'We see,' your sin remains," (John 9:40-41).

Long after the Scriptures were written, the Scribes solidified vowels within the Hebrew Scriptures in an effort to ensure that only a euphemistically traditional rendering could be given. The word "להשכיל" [from "שכל" (ref. 7919)] "*to make wise*" can also mean "שכל" (ref. 7921) "to miscarry, to suffer abortion" with respect to its original consonants and gematria; it tells us of the horrid crime committed in Eden concerning the mother of all humanity who, after sin, was named *Eve* [*Life*].

"שכל" (ref. 7919) = "to be circumspect, intelligent" = "ל+כ+ש" = 30+20+300 = **350**

"שכל" (ref. 7921) = "miscarry; suffer abortion; bereave of children" = "ש+כ+ל" = 30+20+300 = **350**

Satan did not tempt humanity until after Adam's wife was created, for merely deceiving Adam would not have stunted God's first command to humanity, as the battle between good and evil is primarily over what God has said, which is a reason why Satan's first words begin with the first letter of the Hebrew Alphabet, and why those words also sum to the same gematria as the first letter of the Hebrew alphabet. However, once the woman was created by God and impregnated by Adam in accordance with the first command given to humanity (Genesis 1:28), her own willingness to sin in the manner of Satan's temptation led to the very act that defied the first command of God (Genesis 1:28). We can begin to see why she was not named *Eve* [*Life*] until after God promised the Savior.

Satan tricked the woman into disobeying God based on her own desires for wisdom without telling her the consequences of her foolish disobedience. The woman thought the "the tree" was good for food, and she also received everything that Satan promised her – with an extra surprise that Satan failed to mention... just as she failed to mention the Holy Name "Jehovah" regarding His command concerning the "tree" and only identified the Commander as "Elohim," for "Jehovah" is usually viewed in covenant relation to His creation and His Name means something similar to "Eternal, Self-Existent." *Elohim* [*Creator*] gave the command concerning fruitfulness to humans (Genesis 1:28), and it was *Jehovah* [*Eternal*] Elohim Who gave the command concerning the Tree of the Knowledge of Good and Evil (Genesis 2:17). "... Elohim depicts the one true God as the infinitely great exalted One, who created the heavens and the earth, and who preserves and governs every creature," (*Commentary on the Old Testament: Genesis*, Keil & Delitzsch; p. 46). "The name Jehovah... was originally a proper name..." (*Commentary on the Old Testament: Genesis*, Keil & Delitzsch; p. 46); fittingly, it was Jehovah Elohim who gave the proper names of the two central trees apart from the other general trees. Let us observe the commands of *God* [*Elohim* alone & *Jehovah Elohim*] in Genesis 1-3.

Elohim: "'Be fruitful and multiply, and fill the earth and subdue it; and have dominion over the fish of the sea and over the birds of the air and over every living thing that moves upon the earth.' And Elohim said, 'See, I have given you *every plant yielding seed* that is upon the face of the earth, and *every tree with seed in its fruit*; you shall have them for food," (Genesis 1:28-29).

Jehovah Elohim: "You may freely eat of *every tree* of the garden; but of the Tree of the Knowledge of Good and Evil you shall not eat, for in the day that you eat of it you shall surely die," (Genesis 2:17).

Despite English translations (where extra words are sometimes supplied), as a result of the woman's confusion of the Names of God, she also confused His commands; the only "fruit" God bound to commands given to humanity in Scripture until the Fall of man was the human "fruit" that humanity was commanded to produce (Genesis 1:28) and the fruit of which they were allowed to eat (Genesis 1:29). Satan wanted the human fruit consumed "...as one dead, who proceeded from the womb of OUR mother..." (Numbers 12:12) through the human consumption of the forbidden "tree's" fruit. Hence, the woman began her reply to Satan by stating what "Elohim" had said concerning "the tree," when in fact Elohim alone gave no command to humanity in relation to "trees" concerning what they *could not* eat, but that they themselves were to be fruitful and multiply and that they *could* eat of every seed-bearing tree. It was Jehovah Elohim Who gave the command about the "tree" that *could not* be eaten from without sin (Genesis 2:17), and unlike Elohim alone, Jehovah Elohim made no mention of "fruit" at all concerning what was forbidden. Truly, the only "fruit" that was part of a God-given command in this story was human fruit that resulted from human seed and fruit that resulted from vegetation seed. Jehovah Elohim prohibited eating "of the tree" (Genesis 1:17) of the Knowledge of Good and Evil, and He did not limit His command to merely that of the forbidden tree's fruit as is also evident in His accusatory question in Genesis 3:11. Elohim gave humanity "...every plant yielding seed that is upon the face of all the earth, and **every tree with seed in its fruit**..." (Genesis 2:29) to eat; however, Elohim gave "...every beast of the earth, and to every fowl of the air, and to every thing that creepeth upon the earth, wherein there is life," the permission to eat "...every green plant for food," (Genesis 1:30) so as to notice that animals were not bound to eat only *seed-bearing* vegetation like humans were so bound.

"Not only is God called Elohim alone in the middle of this

section, viz., in the address to the serpent, a clear proof that the interchange of the names has reference to their different significations; but the use of the double name, which occurs here twenty times though rarely met with elsewhere, is always significant. In the Pentateuch we only find it in Ex. 9:30; 2 Chron. 6:41, 42; Ps. 84:8, 11; and Ps. 50:1, where the order is reversed; and in every instance it is used with peculiar emphasis, to give prominence to the fact that Jehovah is truly Elohim, whilst in Ps. 50:1 the Psalmist advances from the general name El and Elohim to Jehovah, as the personal name of the God of Israel. In this section the combination Jehovah Elohim is expressive of the fact, that Jehovah is God, or one with Elohim. Hence Elohim is placed after Jehovah. For the constant use of the double name is not intended to teach that Elohim who created the world was Jehovah, but that Jehovah, who visited man in paradise, who punished him for the transgression of His command, but gave him a promise of victory over the tempter, was Elohim, the same God, who created the heavens and the earth," (*Commentary on the Old Testament: Genesis,* Keil & Delitzsch; p. 45).

As is common knowledge, the Scribes euphemized portions of Scripture so as not to read aloud the revolting historical accounts many would prefer to forget – the very reason why the earth became tainted with blood, death, and sorrow, the reason why the blood-covenant entwined with ritual sacrifice was instituted. Obviously, the most appalling history that people would rather forget is the history of the first sin – the horrid story of a stillborn baby boy being birthed in a hideousness that should rather have been an unparalleled beauty. At the same time, the social custom that disallowed the mourning of a *neifel* was edited into the Sacred Text through the insertion of the vowels as "to make wise" was pointed only to agree with the tree of "knowledge" as opposed to the destruction of human "fruit," and had even only this one word been left unpointed (that is, without the vowels), the seemingly ambiguous consonants would have alluded to Adam's dead son. Satan deliberately assaulted this child through calculated words delivered askance, and the child was mourned by our God but forgotten by us. It does not seem consistent that the Lord would not lament this child when considering that the entire earth suffered on account of this one child's demise! – particularly when He sent His only Son (in perfect parallel and in perfect justice) to correct this very error! Rather, it does seem consistent that humans later in history would not lament this child when considering that various Scribes covered the fundamental origin of sin beneath human custom in the name of euphemistic tradition. God's Word is holy. God's Word is for our benefit, and His holy Word has been given to us to guard and to uphold, not to turn into whatever pleases our self-tainted ears – and perhaps this is why Christ is referred to as the "Holy Child" in Acts 4:27.

Traditionally speaking, saying one thing but meaning another proves useful so long as the remembrance of the original sense remains; once the original sense is forgotten or obscured, the other meaning becomes an entity unto itself – though I do not intend to imply anything against metaphorical speech. Tradition is only tradition; good tradition is good, and bad tradition is bad. Unfortunately, people often prefer a tradition over which they have control as opposed to a tradition that they did not make nor over which they can control – even if it for their own good. A mountain road hedged in with guard-rails is hardly the cause of someone's fall, for to defy the guard-rail and to fall to an extent beyond initial intention is only the fault of one willing to set his or her own parameters against sound reason (even if sound reason is temporarily misunderstood). The euphemized renderings of Scripture became the tradition of the people. The euphemized renderings of Scripture obscured the truth as to the fact that Adam and his wife consumed poison ignorantly, thereby killing the very first human procreation. Concerning the blood covenant, the innocent blood of this stillborn infant mingled with the otherwise marital, covenantal blood purely present at birth, resulted in the blood-requirement of the Torah, the same blood requirement that Christ died under as the "*Firstborn* of the Dead" (Colossians 1:18; Revelation 1:5).

It is in remembrance of this slain firstborn *son of Adam* that under the Law of the Torah, "All that first opens the womb is mine, all your male livestock, the firstborn of cow and sheep. The firstborn of a donkey you shall redeem with a lamb, or if you will not redeem it you shall break its neck. **All the firstborn of your sons you shall redeem**. No one shall appear before Me empty-handed," (Exodus 34:19-20). As humans were created on the same "Day" as the cows, sheep, donkeys, lambs, etc. so Coheleth wrote that, "I said in my heart with regard to human beings that God is testing them to show that they are but animals," (Ecclesiastes 3:18). Christ, our Passover (I Corinthians 5:7), rode on a donkey whose neck did not need to be broken, as Christ said, "My yoke is easy, and My burden is light," (Matthew 11:30), and He redeemed us when He said, "Paid in full," (John 19:30) when He fulfilled all of the Torah as "Firstborn of the Dead," (Colossians 1:18; Revelation 1:5) as, "...All the firstborn of your sons you shall redeem. No one shall appear before Me empty-handed," (Exodus 34: 20). "The whole system of the Hebrew rites is one great and complicated allegory, to the study and observance of which all possible diligence and attention were incessantly dedicated by those who were employed in the sacred offices," (*Lectures on the Sacred Poetry of the Hebrews*, Lowth; p. 82). "Much of the Jewish law is employed in discriminating between things clean and unclean; in removing and making atonement for things polluted or prescribed; and under these ceremonies, as under a veil or covering, a meaning the most important and sacred is concealed," (*Lectures on the Sacred Poetry of the Hebrews*, Lowth; p. 83).

"Do you not know this from of old, from setting of Adam on earth? For the exultation of the wicked is but recent; the happiness of the hypocrite lasts but a moment. Though his eminence ascends to heaven and his head touches the clouds, he will perish forever like his own dung; those who had seen him will ask, 'Where is he?' He will fly away like a dream and they will not find him; he will be hustled away like a nighttime vision. The eye that beheld him will not [see him] again; [the people of] his place will not observe him again. His children must appease the poor, and his hands must make restitution for his robbery. His power filled his youth, but it will all lie with him in the dust. Even if evil is *sweet in his mouth* – he hides it under his tongue, he spares it, and will not leave it; yea, keeps holding it in his mouth – yet his food in his belly shall be turned; the gall of asps is within him. He swallows *wealth*, but vomits it; God drives it out from his belly. He shall suck the poison of asps; the viper's tongue shall slay him," (Job 20:4-16). Concerning the Hebrews, "Separated from rest of mankind by their religion and laws, and not addicted to commerce, they were contented with those arts which were necessary to a simple and uncultivated (or rather uncorrupted) state of life. Thus their principle employments were agriculture and the care of cattle; they were a nation of husbandmen and shepherds. The lands had been originally parceled out to the different families; the portions of which (by the laws of the country) could not be alienated by sale, and therefore descended to their posterity without diminution. The *fruits* of the earth, the produce of his land and labor, constituted the *wealth* of each individual," (*Lectures on the Sacred Poetry of the Hebrews*, Lowth; p. 32). Satan wished human "fruit" to be consumed in Eden, "...as one dead, who proceeded from the womb of OUR mother..." (Numbers 12:12), and he received his wish. **There is no forgiveness of sins without the shedding of blood because sin entered Eden and resulted in the shedding of blood**, for Satan was a "murderer from the beginning," (John 8:44). The punishment for sin fit the crime of sin, and God's grace fit the punishment.

[1.12] The first command God gave to humanity is found in Genesis 1:28-29: "Be fruitful and multiply, and fill the earth and subdue it; and have dominion over the fish of the sea an over the birds of the air and over every living thing that moves upon the earth... See, I have given you every plant yielding seed that is upon the face of all the earth, and every tree with seed in its fruit; you shall have them for food." It should be noted that Elohim said to humanity, "See, I have given you every plant yielding seed that is upon the face of all the earth, and every tree with seed in its fruit; you shall have them for food," (Genesis 1:29). God did not say "every tree," but rather "every tree with seed in its fruit," which explains the nature of the Tree of the Knowledge of Good and Evil and Jehovah Elohim's prohibition against it in Genesis 2:17: the Tree of the Knowledge of Good and Evil could not have been a tree that yielded seed – as this concept parallels how the forbidden tree's contents, when consumed by the woman, aborted her fruit with seed in it by a death that defied the first command given to humanity in Genesis 1:28 which was, "Be fruitful and multiply and fill the earth, and subdue it..." Satan did not want humanity to spread about the earth (as we see another attempt to stunt humanity's growth at the Tower of Babel). Satan tempted humanity into stunting the first command of God concerning fruitfulness and multiplication by tempting humanity to take of the forbidden "tree" that could not multiply by its own nature, nor could it aid in human multiplication as it directly inhibited human multiplication. Satan coaxed Eve into the destruction of her "fruit" as she desired the fruit of the forbidden tree, though Eve was ignorant of the fact that the fruit of her womb would eventually be destroyed by her errant decision. The woman became "Eve," the mother of the living, because she began as the mother of death.

When you take a head count of the Children of Israel according to their numbers, every man shall give to Jehovah atonement-money for his soul when counting them..." (Exodus 30:12).

"So when the woman saw that the tree was good for food, and that it was a delight to the eyes, and that the tree was desirable to make one wise, she took of the fruit and ate..."; "to make one wise" is one word in Hebrew and is from "שכל" (ref. 7919). I John 2:16 unlocks the unspoken Textual Reading of Genesis 3:6: "... desire of the flesh, the desire of the eyes, the pride of LIFE... (ref. 979)" and the word "life" here is sometimes translated as "riches," for "life" = "βιος" (ref. 979) = "existence, means of livelihood," as in finances. Human life is a precious and valuable creation of God, so precious that He redeemed it with His own blood.

[1.13] "Now the serpent was subtle above every beast of the field that the Lord God had made, "(Genesis 3:1). God gave humanity dominion over "everything that moves upon the earth," for Adam and his wife (like us) had to actively choose sin because they were given dominion over the tempter. The same truth is found in Genesis 4:7: "... sin is lurking at the door; its desire is for you, but you must master it." We can prostitute ourselves to sin, or we can accept redemption from the Savior. When Eve stated that "The serpent deceived me" in Genesis 3:13 the word "deceive" = "נשא" (ref. 5377) = "א+ש+נ" = 1+300+50 = **351** can also mean to "seduce"; this is the first instance in Scripture that relates sin to whoredom. Notice that "נשא" (ref. 5378) = "to lend on interest; sell on credit" = "א+ש+נ" = 1+300+50 = **351**.

The concept of sin entwined with infidelity is a prevalent concept, as sad cases of idolatry use imagery from Eden as history repeats itself literally: "The Lord said to me in the days of King Josiah: Have you seen what she did, the faithless one, Israel, how she went up on every high hill and under every green tree, and played the whore there? And I thought, 'After she has done all this she will return to Me': but she did not return, and her false sister Judah saw it. She saw that for all the adulteries of that faithless one, Israel, I [God] had sent her away with a decree of divorce; yet her false sister Judah did not fear, but she too went and played the whore. Because she took her whoredom so lightly, she polluted the land, committing adultery with stone and tree," (Jeremiah 3:6-9). Again, "And they shall no more offer their sacrifices unto devils, after whom they have gone a whoring," (Leviticus 17:7) – quite literally in some cases.

"In fulfillment of His own purpose He gave us *birth* by the word of truth, so that we would become a kind of *first-fruits* of his creatures," (James 1:18). The women that were to be purified were placed in the east gate of the court called *Nicanor's* [*Untimely Victory; Conqueror; Victorious*] Gate, and were sprinkled with blood to purify them; in the same way, after the woman accidentally destroyed her firstborn through her willingness to sin – with Adam's approval – we read that Adam was driven out of the eastern portion of the garden in Genesis 3:24. Consider Christ's redemptive reversal of sin's adversity: "...Death has been swallowed up in victory," (I Corinthians 15:54 & Isaiah 25:8).

It is extremely commendable that the Sopherim and Massorites were so diligent in their studies. It is also evident that some of them, at one point or another, had corrupted themselves. Such subtle distinction and separation concerning the knowledge of Scripture caused the Scribes to retain an elite status among the masses. Regarding humanity, wherever a use is possible, an abuse is inevitable.

[1.14] "I said in my heart with regard to human beings that God is testing them to show that they are but animals," (Ecclesiastes 3:18). "The administrators of the law during the second Temple declared that, 'an animal is perfectly sound when it is capable of conceiving and bringing forth young,'" (*Leviticus,* Ginsburg; p. 103). We must distinguish between "test" and "tempt," for God tests, but Satan tempts: "But one is tempted by one's own desire, being lured and enticed by it; then, when that desire has conceived, it gives birth to sin, and that sin, when it is fully grown, gives birth to death. Do not be deceived, my beloved," (James 1:14-16). "The woman said, 'The serpent tricked me, and I ate,'" (Genesis 1:13). By not distinguishing between "testing" and "tempting," Adam blamed God for his own mistakes by declaring defensively, "The Woman whom *You* gave to be with me, she has given to me of the tree, and I ate," (Genesis 3:12). As a matter of legality, "... the mother in case of a miscarriage remains in a state of defilement as many nights as months have elapsed since her conception," (*Leviticus,* Ginsburg; p. 104).

[1.15] "The Hebrew language probably came into existence during the patriarchal period, about 2,000 B.C. The language was reduced to writing about 1,250 B.C., (*Vine's Expository Dictionary of Old and New Testament Words;* Forward – Introduction). According to *Vine's Expository Dictionary,* the oral aspects of the language came first and what became written also became subject to the rules of its redactors, though truly they had no power to diminish the actual Word of God. However, human understanding of the Word of God can be diminished and restricted to the limitations of a pattern devised and practiced by humans. The Scribes' euphemization of the Scriptures came to cause readers to read the Scriptures according to tradition without being altogether aware of what was euphemized.

[1.16] "So when the woman saw that the tree was good for food, and that it was pleasant to the eyes, and the tree was desirable *to make one wise* [להשכיל], she took of its fruit and ate; and she also gave some to her husband, who was with her, and he ate," (Genesis 3:6). It can hardly be thought that the woman saw that the tree was desirable to abort her child. It also can hardly be thought that the "tree was good for food" when that food was poisonous (Job 20), or that it was desirable to "make one wise" when eating of it was so drastically foolish. What she "saw" blurs the lines that framed how she viewed the two principle trees in the garden. Genesis 2:9 tells us that both principle trees, that were named very specifically, were in the "midst" of the garden, and Genesis 2:17 marks these two trees out specifically also. Why then did the woman not mention the name of the "tree" she discussed with the "serpent," and why did she not include the Tree of Life in her statement regarding the "midst" of the garden? Despite the fact that the two principle trees were both in the garden's midst, the woman only nebulously stated that "the tree that is in the midst of the garden" (Genesis 3:3) was prohibited, but the Tree of Life was not prohibited until after human sin and it was in the midst of the garden also. We shall answer these questions later, but it is necessary to point out that only the Word of God is to be trusted without question, for what Adam's wife repeated to Satan was not the Word of God, neither was Satan's question to the woman accurate to the word of God. The woman "saw" various qualities about a tree, but that we have an account concerning what she saw in her own ephemerally perceived reality (if you will) does not mean that what she "saw" was complete or entirely accurate, as I John 2:16 unlocks the unspoken Textual reading of Genesis 3:6:

"... desire of the flesh, the desire of the eyes, the pride of LIFE [or 'riches']..." (I John 2:16).
"... good for food, pleasant to the eyes, desirable TO MAKE ONE WISE..." (Genesis 3:6).

Let us see now what Adam and his wife saw after "their eyes were opened":

"... desire of the flesh, the desire of the eyes, the pride of LIFE [or 'riches']..." (I John 2:16).
"... good for food, pleasant to the eyes, desirable to BEREAVE OF CHILDREN..." (Genesis 3:6).

[1.17] Technically speaking, the term "abortion" can mean either a miscarriage or an intentional killing, though we often use the word "abortion" in but one context. Concerning another word for *abortion*, "...the word מפלת, [is] very usual among the Talmudists for a woman bringing forth an abortion," (*Commentary on the New Testament from the Talmud and Hebraica*, Lightfoot, Vol. 4; p. 269), hence, a miscarriage. Again, as applied to infants, *Webster's New World Dictionary* defines the word "abortion" in these ways:

1:a) any spontaneous expulsion of an embryo or a fetus before it is sufficiently developed to survive; miscarriage

1:b) any deliberate procedure that removes, or induces the expulsion of a living or dead embryo or fetus

2) an aborted embryo or fetus

3) anything immature and incomplete or unsuccessful, as a deformed creature

How cunning was the nature of Satan's deceit! The woman was certainly deceived, but only in that she did not know the consequences of the actions she willingly performed. The woman certainly had a miscarriage (definition 1:a), but the miscarriage was accidental. At the same time, her unintentional miscarriage was the result of her deliberate actions (definition 1:b), and as the description of Numbers 12:12 goes we can understand definition 3. Her ignorant procedure of eating was deliberate, but prior to her deliberate eating of the forbidden tree, she must have been unaware of the consequences and thought that she would become wise ["שכל" (ref. 7919) = "ש+כ+ל" = 30+20+300 = **350**] and not that she would become a manslayer ["שכל" (ref. 7921) = "ש+כ+ל" = 30+20+300 = **350**]. The woman was a manslayer, but Satan, "...was a murderer from the beginning and does not stand in the truth, because there is no truth in Him," (John 8:44). In summary, the woman deliberately ate the fruit, and this deliberate act caused the accidental death of her child. Numbers 12:12 describes the effects of leprosy in terms of an abortive birth; recall the first two miraculous signs given to Moses in Exodus 4 regarding a snake and leprosy.

[1.18] The punishment fit the crime, and the grace fit the punishment. God is perfectly just and perfectly merciful at the same time, and in such perfection, we have no right to consider the story of Christ to somehow randomly account for the seemingly unaccountable. Should any of the story of Christ be considered random or unaccountable in light of the fact that God is perfectly just, then explain to a non-believer versed in an official branch of legality HOW blood, that is not our own, "pays" for anything at all, especially for all eternity, and you may find yourself met with nearly justifiable laughter. Consider that Satan is the Adversary, and that Jesus is the Advocate (I John 2:1) in light of the great Day of Judgment – for these respective titles describe the legal dealings of the most official court. Should Christ have taken any of the 613 laws of Moses to be somehow negligible, then He would not have died in our stead on account of all of those 613 laws for our sakes. Christ never broke a Law of Moses. Christ only broke the inflated laws (like yeast) of the official human administrators, and these traditional laws are not found in the Bible – like when they wanted to stone the woman caught in adultery (John 8) and claimed that such a stoning was commanded by Moses when it was not (compare to Deuteronomy 22 & Numbers 5), and by claiming that Moses commanded something when Moses did not, the woman's accusers became guilty of breaking the ninth commandment concerning "false witness," (Exodus 20:16). Jesus probably wrote the curses required in Numbers 5:23 for such a woman in the ground, which is perhaps why an emphasis is placed on His finger in John 8:6 to remind the Scribes and Pharisees of the word *Torah* which comes from the word "ירא" or "ירה" (ref. 3384) = "to flow as water (i.e. to rain), to lay or throw (i.e. to shoot an arrow); figuratively, *to point (the finger)*, hence, *to teach.*" That is, the curses of Numbers 5:23 are connected to "dust that is in the floor," (Numbers 5:17) and "waters" (Numbers 5:23) in agreement with the origin of the word "Torah" as identified in the adultery case in John 8:6. Jesus continually taught the Torah to the Scribes and Pharisees, and in the adultery case of John 8:6, we might compare the ninth commandment that the Scribes and Pharisees broke in their errant words to the months of a full-term pregnancy in relation to Eve's errant words regarding what Elohim had said (Genesis 3:3). A "mitzvah" is considered a "Torah command" even if it is not Biblical but is rather of Rabbinic origin, and this fact is part of the reason that the officials of Jesus' earthly days claimed that Moses said something when he did not, for they regarded their own rules as necessary to carry out the Torah given to Moses.

[1.19] Christ is described as the "firstborn of the dead" in Colossians 1:18 and Revelation 1:5. The "firstborn of death," (Job 18:13) is an expression that means the cruelest death. What could be crueler than the death of an innocent person? When we think of Adam's firstborn whose death was hushed, before Cain and Able, it is difficult to ignore that Jesus was born as Mary's "firstborn" (Luke 2:7) and was first adorned with "swaddling clothes," i.e. burial clothes. Christ and the Father are One (John

10:30) though They are distinct, and likewise Christ came as the second Adam as well as Adam's firstborn son, i.e. the son of Adam. Consonantally (as well as with respect to Gematria), "Adam" = "אדם" = "man"; Christ is recorded, in Greek, as calling Himself "the Son of Man," though it is nearly impossible to assume that every time He referred to Himself as such that He spoke such a description in the Greek tongue (if He even used Greek at all). Let us remember that Jesus was wound in linen cloths or bandages after He was taken down from the cross – cloths/bandages similar to those used for swathing the bodies of the wealthy ("... He made His grave with the wicked, and with the rich in His death..." Isaiah 53:9), as it was Joseph of Arimathaea, a "rich man," (Matthew 27:57), along with *Nicodemus* [*Innocent Blood; Victor*], who took Jesus' body, wrapped It, and laid It in a garden tomb (John 19:41). The cloths/bandages with which Jesus' Body was wound when He died point us back to the cloths with which He was wrapped when He was born. These "swaddling cloths" are described in Luke 2:7 by the medical term "σπαργανοω" (ref. *4683*) = "to swathe"; we can see birth and death intertwined – especially considering that the mangers in Israel were to be found in caves, just as the body of Christ was laid in a freshly hewn cave (John 19:41).

Christ, being "Firstborn of the Dead" (Colossians 1:18 & Revelation 1:5) was specifically identified as such by the Angel of the Lord: "*This will be a sign to you*: You will find a baby wrapped in swaddling clothes, lying in a manger," (Luke 2:12), for such garments and in such a location were a Heavenly "sign" and not some arbitrary point of observation. As angels are often beautifully compared to heavenly lights, likewise, the Magi followed a star to find Christ, and the stars were made, *"for signs,* and for seasons, and for days, and years," (Genesis 1:14): "signs" is named first, and we can observe why Satan specifically wanted to pervert legitimate astronomy into the falsehood of astrology; consider the question, "When did Christ die?" and observe the host of discrepancy. Concerning the stars, the famous pictures drawn around them do not suggest the shape of those clusters, but the star maps reflect the ancient names of the stars found within those clusters (just try finding a lion amongst all those brilliant dots...). "He determines the number of the stars; He gives to all of them their names," (Psalm 147:4).

[1.20] When Christ resurrected from the cave-tomb in the garden, "...Mary stood outside the tomb crying. As she wept, she bent over to look into the tomb and saw two angels in white, seated where Jesus' body had been, one at the head and the other at the foot," (John 20:11-12). The situation of the angels seated at opposing ends of where the body of Jesus was laid points us back to the Ark of the Covenant in Exodus 25:17-20: "Make an atonement cover of pure gold... And make two cherubs out of hammered gold at the ends of the cover. Make one cherub on one end and the second cherub on the other: even the mercy seat shall you make the cherubs on the two ends thereof. The cherubs are to have their wings spread upward, overshadowing the cover with them." In the same way that the mercy seat had cherubs positioned on either end, the mercy can be perceived by the situation of the angels in Jesus' tomb. The Ark of the Covenant held the Testimony of God, the jar of manna, and Aaron's staff that budded anew enclosed by the lid with the mercy seat and the cherubs. Similarly, the stone rolled before the opening of Christ's tomb was rolled away, as He, the "Word," (John 1:1), the "Bread of Life" (John 6:35) died on the cross and rose anew as "the bright Morning Star," (Revelation 22:16).

[1.21] When we take into account the immediacy with which Christ says that He will return (Revelation 16:15), that He is coming "quickly" (Revelation 22:7,12,20), coupled with His blessing to him who "stays awake" (Revelation 16:15), it becomes difficult to ignore the constellations in light of Scriptures like Hebrews 1:13: "...Sit at My right hand until I make Your enemies a footstool for Your feet," (compare to Psalm 110:1), for the constellation *Cepheus*: "The Greek name by which he is now known, *Cepheus*, is from the Hebrew, and means *the branch*, and is called by Euripides *the king*," (*Witness of the Stars,* Bullinger; p. 103). This text seeks not to be foolish by attempting to predict the chronology of the end times, but it is interesting to note that the ancient drawing around the stars of Cepheus depicts that his foot will stand atop the crown of the sky in the near future (relatively speaking, as indicated by the North Celestial Pole because of Precession), and that Cepheus' brightest star is called *Al Deramin* [*Coming Quickly*] and it has another star called *Al Phirk* [*The Redeemer*]. The constellation of "The King" or "The Branch" stands next to the constellation of "Leviathan" (for all of the serpentine star maps discuss the same being), and the constellation that the Jews called the "Little Winnowing Fan" (Little Dipper) is near Cepheus and Leviathan, for Jesus said,

"...Satan has demanded to sift all of you like wheat," (Luke 22:31), and John the Baptist described the Savior by saying, "His winnowing fan is in His hand, to clear His threshing floor and to gather the wheat into His granary..." (Luke 3:17). "...*Bread* is very frequently used in the Jewish writers for *doctrine*," (*Commentary on the New Testament from the Talmud and Hebraica,* Lightfoot, Vol. 3; p. 307-308). "I tell you the truth, it is not Moses who has given you the bread from Heaven, but it is My Father Who gives you the true bread from Heaven. For the bread of God is He Who comes down from Heaven and gives life to the world," (John 6:32). It is also interesting to note that some of the names of the Hebrew letters are also reminiscent of various star names.

[1.22] Hebrew letters have important names. The name of a given Hebrew letter uttered aloud also happens to be a Hebrew word (or words) that conveys various concepts. The shapes of Hebrew letters are the simplification of ancient pictographs from which both Hebrew and Greek developed into their own independent alphabetic systems. Though the original Hebrew Scriptures lacked vowels (as we know them currently), the original Hebrew Scriptures were hardly lacking, and they presented a more expansive and descriptive system of communication far above anything that we have understood today. The original Hebrew Text was and is a Text of perfection uncolored by any human mark.

By recalling the History of the Hebrew Scriptures prior to the vowels with which it is copied and pronounced today, we can understand that the fruit of the "Tree" of the Knowledge of Good and Evil contained "rosh" = "ראש" or "רוש" (ref. 7219) which, in its most literal sense, is rendered "gall" (like the liquid Christ drank as He hung on the tree in John 19:30) or "poison," and in a figurative sense is rendered "venom of the serpent." Let us consider how the wine of Christ's New Covenant is the exact opposite of that wine discussed in Deuteronomy 32:32-33 which may indicate why the "serpent" tempted Eve with the "tree": "Their vine comes from the vinestock of Sodom, from the vineyards of Gomorrah; their grapes are grapes of poison, their clusters are bitter; their wine is the poison of serpents, the cruel venom of asps." That the "tree" of the knowledge of Good and Evil was a "vine-tree," similar to "vine-tree" discussed in Ezekiel 15, is old news to Jews, though I can guess that it might be considered new news to Christians. We can see Satan's divisive intentions in his numerous efforts to continually arouse enmity between Jews and Christians. Given the information above, it is difficult to argue these words: "The Talmud and Midrash record a dispute regarding the species of the Tree of Knowledge. According to one view, it was a grapevine..." (*Baal Ha Turim*, Gold; p. 1397). Again, "... the tree from which Adam ate [was a grape vine, as the Midrash derives from the verse,]... their grapes are grapes of gall (Deuteronomy 32:32)," (*Baal Ha Turim*: brackets by Gold; p. 1397). "And to the passage of the [wife suspected of faithlessness], the Torah juxtaposed the passage concerning a Nazirite, because the tree from which Adam ate [was a grapevine, as the Midrash derives from...,] their grapes are grapes of gall (Deuteronomy 32:32)," (*Baal Ha Turim*; p. 1396). Regarding Luke 1:15, John the Baptist was to be as a Nazarite: "He must never drink wine or strong drink; even before his birth he will be filled with the Holy Spirit." Notice how "wine" and "strong drink" are differentiated. Dr. Lightfoot said, "Whilst I a little more narrowly consider that severe interdiction by which the Nazarite was forbidden the total use of the vine, not only that he should not drink of the wine, but no so much as taste of the grape, not the pulp nor stone of the grape, no, not the bark of the vine; I cannot but call to mind... [whether] the vine might not be the tree in paradise that had been forbidden to Adam, by the tasting of which he sinned. The Jewish doctors positively affirm this without any scruple [*Sanhedrin* fol. 70.1]," (*Commentary on the New Testament from the Talmud and Hebraica*, Lightfoot, Vol. 3; p. 19). However, wild vines do not produce "grapes" like those of trained vines intended for wine (like that of the New Covenant), and the "grapevine" in discussion is probably more closely linked to this Scripture: "When Elisha returned to Gilgal, there was a famine in the land. As the company of prophets was sitting before him, he said to his servant, 'Put the large pot on, and make some stew for the company of prophets.' One of them went out into the field to gather herbs; he found a wild vine and gathered from it a lapful of wild gourds, and came and cut them up into the pot of stew, not knowing what they were. They served some for the men to eat. But while they were eating the stew, they cried out, "O man of God, there is death in the pot!" (II Kings 4:38-40).

[1.23] "When the cloud went away from over the tent, Miriam had become leprous, as *white* as snow. And Aaron turned towards Miriam and saw that she was leprous. Then Aaron said to Moses, 'Oh, my lord, do not punish us for a sin that we have so foolishly committed. Let her not be as one dead, who proceeded from the womb of OUR mother, and half of OUR flesh be consumed," (Numbers 12:10-12). In an abbreviated way:

"עץ־הגפן" (ref, 6086-1612) = "vine-tree" = "ע+ץ+ה+ג+פ+ן" = 50+80+3+5+90+70 = **298**

"רצח" (ref. 7523) = "to dash in pieces, i.e. kill (a human being); to murder" = "ר+צ+ח" = 8+90+200 = **298**

"צחר" (ref. 6713) = "to dazzle; sheen, whiteness, white" = "צ+ח+ר" = 200+8+90 = **298**

"צחר" (ref. 6715) = "white" = "צ+ח+ר" = 200+8+90 = **298**

"צרח" (ref. 6873) = "shrill, cry, roar" = "צ+ר+ח" = 8+200+90 = **298**

"חרץ" (ref. 2757) = "incisure, incised; a threshing-sledge (with sharp teeth)" = "ח+ר+ץ" = 90+200+8 = **298**

"חרץ" (ref. 2782) = "to point sharply, i.e. to wound; to decide, decree, determine" = "ח+ר+ץ" = 90+200+8 = **298**

"חרץ" (ref. 2783) = "the loin (as the seat of strength)" = "ח+ר+ץ" = 90+200+8 = **298**

"חרץ" (ref. 2784) = "a fetter, pain, band" = "ח+ר+ץ" = 90+200+8 = **298**

"חצר" (ref. 2690) = "to surround with a stockade" = "ח+צ+ר" = 200+90+8 = **298**

"חצר" (ref. 2691) = "a yard (as enclosed by a fence)" = "ח+צ+ר" = 200+90+8 = **298**

"רחץ" (ref. 7635) = "to attend upon, trust" = "ר+ח+ץ" = 90+8+200 = **298**

"He shall suck the poison of asps; the viper's tongue shall slay him," (Job 20:16). The viper's *tongue* shall slay him; in Genesis 3, the serpent *said*...

[1.24] Christ atoned for the innocent blood that was shed in Eden, as He also atoned for all of us by His blood, for He lived in the stead of the innocent firstborn child of Adam who was born before Cain and Able. "For of a truth against Thy holy Child Jesus, Whom thou hast anointed, both Herod, and Pontius Pilate, with the Gentiles, and the people of Israel, were gathered together," (Acts 4:27).

The Greek New Testament describes the veiled intricacies of the Hebrew Old Testament history perfectly, as it is clear that the New Testament is not some mere continuation, but the New Testament is the glorious unveiling of the mysteries of the words and history of the Hebrew Scriptures through Christ. "Since, then, we have such a hope, we use great plainness of speech, not like Moses who put a veil over his face to keep the people of Israel from gazing at the end of the glory that was being set aside. But their minds were hardened. Indeed, to this very day, when they hear the reading of the old covenant, that same veil is still there, since only in Christ is it set aside. Indeed, to this very day whenever Moses is read, a veil lies over their minds," (II Corinthians 3:12-15).

We can see why Christ was so angry at the Scribes: Christ was living out the Written Law to the shame of the oral law, and prior to His earthly actions and words, the people did not know the Written Law as they could have known it largely because of the imposing limitations placed on the people by the religious elites. However, a select few were privileged to know the dark history of Eden, though their knowledge became, once again, covered by other resulting traditions: "What has been is what will be, and what has been done is what will be done; there is nothing new *under the sun*," (Ecclesiastes 1:9). Yet, in the end, "...there will be no more night; they need no lamp or *sun*, for the Lord God will be their light..." (Revelation 22:5).

[1.25] "Then He [Jesus] said to them, 'These are My words that I spoke to you while I was still with you – that everything written about Me **in the law of Moses, the prophets, and the Psalms** must be fulfilled.' Then He opened their minds to understand the Scriptures, and He said to them, 'Thus it is written, that the Messiah is to suffer and rise from the dead on the third day, and that repentance and forgiveness of sins is to be proclaimed from Jerusalem," (Luke 24:44-47). The first sin resulted in the slaying of *Adam's* firstborn son, before Cain and Able were born, which specifically explains why Christ, The Son of *Man*, did what He did in the way that He did it. Adam's firstborn son was born dead as the result of Eve's consumption of "ראש" (ref. 7219) = "a poisonous plant; poison (even of serpents):- gall," which is a reason why such an emphasis is made in the Gospels that Christ did not drink this poison until "...Jesus, knowing that all things were now accomplished, that the Scripture might be fulfilled [Psalm 22:15], saith, 'I thirst'..." (John 19:28), for once He drank this poison (John 19:30), He died ultimately of this drink, on a tree, in congruence with the death of Adam's firstborn son: "For this reason the Father loves me, because I lay down my life in order to take it up again. No one takes it from Me, but I lay it down of my own accord. I have power to lay it down, and I have power to take it up again. I have received this command from my Father," (John 10:18).

"It was the custom towards those that were condemned by the Sanhedrim to allow them a cup, but it was of wine mingled with myrrh or frankincense; that by drinking that their brains might intoxicate, and themselves become the more insensible of their torments, and less apprehensive of their death," (*Commentary on the New Testament from the Talmud and Hebraica,* Lightfoot, Vol. 3; p. 434). Notice how Christ bravely refused the cup that would make Him less apprehensive of His death before He was hung (Matthew 27:34 & Mark 15:23) so that He was fully conscious of His pain when He was hung, and that He refused a drink as His crucifixion was unfolding (Luke 23:36); but notice also how, "After this, Jesus, knowing that all things were now accomplished, that the Scripture might be fulfilled, saith, 'I thirst.' Now there was set a vessel full of sour wine [*or vinegar*]: and they filled a sponge with the wine [*or vinegar*], and put it upon hyssop, and put it to His mouth. When Jesus therefore had received the wine [*or vinegar: possibly in connection with Matthew 27:48*], He said, "*Paid in full,*" and He bowed His head, and gave up the ghost," (John 19:28-30). Notice also how the gold, frankincense, and myrrh of the Magi sorcerers (if you will) was given to the Infant King Who's first articles of clothing were burial clothes in relation to the "sour wine" that Jesus drank only after "all things were now accomplished" in relation to His statement "Paid in full." King James uses the word "vinegar" and the N.R.S.V. uses "sour wine" in John 19 to discuss the same thing. In order for both perfect justice and perfect grace to mingle flawlessly on the cross, Christ, being the Second *Adam* and the Son of *Man* in relation to His Oneness with the Father (John 10:30), drank "ראש" (ref. 7219) = "poison (even of serpents):- gall," to die the death of Adam's firstborn son in connection with a "tree." In parallel agreement with gall and vinegar, the word "vinegar" = "חמץ" (ref. 2558) = "ץ+מ+ח" = 90+40+8 = **138** is connected to these terms:

"חמץ" (ref. 2556) = "a prim. root; to be pungent; i.e. in taste (sour, i.e. lit. *fermented*, or figuratively *harsh*), in color (dazzling):- cruel (man), dyed, be grieved, *leavened*" = "ץ+מ+ח" = 90+40+8 = **138** [...*beware the yeast of the Pharisees (Luke 12:1-2)*.]

"חמץ" (ref. 2557) = "ferment, (figuratively) extortion:- leaven, leavened (bread)" = "ץ+מ+ח" = 90+40+8 = **138**

"מצח" (ref. 4696) = "the forehead, *brow*" [*He bowed His head and gave up the ghost (John 19:30)*.] = "ח+צ+מ" = 8+90+40 = **138**

"מחץ" (ref. 4272) = "(figuratively) to subdue or destroy:- dip, *pierce* (through), smite" = "ץ+ח+מ" = 90+8+40 = **138** [*One of the soldiers with a spear pierced His side (John 19:34)*.]

[1.26] The purpose of any tradition is to remember something in unity; if that something is forgotten, the purpose of the tradition loses its intended meaning, and the tradition becomes an entity unto itself. Let us not attempt to match the Holy Scriptures to our personal theology and tradition, for it is our immovable duty to match our personal theology and tradition to the Holy Scriptures, as Jesus said, "that all of them may be one, Father, just as You are in Me and I am in You. May they also be in Us so that the world may believe that You have sent Me," (Luke 17:21), for God said, "Let Us make man in Our image, after Our likeness..." (Genesis 1:26).

It is also beneficial to keep in mind that adults communicate the same truths to other adults as well as to children; however, the children's version of those truths is of a simplified format. That is, a formal lecture on the topic of honesty delivers the same essential message as a parent-to-child lesson on honesty, though the levels of intensity regarding the same subject vary with respect to the capacity of the audience. Consider a parent speaking to a child, and then consider the Almighty speaking to us. Consider also human elites speaking to commoners, and think of the conceit so often found in human elites. In both instances of elite adulthood and of beautiful childhood, a correct maturation process is expected regardless of age or position. Humanity was first created from the dust of the ground, and vegetation was caused to *spring up* from the earth on "Day" Third of Creation by Elohim. As vegetation is supported, pruned, fed, etc., so humanity is to exist likewise.

King Solomon was the wisest man to ever live, so we can imagine what effort he must have taken to speak to others.

When we consider the Garden of Eden account in Genesis 2-3 with respect to the Creation account of Genesis 1-2, let us consider King Solomon's understanding and communication: "God gave Solomon very great wisdom, discernment, and breadth of understanding as the sand on the seashore, so that Solomon's wisdom surpassed the wisdom of all the people of the east, and all the wisdom of Egypt. He was wiser than anyone else, wiser than *Ethan* [*Perplexity*] the *Ezrahite* [*Sprung Up (as arising out of the soil)*], and *Heman* [*Right-handed*], *Calcol* [*Sustenance; Comprehended*], and *Darda* [*Dwelling of Knowledge*], children of *Mahol* [*Exultation*]; his fame spread throughout all the surrounding nations.

Solomon composed 3,000 proverbs, and his songs numbered 1,005. He would speak of trees, from the cedar that is in the *Lebanon* [*Very White*] to the hyssop that grows in the wall; he would speak of animals, and birds, and reptiles, and fish," (I Kings 4:29-33) – like all that was created in Genesis 1 & 2 so that people might gain in understanding: "Let Us make man in Our image, after Our likeness; and let them have dominion over the fish of the sea, and over the birds of the air, and over the cattle, and over all the wild animals of the earth, and over every creeping thing that creeps upon the earth," (Genesis 1:26). "Now the serpent was subtle above every beast of the field that the Lord God had made"; and "...sin is lurking at the door; its desire is for you, but you must master it," (Genesis 4:7).

SECTION II

ב
THE LOCK

"While in their joy they were disbelieving and still wondering, He said to them, 'Have you anything here to eat?'" (Luke 24:41).

[2.1] Let us reflect on the Biblical concept of "eating and drinking": "... O Mortal, eat what is offered to you; eat this scroll... Then I ate it; and in my mouth it was as sweet as honey," (Ezekiel 3:1-3); "Your words were found, and I ate them, and your words became to me a joy and the delight of my heart; for I am called by your Name, O Lord, God of Hosts," (Jeremiah 15:16); "In the beginning was the Word, and the Word was with God, and the Word was God... What has come into being in Him was life, and the life was the light of all people," (John 1:1-4); "...I am the bread of life. Whoever comes to Me will never be hungry, and whoever believes in Me will never be thirsty," (John 6:35); "So Jesus said to them, 'Very truly, I tell you, unless you eat the flesh of the Son of Man and drink his blood, you have no life in you," (John 6:53); "Whatsoever soul it be that eateth any manner of blood, even that soul shall be cut off from his people," (Leviticus 7:27); "...you drank fine wine from the blood of grapes," (Deuteronomy 32:14); "דם" (ref. 1818) = "*blood* (as that which when shed causes death) of a man or animal; by analogy, *the juice of the grape*, figuratively bloodshed (i.e. drops of blood); "Then Moses and *Aaron [A Shining Light; A Mountain of Strength; Enlightened Teaching]* Nadab, and Abihu, and 70 of the elders of Israel went up, and they saw the God of Israel. Under His feet there was something like a pavement of sapphire stone, like the very heaven for clearness. God did not lay His hand on the chief men of the people of Israel; also they beheld God, and *THEY ATE AND DRANK*," (Exodus 24:9-11).

[2.2] *Webster's New World Dictionary* defines "myth" in this way: "a traditional story of unknown authorship, ostensibly with a historical basis, but serving usually to explain some phenomenon of nature, the origin of man, or the customs, institutions, religious rites, etc. of a people; myths usually involve the exploits of gods and heroes." *Webster's New World Dictionary* defines "legend" in this way: "a story handed down for generations among a people and popularly believed to have a historical basis, although not verifiable." It is no secret that oral transmission from one person to another evinces a rapid degeneration of accuracy whereby omission and augmentation decorate accounts beyond the precision and purpose of their initial design, as even children's games display this common knowledge. Often, there appears to be a traditional preference for the magical over an adherence to the historically miraculous. As we have examined the legendary 40-day flood fable that developed around the historical year-long flood period of Noah's day, let us again take into account the Biblical concepts of "eating and drinking."

"The word that came to Jeremiah from the Lord in the days of King *Jehoiakim* [*The Lord Will Set Up*] son of *Josiah* [*Jehovah Supports*] of Judah: Go to the house of the *Rechabites* [*Horsemen*], speak with them, and bring them to the house of the Lord, into one of the chambers; then offer them wine to drink. So I took Jaazaniah son of Jeremiah son of Habazziniah, and his brothers, and all his sons, and the whole house of the Rechabites. I brought them to the house of the Lord into the chamber of the sons of Hanan son of Igdaliah, the man of God, which was near the chamber of the officials, above the chamber of Maaseiah son of Shallum, keeper of the threshold. Then I set before the Rechabites pitchers full of wine, and cups; and I said to them, 'Have some wine.' But they answered, We will drink no wine, for our ancestor Jonadab son of Rechab commanded us, 'You shall never drink wine, neither you nor your children; nor shall you ever build a house, or sow seed; nor shall you plant a vineyard, or even own one; but you shall live in tents all your days, that you may live many days in the land where you reside.' We have obeyed the charge of our ancestor Jonadab son of Rechab in all that he commanded us, to drink no wine all our days, ourselves, our wives, our sons, or our daughters, and not to build houses to live in. We have no vineyard or field or seed; but we have lived in tents, and have obeyed and done all that our ancestor Johadab commanded us... Then the word of the Lord came to Jeremiah: Thus says the Lord of hosts, the God of Israel: Go and say to the people... Can you not learn a lesson and obey My words? says the Lord. The command has been carried out that Jonadab son of Rechab gave to his descendants to drink no wine; and they drink none to this day, for they have obeyed their ancestor's command. But I Myself have spoken to you persistently, and you have not obeyed Me," (Jeremiah 35:1-14).

How strange it is that the God's words were ignored, but that an entirely human tradition was kept. The *Rechabites* [*Horsemen*] who kept their human traditions were set up to teach God's people about their own faulty actions. It is ironic that it is written, "If you have raced with foot-runners and they have wearied you, how will you compete with horses?" (Jeremiah 12:5).

[2.3]   Tradition, in and of itself, is but a neutral entity designed for the purposes of celebratory remembrance and uniformity. Good tradition is good, and bad tradition is bad. There is the tradition that celebrates the annual remembrance of a marriage, and there is the tradition that degrades a fiancé immediately prior to marriage. There are Biblical traditions, and there are non-Biblical traditions that originate partially from the lessons of the Bible. The point of a tradition is to remember something, but once memory fails, such a tradition becomes an entity unto itself. When we consider Eden along with the trees and vines of its grounds, let us also consider this Holy Tradition:

"For I received from the Lord what I also handed on to you, that the Lord Jesus on the night He was betrayed took a loaf of bread, and when He had given thanks, He broke it and said, 'This is My body which is *broken* on behalf of you' this do for remembrance of Me.' In the same way, He took the cup also, after supper, saying 'This cup is the new covenant in My blood. Do this, as often as you drink it, in remembrance of Me.' For as often as you eat this bread and drink the cup, you proclaim the Lord's death until He comes," (I Corinthians 11:23-26). Why did Paul state that Christ said His body was "broken" in light of the Gospel references: "Take, eat; this is My body," (Matthew 26:26); "Take, eat: this is My body," (Mark 14:22); "This is My body *given* for you; do this in remembrance of Me," (Luke 22:19)? "...And indeed the bread which I will *give* is My flesh, which I will *give* for the life of the world," (John 6:51) Consider that, "These things occurred so that the Scripture [Psalm 34:20] might be fulfilled, 'None of

His bones shall be *broken*,' and again another passage of Scripture [Zechariah 12:10] that says, 'They will look on the One Whom they have pierced,'" (John 19:36-37). As we are assured, the Holy Spirit is the True Author of Scripture, for, "So we have the prophetic message more fully confirmed. You will do well to be attentive to this as to a lamp shining in a dark place, until the day dawns and the morning star rises in your hearts. First of all you must understand this, that no prophecy of Scripture is a matter of one's own interpretation, because no prophecy ever came by human will, but men moved by the Holy Spirit spoke from God," (II Peter 1:19-21). So the Apostle Paul must have written "broken" for a specific reason... that is, Christ is our Passover (I Corinthians 5:7), but concerning the Passover lamb, "...you shall not break a bone in it," (Exodus 12:46). Why then did the Apostle Paul indicate that Christ's body was "broken" for us? – perhaps to link the concepts behind new moon and full moon as in Exodus 12. "For there is one God; there is also one mediator between God and humanity, Christ Jesus, Himself human, Who gave Himself as a ransom for all – this was attested at the right time," (I Timothy 2:5-6). Indeed, the Lord's Supper is no small tradition, but it is the grand remembrance, the sublime reenactment, the solemn celebration of our Savior's eternal love for us.

[2.4] The word "vintage" refers to "the crop or yield of a particular vineyard or grape-growing region in a single season, with reference either to the grapes or to the wine made from them," (*Webster's New World Dictionary*).

"'Who is this that comes from *Edom* [*Red*], from *Bozrah* [*A*

Vintage; A Sheepfold] in garments stained crimson? Who is this so splendidly robed, marching in his great might?' 'It is I, announcing vindication, mighty to save.' 'Why are your robes red, and your garments like theirs who tread the wine press?' 'I have trodden the wine press alone, and from the peoples no one was with me? I trod them in my anger and trampled them in my wrath; their juice spattered on my garments, and stained all my robes. For the day of vengeance was in my heart, and the year for my redeeming work had come. I looked, but there was no helper; I stared, but there was no one to sustain me; so my own arm brought me victory, and my wrath sustained me. I trampled down the peoples in my anger, I crushed them in my wrath, I poured out their lifeblood on the earth," (Isaiah 63:1-6).

"דם" (ref. 1818) = "*blood* (as that which when shed causes death) of a man or animal; by analogy, *the juice of the grape*; figuratively bloodshed (i.e. drops of blood).

Notice how Christ was mocked being dressed in a white robe under Herod (Luke 23:11) and in a purple robe under Pilate (John 19:5). Concerning the righteous follower of God, "These are they who have come out of the great tribulation; they have washed their robes and made them white in the blood of the Lamb," (Revelation 7:14). The blood (red) of the Lamb made the robes white, for it is written, "Come now, let us reason together, says the Lord: though your sins are like scarlet, they shall be like snow; though they are red like crimson, they shall become like wool; If you are willing and obedient, you shall eat the good of the land; but if you refuse and rebel, you shall be devoured by the sword; for the mouth of the Lord has spoken," (Isaiah 1: 18-19). How can a blade actually "devour" anything, though it certainly can "pierce" many things, as Zechariah 12:10 says, "They will look on the One Whom they have pierced," as Christ, the Second Adam, was speared in His side for His Bride, in relation to the fact that the first Adam's bride was made from his rib. "And I heard as it were the voice of a great multitude, and as the voice of many waters, and as the voice of mighty thunderings, saying, 'Alleluia: for the Lord God Omnipotent reigneth. Let us be glad and rejoice, and give honor to Him: for the marriage of the Lamb is come, and His wife hath made herself ready,' And to her was granted that she should be arrayed in fine linen, clean and white: for the fine linen is the righteousness of the saints," (Revelation 19:6-8). As for the "fine linen," it is a bit more than doubtful that righteousness will literally become an actual garment like one that touches actual human flesh.

[2.5] It should be understood that under no circumstance was actual blood that flows through veins ever to be consumed according to the Scriptures, as it was considered a dire abomination, particularly to the Jews: "Whatsoever soul it be that eateth any manner of blood, even that soul shall be cut off from his people," (Leviticus 7:27). "Ye shall not eat anything with the blood; neither shall ye use enchantment, nor observe times," (Leviticus 19:26). Concerning the common Jewish manner of calling "wine" by the name of "blood," the only time "blood" was permitted to be consumed was when it issued from grapes: "...you drank fine wine from the blood of grapes,"

(Deuteronomy 32:14); thus, "blood," i.e. *wine* was to be consumed – not literal blood. Christ fulfilled all 613 laws of the Torah. In Jesus' earthly days, the concept of eating the flesh and blood of a deity would have stimulated the interest of Bacchus worshippers, and would also have provided them with the truest signification of what they had themselves misunderstood {1}. "And whatsoever man there be of the house of Israel, or of the strangers that sojourn among you, that eateth any manner of blood; I will even set my face against that soul that eateth blood, and will cut him off from among his people. For the life of the flesh is in the blood: and I have given it to you upon the altar to make atonement for your souls: for it is the blood that maketh atonement for the soul," (Leviticus 17:10-11).

Dr. Lightfoot pointed out the following concerning John 6:53: "There was nothing more common in the schools of the Jews than the phrases of 'eating and drinking' in a metaphorical sense. And surely it would sound very harsh, if not to be understood here metaphorically, but literally. What! To drink blood? a thing so severely interdicted the Jews once and again. What! to eat man's flesh? a thing abhorrent to human nature; but above all abhorrent to the Jews... Bread is very frequently used in the Jewish writers for *doctrine*," (*Commentary on the New Testament from the Talmud and Hebraica,* Lightfoot, Vol. 3; p. 307-308). "Wisdom" is personified in the Proverbs, and she says, "Come, eat of my bread and drink of the wine I have mixed," (Proverbs 9:5), for consuming such a doctrine is beneficial as "...wisdom gives life to the one who possesses it," (Ecclesiastes 7:12); Christ said, "...I am the bread of life. Whoever comes to Me will never be hungry, and whoever believes in Me will never be thirsty," (John 6:35) {2}.

Consider Luke 24:41-45: "... He [Jesus] said to them, 'Have you anything here to *eat?*' They gave Him a piece of broiled fish, and He took it and ate it in their presence. Then He said to them, '*These are My words* that I spoke to you while I was still with you – that *everything written* about Me in the Law of Moses, the prophets, and the Psalms must be fulfilled.' Then *He opened their minds to understand the Scriptures..*" "Your words were found, and I ate them, and your words became to me a joy and the delight of my heart; for I am called by your Name, O Lord, God of Hosts," (Jeremiah 15:16) – can it be that Jeremiah ate the actual surface that he wrote on so that the words on it went into his stomach? Should we take the expression of "eating" flesh and "drinking" blood in a humanly physical sense (by deliberately rejecting the explicit commands of the Torah), then we might also assume that Christ was an actual vine because He called Himself the "True Vine" (John 15:1); but how can a "vine" also be "bread," for Christ called Himself the "Bread of Life" (John 6:35). He was no more a walking loaf than He was a talking vine. When recalling that Christ called Herod a "fox" (Luke 13:32), we cannot possibly assume that Herod had a tail and fur... and as such, it may prove beneficial to reflect on the "serpent" of Genesis 3.

"In the first place, the Hebrew poets frequently make use of imagery borrowed from common life, and from objects well known and familiar. On this perspicuity of figurative language will be found in a great measure to depend; for a principle use of metaphors is to illustrate the subject by a tacit comparison," (*Lectures on the Sacred Poetry of the Hebrews*, Lowth; p. 60). Consider Jeremiah 2:21: "Yet I planted you as a choice vine, from the purest stock. How then did you turn degenerate and become a wild vine?" "You plant them, and they take root; they grow and bring forth fruit; you are near in their mouths yet far from their hearts," (Jeremiah 12:2).

Dr. Bullinger pointed out the following concerning John 6:53: "'eat... drink', &c. The Hebrews used this expression with reference to knowledge by the... [*figure of*] Metonymy (of the Subject)... where it is put for being alive; so eating and drinking denoted the operation of the mind in receiving and 'inwardly digesting' truth or the words of God. See Deut. 8:3, and cp. Jer. 15:16. Ezek. 2:8. No idiom was more common in the days of our Lord. With them as with us, eating included the meaning of enjoyment, as in Ecc. 5:19; 6:2; for "riches" cannot be eaten... The Lord's words could be understood thus by hearers, for they knew the idiom; but of 'the eucharist' they knew nothing, and could not have thus understood them. By comparing vv. 47 and 48 with vv. 53 and 54, we see that believing on Christ was exactly the same thing as eating and drinking Him," (*Companion Bible*, Bullinger; p. 1532). Observe Job 12:11:

"Doth not the *ear* test **words**, As the *palate* tasteth **food**? (Compare to Job 34:3.) "He humbled you by letting hunger, then by *feeding you* with manna, with which neither you nor your ancestors were acquainted, in order *to make you understand* that one does not live by bread alone, but by everything that emanates from the mouth of the Lord," (Deuteronomy 8:3). Hence, the human consumption of the Heavenly manna was paralleled to what comes out of God's mouth for our sustenance by righteous mental faculty entwined with righteous faith; conversely, consider why the "serpent's" words were so venomous in Genesis 3. "'But thou, son of man, hear what I say unto thee; be not thou rebellious like that rebellious house: open thy mouth, and eat that I give thee.' And when I looked, behold, a hand was sent unto me; and, lo, a roll of a book was therein," (Ezekiel 2:8-9) – can it be that Ezekiel ate an actual scroll so that the words on it went into his stomach?

We can see the juxtaposition of sacrificial flesh and knowledge through the figuration of Antithetical Parallel in the Book of Hosea where it is written –

"For I desire **steadfast love** and not **sacrifice**,
the *knowledge of God* rather than *burnt offerings*," (Hosea 6:6).

Observe how "steadfast love" (line 1) and "knowledge of God" (line 3) are paralleled to each other in opposition to the "sacrifice" (line 2) and "burnt offerings" (line 4) that are paralleled to each other.

The pagan god Bacchus was worshipped prior to the birth of Jesus, and the priests of Bacchus were known for wine-making magic. "Bread and/or wine, tangible emblems of divine care for mortals, played important roles in some Greco-Roman mystery religions, where food and beverage emblematic of earth's fecundity furnished sacred dining tables at which initiates communed with their gods," (*Classical Mythology*, Harris & Platzner; p. 507). "Even as a baby, Dionysus's [Bacchus'] presence causes a huge vine – inhabited by nesting birds, the Great Goddess's serpent, and other symbols of the life force – to spring up and shelter him," (*Classical Mythology*, Harris; p. 234). "Dionysus [Bacchus] is commonly identified with other male fertility gods of the ancient Near East, including the Mesopotamian and Syrian Tammuz (Dumuzi), whose name means 'proper son,' the true offspring of divinity; the Near Eastern Adonis (a Semitic term meaning 'lord,' or 'master'); and the Egyptian Osiris... All of these youthful figures have similar stories: they undergo a violent death – typically by being torn asunder – descend into the Underworld, and are ultimately reborn as immortal beings," (*Classical Mythology*, Harris; p. 230).

The fables regarding Bacchus have no particular time-stamp on them so that such accounts cannot possibly be validated, whereas the Scriptures give us very deliberate time-stamps (as time cannot be told without the celestial bodies). The beauty of celestial accounting via literary record is that the patterns of the heavens are cyclic; as long as one knows the patterns, one can go back to the precise date of a given historical event known to occur beneath a given celestial event. Consider II Peter 1:19: "We have also a true word of prophecy; you do well when you look to it for guidance, as you look to the lamp that shines in a dark place until the dawn of day, when the sun will shine in your hearts."

[2.6] "And God said, 'Let luminaries be in the expanse of the heavens, to divide between the day and the night. And let them be for signs and for seasons and for days and years," (Genesis 1:14). The word "luminaries" = "מארה" (ref. 3974) = "a chandelier; bright, light," and this definition is similar to the word "מאורה" (ref. 3975) = "something *lighted*, i.e. an *aperture*; by implication, *a crevice or hole of a serpent*:-den." Observe how it was the chief CUP bearer who had a dream about a VINE in Genesis 40:9; reflecting pools were sometimes used by the ancients to study the stars; consider also the ancient magical practice of diving by cups that the righteous Joseph feigned in Genesis 44:5: "Is it not from this that my lord drinks? Does he not indeed use it for *divination* [ref. 5172]?"

"נחש" (ref. 5172) = "to hiss, whisper a (magic) spell, to prognosticate, enchanter, diligently observe, learn by experience" = "ש+ח+נ" = 300+8+50 = **358**

"נחש" (ref. 5173) = "an incantation, augury, enchantment" = "ש+ח+נ" = 300+8+50 = **358**

"נחש" (ref. 5175) = "a serpent" = "ש+ח+נ" = 300+8+50 = **358**.

We may notice why the "serpent" desires to continually pervert the study of the heavens into Satanic astrology or scientific astronomy that disregards God altogether, for by doing so, historical record becomes tainted by traditional legend, cultural myth, and the strange notion that Scriptures and science are somehow at odds with each other – even though the One who wrote the Scriptures is the same One who created scientific law.

[2.7] "And he poured of the anointing oil upon Aaron's head, and anointed him, to sanctify him," (Leviticus 8:12); "This profuse pouring of oil was repeated at the consecration every successor to the high priesthood, whilst the common priests were simply anointed, or were simply marked with the finger on the forehead on their first installation, and this anointing descended with them for all futurity." (*Leviticus*, Ginsburg; p. 57). Accordingly, "a woman came to Him [Jesus] with an alabaster jar of very expensive perfume, which she poured on His head as He was reclining at the table." When the disciples saw this, they were indignant. 'Why this waste?' they asked. 'This perfume could have been sold at a high price and the money given to the poor.' Aware of this, Jesus said to them, 'Why are you bothering this woman? She has done a beautiful thing to Me. The poor you will always have with you, but you will not always have Me. When she poured this perfume on My body, she did it to prepare Me for burial (Matthew 26:7-12). Burial? Such a profuse pouring of oil was the sign of a new high priest – but it also corresponded to Leviticus 8:33 on which Dr. Ginsburg recalled the facts that, "... on each of these seven days the same sacrifices are to be repeated, the sin offering, the burnt offering, and the consecration offering are to be offered up, and Aaron and his sons, as well as their garments, are to be sprinkled with the sacrificial blood and the anointing oil..." (*Leviticus*, Ginsburg; p. 62); hence, "It was fitting that God, for Whom and through Whom all things exist, in bringing many children to glory, should make the pioneer of their salvation perfect through sufferings," (Hebrews 2:10). "Since, therefore, the children share flesh and blood, He Himself likewise shared the same things, so that through death He might destroy the one who has the power of death, that is, the devil, and free those who all their lives were held in slavery by the fear of death. For it is clear that He did not come to help angels, but the descendants of Abraham. Therefore, He had to become like His brothers and sisters in every respect, so that He might be a merciful and faithful high priest in the service of God, to make a sacrifice of atonement for the sins of the people. Because He himself was tested by what He suffered, He is able to help those who are being tested," (Hebrews 2:11-18).

Since we have all sinned, Christ, through His infinite mercy and boundless love, died in our stead in order to pay the penalty for our mistakes. We know that God is love, we know that sin leads to death, and we also know that there is no forgiveness of sin without the shedding of blood. We know that God Almighty loves His creation, and we know that Jonah 4:11 reveals God's fondness for His animals: "And should I not be concerned about *Nineveh* [*Offspring's Habitation*], that great city, in which there are more than a hundred and twenty thousand persons who do not know their right hand from their left, and also many animals?" Why then did God command that His animals be slain for His peoples' redemption? "Your righteousness is like the mighty mountains, your judgments are like the great deep; you save humans and animals alike, O Lord," (Psalm 36:6).

[2.8] The Garden of Eden story in Genesis 3 is the fundamental building block on which all of the remaining Holy Scriptures are constructed. Had Adam and his wife not sinned, there would be no need for God to prophesy about the Savior in Genesis 3:15. We also understand that perfect love casts out fear (I John 4:18). Why then does Proverbs 1:7 tell us that "The fear of the Lord is the beginning of knowledge," if we desire to love God perfectly when perfect love casts out fear? We know that Adam and his wife (who was named "Eve" only after God pronounced His judgments) covered themselves with fig leaves, but of all materials, why did the two humans choose the fig leaf, and why did God reject this attempt and provide them with coverings of skin? Again, in the Holy Scriptures, a specific, explanatory formula imbues every page of the Holy Bible by way of a blood requirement; the formula is as follows: the punishment for sin perfectly fits the crime of sin, and God's grace perfectly fits the punishment; this is the pattern that led to Christ's crucifixion. If the formula were not so, there would be no need for Christ to fulfill the whole Law, as He did not break even one of the 613 laws of the Torah, though He did intentionally break national laws that existed independently of the Torah (and He proved such an independence through his accordance with the Torah).

[2.9] Dr. Ginsburg pointed out in his introduction to his translation of Jacob Ben Chajim's *Introduction to the Rabbinic Bible*, "Owing to the extreme sacredness with which the letter of the text was regarded, and believing that the multifarious legal enactments which were called forth by the ever-shifting circumstances of the commonwealth, the sacred legends which developed themselves in the course of time, and all the ecclesiastical and civil regulations, to which an emergency may at any time give rise, are indicated in the Bible by the superfluous letter, or the redundant word, or the repetition of a phrase, or the peculiarity of a construction, the greatest care has been taken, since the beginning of the Christian era, to mark every peculiarity and phenomenon in the spelling and construction of the words in the Scriptures, so that 'one jot or one tittle shall in no wise pass from the law,'" (p. 14-15). A Christian may be inclined to ask, "What "sacred legends?" Notice how the Christian era was after the time when the Sopherim (Scribes; Numberers) began to "edit" the Scriptures. Dr. Ginsburg's words illustrate how those in the Christian era had received the edited tradition of the Scriptures prior to receiving the original Scriptures – along with developed, and developing, legends. "To facilitate still further the study of the unpointed consonants on the part of the laity, the Scribes gradually introduced into the text the *matres lectionis* which also served as vowel-letters. But in this branch of their labors as is the case in the other branches, the different Schools which were the depositories of the traditions as to the import of the text, exhibited considerable diversity of opinion owing to the fact that the traditions themselves were not uniform. So great indeed was this diversity of opinion about the respective traditions and the import of the text of Scripture *circa 300 B.C.* that it gave rise to the division of the people into the two national sects the Pharisees and the Sadducees," (*Introduction to the Massaretico-Critical Edition of the Hebrew Bible*, Ginsburg; p. 299). As far as "*circa 300*

B.C." it was near this time in history that the Septuagint, the famed Greek version of the Hebrew Scriptures, was written (*The Septuagint*, Brenton; p. ii).

[2.10] Again, Dr. Ginsburg pointed out the fact that, "To understand... the exegetical rules of the ancient Rabbins, the Bible never repeats a word twice without designing to convey thereby a special meaning. Accordingly, if a thing is repeated twice, and the repetition appears superfluous, it is explained as implying more than one statement would convey. But if the repetition cannot be explained as implying inclusion, it is taken to denote exclusion. This rule is called 'inclusion after inclusion, effecting exclusion,'" (*Introduction to the Rabbinic Bible,* Jacob Ben Chajim; p. 60). Many of the human traditions built around the Scriptures hinged on the personal explanative abilities or inabilities of its officials. The tradition of the Holy Word of God Almighty appeared to hinge on teachers' abilities to explain the entirety of Scripture. We can understand this warning: "Not many of you should become teachers, my brothers and sisters, for you know that we who teach will be judged with a greater strictness. For all of us make many mistakes..." (James 3:1). Anyone, whether novice or sage, can read the Jewish fathers and see their squabbles concerning what words were changed, omitted, added, permutated, abbreviated, etc.

[2.11] Let us ponder the order of the Pharisees. The sect of the Pharisees became so detached from reality that one of their divisions was called "A Pharisee that lets out his blood": this type of Pharisee "'... shows himself such a one as if his eyes were hood-winked, that he might not look upon a woman; and here upon dashed his head against the walls, and let out his blood.' The Aruch writes, 'pressed up himself against the walls, that he might not touch those that passed by, that by dashing he fetched blood of himself,'" (*Commentary on the New Testament from the Talmud and Hebraica*, Lightfoot; Vol. 2, p. 74). Many Pharisees believed that the actions described above were admirable, reverent, and to be imitated.

The Lord Jesus said, "Woe to you, Scribes and Pharisees, hypocrites! For you are like white-washed tombs, which on the outside look beautiful, but inside they are full of the bones of the dead and all kinds of filth. So you also on the outside look righteous to others, but inside you are full of hypocrisy and lawlessness. Woe to you, Scribes and Pharisees, hypocrites! For you build the tombs of the prophets and decorate the graves of the righteous..." (Matthew 23:27-29). The Jews of Jesus' earthly days used to paint sepulchers with chalky whitewash in the likeness of bones so that when others saw the bone-white tombs they might avoid them because tombs contain impurity, though they appeared brilliant. Like the Magi, the Pharisees often wore white as a symbol of purity, as bright garments are beautiful to behold. The outward appearance of "whiteness" is paralleled to the direct indication of the whiteness used to mark tombs. Ironically, the very color some of the Pharisees wore to mark their moral purity was also used to mark the impurity of tombs. The concepts behind the color white are manifold, as they apply to both good and evil. Once again we see how evil is but a counterfeit of good; evil is but a camouflaged parasite, and goodness is the resilient, brilliant host.

Goodness has no evil in it and exists independently as the standard, but evil is dependant and far weaker than goodness; to illustrate this point, let us contemplate Psalm 51:7-9:

> "Cleanse me with hyssop, and I will be clean;
> wash me, and I will be whiter than snow.
> Let me hear joy and gladness;
> let the bones you have crushed rejoice.
> Hide your face from my sins
> and blot out all my iniquity."

Hyssop is an aromatic plant of the mint family and produces white flowers; it was used for purification rituals (consider Passover in relation to the branch given Jesus to drink from on the cross). Hyssop being mentioned in the first line explains the second line through Synonymous Parallel concerning the pure whiteness of snow. However, the fourth line of this very Psalm discusses "bones," and by recognizing unclean, white bones the "whitewashed tomb" comment becomes more vivid. Psalm 51 depicts David asking to be purified that he may be whiter than snow, but he also acknowledges that God crushed his bones (which are also white) for his sin. The sixth line ties the second line to the fourth line by the discussion of iniquity, for David's bones were righteously crushed (figuratively) and he sought purification, hence the hyssop with its white flowers. The color white can signify both evil and righteousness; Miriam became leprous, as "white as snow," in Numbers 12; yet, "...and behold, if the leprosy have covered all his flesh, he shall pronounce him clean that hath the plague: it is all turned white: he is clean,"

(Leviticus 13:13). Christ's hair is white according to Revelation 1:14.

[2.12] The Written Law describes the actual letters and words of the Hebrew Scriptures. The oral Law describes the traditions of elders. Let us consider, again, the words of Dr. John Lightfoot: "R. Judah, who first removed the university to Tiberias, sat also in Zippor for many years, and there died: so that in both places were very famous schools. He composed and digested the Mishnaioth into one volume. 'For when he saw the captivity was prolonged... and the scholars to become faint-hearted, and the strength of wisdom and the cabala to fail, and the oral law to be much diminished, – he gathered and scraped up together all the decrees, statutes, and sayings of wise men..." (*Commentary on the New Testament from the Talmud and Hebraica*, Lightfoot; Vol. 1, p. 160-161). If the oral law is the same now as it was when the Written Law was given to Moses on Sinai, how then could the oral law have been "much diminished?" Had the knowledge of the oral law remained consistent from Sinai, it would not have become "diminished" at all. God's Word is immovable. Humanity's mind is movable.

A significant portion of the tradition of the Hebrew Scriptures, as we know it, can be summed up this way: the oral law completes the Written Law; at the same time, "Massorah [Rubric 1.8] exists independently of halakhah (rabbinic law)..." (*J.P.S. Tanakh*, p. ix). "The Masoretic text dominated Old Testament studies in the Middle Ages, and it has served as the basis for virtually all printed versions of the Hebrew Bible," (*Vine's Expository Dictionary of Old and New Testament Words*, Forward – Introduction). The very reading of the Hebrew Scriptures is divided, and on such divisions it has been translated. "And if a house is divided against itself, that house will not be able to stand," (Mark 3:25), but at the same time, "...not one letter, not one stroke of a letter, will pass from the law until all is accomplished," (Matthew 5:18). The divisions imposed on Scripture (whether accidental or deliberate) have carved a giant canyon between those who would otherwise join hands in unity; at the same time, the very Word under discussion binds those who are opposed to each other because they share a common hope. May God have mercy on us all.

Reflecting on the immense conflict between Christ and the Pharisees, it is striking to note that the Pharisees' main doctrine was that the oral law (the traditions of the elders) completed the Written Law (the Scriptures). Concerning the many historical trials and ardors imposed against the Jews by various ruling officials, "Their corrupt and unwise handling of Jewish affairs was one of the chief causes of the war of 66 which led to the destruction of Jerusalem in 70 CE, and to the subsequent decline of the Sadducees, the extinction of the Zealots in Masada in 74, the disappearance of the Essenes, and the survival and uncontested domination of the Pharisees and their rabbinic successors," (*The Complete Dead Sea Scrolls*, Vermes; p. 53).

"Torah interpretation was entrusted to the priests and Levites during the first two or three centuries following the Babylonian exile. Ezra and his colleagues, the ancient scribes of Israel, 'read from the book of the Law... made its sense plain and gave instruction in what was read'. In this passage from the Book of Nehemiah viii, 8, Jewish tradition acknowledges the institution of a regular paraphrase of Scripture known as Targum, or translation into the vernacular of the members of the congregation. When the parties of the Pharisees, Sadducees, Essenes, etc., came into being with their different convictions, they justified them by interpretations suited to their needs," (*The Complete Dead Sea Scrolls*, Vermes; p. 69).

Does this mean that our English Bibles are flawed because most of the Pharisees were corrupt? Yes, in the sense that there are blatantly altered passages, additional words, and omitted words within it; no, in that the New Testament elucidates where these alterations are, as the various catalogues of the Old Testament attest to these facts as well. Scripture still stands in an untainted and pristine immovability, but the way it is read and carried out is often from the minds of people. Specifically, our English Old Testaments are more limited (seemingly) to what was said about them by many of the greatest scholars more so than they are errant by false transmissions; perhaps a better way to state this point is that we are only reading the introductory version of the Old Testament, the initial teaching-tool of the masters. The Bible safeguards against corruption by providing the New Testament along with the fact that Jeremiah (Old Testament) tells us that the Scribes erred. It is therefore necessary to read where the Old Testament has been altered so that we may explicitly understand why Christ died for what He did in truth and integrity – for without recognizing the immensity of the effects produced by the alterations of the Scribes, there proves little consistency in understanding why the greatest Torah Scholars wanted Christ dead.

Consider the history of even the stylistic formats of the Scriptures: "The Jews, by their own confession, are no longer, nor have been indeed for many ages, masters of the system of the ancient meter. All remembrance of it has ceased from the times in which the Hebrew became a dead language; and it really seems probable that the Masorites, (of whom so little is known,) who afterwards distinguished the sacred volumes by accents and vowel points, as they are now extant, were possessed of so trifling and imperfect a knowledge of this subject, that they were even incapable of distinguishing what was written in meter from plain prose. For when, according to their manner, they marked certain books as metrical, namely, the Psalms, the Proverbs, and the book of Job; they accounted others, which are no less evidently metrical, absolutely prosaic, such as the Song of Solomon, and the Lamentations of Jeremiah, and consequently assigned to them the common prose accent only," (*Lectures on the Sacred Poetry of the Hebrews*, Lowth; p. 191).

[2.13] Those saved in Christ are "born again," (John 3), and as we are to be born again, Christ told us that we are to "become like children," (Matthew 18:2) – not in immaturity, for if we were supposed to revert away from mature knowledge, then the Scriptures would not say: "Whom shall He teach knowledge? And whom shall He make to understand doctrine? Them that are weaned from the milk, and drawn from the breasts," (Isaiah

28:9) or "Brothers and sisters, do not be children in your thinking... but in thinking be adults," (I Corinthians 14:20). By being complacent and believing that we are not meant to know the details of Scripture – the very word that God gave us to guide us and to guard us, as He Himself is referred to as the "Word" in John 1 – we reject the specific record of salvation that was meticulously ordained to feed us daily with the knowledge of the hope that is within us. "Massorah exists independently of halakhah (rabbinic law). The early medieval masters of the biblical text who developed this documentation are known in English as 'masoretes' [*Massorites*]. Many masoretic annotations seem designed to reduce loss or distortion in transmission of the text," (*J.P.S. Tanakh*, p. ix). "At first the Massorah was transmitted by word of mouth. Moreover we do not posses old manuscripts from the early days when the text was first handed down, because copies no longer in use were kept in the Genizah (storeroom) of the synagogue and buried ceremonially from time to time, in order to guard against any profanation of the sacred scriptures," (*The Old Testament*, Weiser; p. 361).

The Transmission of the Hebrew Scriptures is called the "Massorah" (מסורה) or the "Massoreth" (מסורת). The Massorites existed apart from the strictures of the Rabbis, although it seems improbable for the influences of both the Rabbis and the Massorites to have been entirely mutually exclusive. As various Bible translations came from the Massoretic Text, it should be noted that the Massorites themselves were not entirely unified, for there were varying schools of Massorites who reckoned the Scriptures differently. For instance, the Eastern Massorites employed simpler vowel-signs in a less complicated system than the Western Massorites. The Eastern Massoretic system, because of its relative simplicity, was considered difficult to decipher with respect to interpretive intricacy. "The Massorah, which developed Talmudic traditions, gradually came under Western influences and there emerged finally a mixed type which obliterated the characteristics of the Eastern Massorah," (*The Old Testament*, Weiser; p. 362).

[2.14] "At first the Massorah was transmitted by word of mouth (*The Old Testament*, Weiser; p. 361); "The correlative term to מסורה [*Massorah*] is קבלה Qabbalah... expressing properly whatever has been *received* by tradition. Technically, however, the latter word [Qabbalah] is restricted to matters of esoteric doctrine and theology, and gives a name to the great mass of speculative philosophy and mysticism of the later Rabbis," (*Introduction to the Ginsburg Edition of the Hebrew Old Testament*, Geden & Kilgour; p.48-49). Despite the correlative nature of the terms "Massorah" and "Qabbalah (Cabala, Kabala, Kabbalah)," there is a significant distinction between them. Regarding the doctrines of Qabbalah (of which the author of this book despises), what probably began with decent intentions ended with shameful deceit.

A famous Kabalistic text, the *Sohar* is bound to this historical account: "The very existence of the Sohar, according to the confession of the staunch Kabbalist, Jehudah Chajoth (flourished 1500), was unknown to such distinguished Kabbalists as Nachmanides (1195-1270) and Ben-Adereth (1234-1310)... That Moses de Leon, who first published and sold the *Sohar*, as the production of R. Simon b. Jochai, was himself the author of it, was admitted by his own wife and daughter, as will be seen from the following account in the *Book Juchassin*, (p.p. 88, 89, 95, e. Filipowski, London, 1857), which we give in an abridged form. When Isaac of Akko, who escaped the massacre after the capture of this city (A.D. 1291), came to Spain and there saw the *Sohar*, he was anxious to ascertain whether it was genuine, since it pretended to be a Palestine production, and he, though born and brought up on the Holy Land, in constant intercourse with the disciples of the celebrated Kabbalist, Nachmanides, had never heard a syllable about this marvelous work. Now, Moses de Leon, whom he met in Valladolid, declared to him a most solemn oath that he had at Avila an ancient exemplar, which was the very autograph of R. Simon ben Jochai, and offered to submit it to him to be tested. In the meantime, however, Moses de Leon was taken ill on his journey home, and died at Arevolo, A.D. 1305. But two distinguished men of Avila, David Rafen and Joseph de Avila, who were determined to sift the matter, ascertained the falsehood of this story from the widow and daughter of Moses de Leon. Benig a rich man and knowing that Moses de Leon left his family without means, Joseph de Avila promised that if she would give him the original MS. of the *Sohar* from which her husband made the copies, his son should marry her daughter, and that he would give them a handsome dowry. Whereupon the widow and daughter declared, that they did not possess any such MS., that Moses de Leon never had it, but that he composed the *Sohar* from his own head, and wrote it with his own hand. Moreover, the widow candidly confessed that she had frequently asked her husband why he published the production of his own intellect under another man's name, and that he told her that if he were to publish it under his own name nobody would buy it, whereas under the name of R. Simon b. Jocahi it yielded him a large revenue. This account is confirmed in a most remarkable manner by the fact that... [the] *Sohar* contains whole passages which Moses de Leon translated into Aramaic, from his other works, as the learned Jellinek has demonstratively proved," (*The Kabbalah*, Ginsburg; 171-174).

Regarding the relationship between the terms "Kabala" and "Massorah," it is probable that Kabala (or what pre-dated Kabala and its famous doctrines that pretend to be older than they are) began as the recognition of recondite Biblical phenomena, and this recognition, propelled by wonder concerning the grandeur of Scripture, spawned a search for deeper Biblical meaning beyond the traditional sense of study – a search that later became a system unto itself, as is prone to happen with oral tradition that usually becomes legend and myth when enough time elapses. For instance, "Massorah" means "transmitted; to deliver into the hands of another" and "Kabala" means "received." The Apostle Paul said, "For I handed on to you as of first importance what I in turn had received: that Christ died for our sins in accordance with the Scriptures," (I Corinthians 15:3). However, the Sohar, among the main texts of Kabalah, was composed by one Moses de Leon long after the death of the Apostle Paul.

[2.15] The Sopherim replaced the Name ("Jehovah" or "YHWH" or יהוה) 134 times in the Scriptures with

"Adonai." In all fairness, these 134 alterations were mostly authorized out of extreme reverence (but mistaken reverence) for this Holy, unspeakable Name in an effort to prevent blasphemy against the Name of God Almighty. However, the mistakenly reverent nature of the intentions that fueled such alterations grew contrary to the fact that the act of naming is always an act of superiority (Genesis 2:20), for God named Adam, and Adam named the animals. Furthermore, by similar editing choices, the numeric sequence of the flawless Scriptures became lost.

[2.16] As far as we are currently aware, a definitive Hebrew Bible Text no longer exists, so the entire syntactic gematria of the entire Hebrew Bible cannot be determined even by a computer because there is no one manuscript that settles all of the disputes. How thankful we are obliged to be for the New Testament that settles the thematic disputes regarding the Hebrew Scriptures! Various Hebrew transmissions that disagree with each other at points exist along side each other in contention. We should recognize that there is hardly any book of any genre without the occasional misprint, or scribal (typographical) error, though we should also remember that the Holy Scriptures were given to Moses flawlessly – absolutely flawlessly. The flawlessness of the Scriptures became copied in a flawed manner. A simple way of understanding scribal error can be achieved if one attempts to copy a document of only several pages by hand or by typing; one might often notice one's own errors very quickly as goes the nature of copying itself (as I attest of myself) – but this matter is entirely different than deliberate alteration. The Biblical manuscripts that remain, which are copies of transmissions, place a translator/publisher in a vexing position that forces one to choose one textual variant over another, and such a dilemma is a burden left to the "correction" of another editor/translator/publisher who attempts the same task. The best a publisher can produce is a defensible version of the Scriptures. The Word of God has not passed away, nor is The Word in a state of erosion. Human error within transmitted copies of the Text has placed the occasional hurdle before us; thank God for His mercy.

[2.17] Again, there is a distinction between the oral law and the Written Law. Satan manipulated human conception of the oral law (the pure Oral Law from the mouth of God) in order to deceive Adam and Eve. If the tradition today were the exact same as it was during the time of Moses, or even the time of Ezra, there would be no disagreement as to what was said originally at Sinai when the Torah was declared to Moses from God and to the people from Moses, nor would there be the translational variants we observe today. The oral law, the legal commentary on the Torah, extends from the initial reading of the Torah, whereas the Written Law is the infinite reading of the Torah.

The *J.P.S. Hebrew-English Tanakh* records that, "Jewish translators were also influenced by the widely held view that, along with the Written Law... God had given Moses on Mount Sinai an oral Law... as well; so that to comprehend God's Torah fully and correctly, it was essential to make use of both. Thus, when a translation of the Hebrew Bible into the Judeo-Arabic vernacular was deemed necessary for Jewry in Moslem countries toward the end of the first millennium, the noted philologian, philosopher, and community leader Saadia Gaon (882-942) produced a version that incorporated traditional Jewish interpretation but was not based on a word-for-word translation; at the same time, it was a model of clarity and stylistic elegance. The present version is in the spirit of Saadia," (*J.P.S. Tanakh*; p. xxii).

Nehemiah 8:8 records, "So they read in the book of the Law of God distinctly, and gave the sense, and caused them to understand the reading." The fact that the Law was read "distinctly" illustrates a traditional reading, which, during Ezra's time, like Moses' time, was correct – though it can hardly be assumed that this reading was the defining end of the Scriptures and not but the correct beginning of the Scriptures, for what is spoken aloud cannot account for every allusion of Scripture that is most speedily perceived through the eye. Consider Psalm 19:1-4: "The heavens are telling the glory of God; and the firmament proclaims His handiwork. Day to day pours forth speech, and night to night declares knowledge. There is no speech, nor are there words: their voice is not heard; yet their voice goes out through all the earth, and their words to the end of the world." Psalm 19 explains that the celestial bodies speak resoundingly, though they are silent; they have a voice that heard in one way but not heard in another way. "Open my eyes, so that I may behold wondrous things out of Your law," (Psalm 119:18), for the "eyes" are to be opened in order to perceive that which is not heard with the ears.

[2.18] "Who is as the wise man? And who knows the

interpretation of a thing? A man's wisdom makes his face to shine and the boldness of his face shall be changed," (Ecclesiastes 8:1). The description of "interpretation" coupled with a face that "shines" brings us to Moses in Exodus 34 concerning the recording of the commands and characteristics (Exodus 34:5-7) of God. "Moses came down from Mount Sinai. As he came down from the mountain with the two tablets of the covenant in his hand, Moses did not know that the skin of his face shone because he had been talking with God. When Aaron and all the Israelites saw Moses, the skin of his face was shining, and they were afraid to come near him. But Moses called to them; and Aaron and all the leaders of the congregation returned to him, and Moses spoke with them. Afterward all the Israelites came near, and he gave them in commandment all that the Lord had spoken with him on Mount Sinai. When Moses had finished speaking with them, he put a veil on his face; but whenever Moses went before the Lord to speak with Him, he would take the veil off, until he came out; and when he came out, and told the Israelites what he had been commanded, the Israelites would see the face of Moses, that the skin of his face was shining; and Moses would put the veil on his face again, until he went in to speak with Him," (Exodus 34:29-35).

The Apostle Paul wrote, "Since, then, we have such a hope, we use great plainness of speech, not like Moses who put a veil over his face to keep the people of Israel from gazing at the end of the glory that was being set aside. But their minds were hardened. Indeed, to this very day, when they hear the reading of the old covenant, that same veil is still there, since only in Christ is it set aside. Indeed, to this very day whenever Moses is read, a veil lies over their minds," (II Corinthians 3:12-15). Christ said, "For nothing is hidden that will not be disclosed, nor is anything secret that will not become known and come to light. Then pay attention to how you listen; for those who have, more will be given; and from those who do not have, even what they seem to have will be taken away," (Luke 8:17-18).

Moses was equipped with superior wisdom (as he was taught by the One teacher Who instructed the Apostle Paul) in comparison to the remaining Israelites; he was the one who received the Torah personally, and having supped with God, Moses' face shined. Moses, by digesting the interpretive knowledge that God imparted to him, served as the example of Coheleth's teaching: "Who is as the wise man? And who knows the interpretation of a thing? A man's wisdom makes his face to shine, and the boldness of his face shall be changed," (Ecclesiastes 8:1).

[2.19] The Torah was written originally in the vowel-lacking style. Without vowels, the word "בכר" can mean "camel" (ref. 1070) or "to burst from the womb; to bear early fruit (of a woman or of a tree)" (ref. 1069) out of context, and can connect all of these concepts by Gematria; these letters are "ר+כ+ב" = 200+20+2 = **222**. When we reflect on the importance of the constellations to the Jews for the purposes of agricultural/seasonal indicators, it is difficult to ignore the fact that when the Savior was prophesied in Genesis 3:15, the constellations of Hercules and Draco were identified: "He shall bruise thy head, and thou shalt bruise His heel." The constellation Hercules, "...is one of the oldest sky figures, although not known to the first Greek astronomers under that name, – for Eudoxos had Ενγουνασι; Hipparchos... *Bending on his knees*... Aratos added to these designations... *the Kneeling One*," (*Star Names*, Allen; p. 239) as the constellation we now refer to as "Hercules" was organized in its ancient map to depict a mighty warrior on bended knee (due to a wounded heel) in preparation to smash the head of a serpent and a vine held in one of his hands by a piece of wood in his other hand. In a similar way, "ברך" (ref. 1288) = "to kneel" = "ב+ר+ך" = 20+200+2 = **222**; "ברך" (ref. 1290) = "knee" = "ב+ר+ך" = 20+200+2 = **222**, as the constellations indicate time-periods similar to our present-day analog clocks, for "כבר" (ref. 3528) = "extent of time; long ago, formerly, hitherto:- already, (seeing that which), now" = "כ+ב+ר" = 200+2+20 = **222**.

The vowelized Scriptures distinguish between all of the definitions of words constructed of the same letters in the same order so that only one definition is communicated when reading the Hebrew Text aloud. As a given word occurs syntactically, a sense is perceived, and the inserted vowels capture that particular sense. However, Jesus often made His points in His teachings and arguments by the allusions of Hebrew – a fact that shows the incomprehensible mind of God, for, in order to teach and argue this way, Christ must have had the entire Hebrew dictionary memorized along with whatever languages He spoke, taught, and argued within depending on His audience, a fact that accounts for His heavenly mastery of those languages as well, a fact that illustrates His deity in relation to the fact that He must have had the all the Scriptures perfectly memorized, which, altogether, is a superhuman feat. We can appreciate why the New Testament is written in Greek, by the rules and allusions of the Hebrew Written Law as opposed to the oral law of the Pharisees. The traditions of the Pharisees are not defined by the Law Moses gave, for they are off-shoots only somewhat based on the Torah, and the ends of these offshoots often contradict the Torah.

No human can possibly adhere to every one of the 613 regulations of the Written Law completely, nor can any human cognize every allusion of every word simultaneously as one reads the Scriptures. Thank God for the New Testament as it records the fulfillment of the 613 standards by God in the form of a Man. No mere human can account for each expansive concept and allusion at all times when reasoning on-demand, which is a reason why none of the Jewish elites could ever conquer Christ in an argument. The idioms and descriptions of the Greek New Testament reflect Hebrew. Again, the Reverend Alfred S. Geden, M.A., D.D. and the Reverend R. Kilgour, D.D. of the London British and Foreign Bible Society remarked in *Introduction to the Ginsburg Edition of the Hebrew Old Testament* (p. 54) that, "It is not always possible to determine with certainty how the [actual Text of the Hebrew Bible] was intended to be pronounced; but that it represents in many instances a text older and more correct than the [traditional reading] is unquestionable." Christ fulfilled every one of the Torah Laws by not breaking them and by openly demonstrating their applications through His teachings (the true Oral Law), and He did so in a manner that broke the oral laws of the Jewish elites and that exposed these artificial regulations to be fraudulent and against the true traditions of God for His people.

[2.20] Again, regarding the specific regulations of the Torah, as in the Book of Leviticus (for example), "The whole system of the Hebrew rites is one great and complicated allegory, to the study and observance of which all possible diligence and attention were incessantly dedicated by those who were employed in the sacred offices," (*Lectures on the Sacred Poetry of the Hebrews*, Lowth; p. 82). "Much of the Jewish law is employed in discriminating between things clean and unclean; in removing and making atonement for things polluted or prescribed; and under these ceremonies, as under a veil or covering, a meaning the most important and sacred is concealed, (*Lectures on the Sacred Poetry of the Hebrews*, Lowth; p. 83). We can understand easily why there was such a fierce contention concerning how the Scriptures should be read and how the readings should be carried out, for the Scriptures were intended to imbue every part of private, social, political, and religious life, facets of life that were originally intended to be one consistent whole.

[2.21] The "Ten Nequdoth of the Torah," which are words so marked as to be canceled in reading (*Ten Nequdoth of the Torah*, Butin; p. 117), point to uncertainty left open to possible amendment: "... our last and apparently most direct argument, is derived from the meaning attributed to the Points by the Jewish tradition... The earlier Jewish writings are the reproduction of the oral lessons given in the Jewish schools and academies, as is evident from the fact that the authority of some Rabbi or Rabbis is generally given," (*The Ten Nequdoth of the Torah*, Butin; 15). Consider "… the age of the Massoretes in general terms [extended] from about the fourth to sixth centuries of our common era or even later; and we are not always certain of the meaning which they intended to convey by some of the diacritical signs employed," (*The Hebrew Old Testament*, Ginsburg; p. 55). It should be noted that, "The aim of the Massorah may be to preserve the text, but it preserves the text with all the peculiarities which the ancients had already noticed…" (*The Ten Nequdoth of the Torah*, Butin; 17). Dr. Butin placed a chronology on the Ten Nequdoth of the Torah claiming that, "Everything tends to show that the Nequdoth should be ascribed, at the latest, to the very dawn of the Christian era, and probably to a still more remote antiquity," (*The Ten Nequdoth of the Torah*, Butin; 24).

The Massorah Magna is the writing on the actual pages of the Hebrew Scriptures written above and below the Text; the Massorah Parva is the writing on the side margins of the Text, and between the columns of the Text; together, these two form part of the fence of the Scriptures. The word "Massorah" (or Transmission) indicates "to deliver into the hands of another," and it was a painstaking, meticulous compilation that recorded the mysterious phenomena of patterns and peculiarities in the Hebrew Scriptures. Such recorded phenomena is to be observed along with the alternate readings called "Severin," the "15 Extraordinary Points of the Sopherim" of which there are the "Ten Nequdoth of the Torah," and with the "18 Emendations of the Sopherim" (which were places the Scribes admittedly altered and marked as such), the

134 altered passages where the Name "Jehovah" was changed to "Adonai," the omission of words found in the Text, and the insertion of words not found in the Text. The Massorah was designed to lock a masterful tradition on top of the Holy Scriptures. The Massorah is considered by some to be the most intricate lock ever constructed by human cognition. Let the reader's opinion be as it may be.

[2.22] Without vowels in the Hebrew Scriptures, two readers can look at one word and each reader can pronounce the one word differently, but by being well acquainted with the traditional accounts of Scripture, the vowel-lacking Torah Scrolls are read with ease by fluent Hebrew readers. As an example, if we were to consider the difficulties of Hebrew in English, we could consider the letters "r" and "d." If we read the original Scriptures and came to a word that read "rd" (without being familiar with the contents of Scripture) as those letters stand out of context, we would have little way of determining if the word is "red," "read," "reed," "rude," or "raid," etc. other than by the context of the passage. The Scribes invented a system of vowels long after the Scriptures were written. In other words, what the Scribes said the Scriptures communicated is how the various interpretive recording traditions built around the Word of God became eventually written; this was part of the reason that ancient versions of the Scriptures do not perfectly align with our present-day Old Testaments.

[2.23] We may recall that some English Bibles render Genesis 1:1-2 to say, "In the beginning, *when* God created the heavens and the earth, the earth was formless and void..." (Genesis 1:1-2), but such a render contradicts Isaiah 45:18 that boldly states that, "For thus says the Lord, Who created the heavens (He is God!), who formed the earth and made it (He established it; He did not create it a chaos, He formed it to be inhabited!)"; to this point, the Hebrew states that "In the beginning, Elohim created the heavens and the earth," in 7 words and 28 letters. The tradition that claims an initial chaos, whereby God created life out of chaos, is not found in the Scriptures and is but the product of human forgetfulness by way of oral transmission that resulted in legend and myth. Various creation myths describe primeval waters where deities battled through chaos, and whereby the victor defeated the chaos and created something out of it. In Greek thought, Zeus battled Typhon {3} and, upon Zeus' victory, Zeus established the present order of the world; this thought merely reflects forgetfulness that finds it roots in the truth of Scripture. Holy Scripture was written down flawlessly on Sinai after human tradition bent away from the truths known in primitive history. On account of a great diversity of the oral traditions that were systems unto themselves (and that greatly affected religious, social, private, and political behavior), it became more than necessary to reinstate what had been forsaken. Contrarily, myth is but tradition whose source-information becomes inflated on account of what has been forgotten. Myth is similar to possessing segments A, B, and D; the missing C segment is semi-reconstructed (at best) or invented (at worst) to compensate for the noticeable loss in the sequence, and because of the reshaped C segment, myth begins to spread over the original truth like a wild vine.

[2.24] The original Scriptures were written as an unbroken sequence whereby every letter was equidistant to another so that there were no breaks between words. The ancient Scribes divided the continuous sequence into individual words, but the ancient Scribes disagreed as to exactly how the letters should be broken apart into individual words. The varying traditions that grew out of the disagreements concerning the correct division of Scripture was no small matter: "To facilitate still further the study of the unpointed consonants on the part of the laity, the Scribes gradually introduced into the text the *matres lectionis* which also served as vowel-letters. But in this branch of their labors as is the case in the other branches, the different Schools which were the depositories of the traditions as to the import of the text, exhibited considerable diversity of opinion owing to the fact that the traditions themselves were not uniform. So great indeed was this diversity of opinion about the respective traditions and the import of the text of Scripture *circa 300 B.C.* that it gave rise to the division of the people into the two national sects the Pharisees and the Sadducees," (*Introduction to the Massaretico-Critical Edition of the Hebrew Bible*, Ginsburg; p. 299).

[2.25] Even the very names of Biblical letters are extremely important as they can indicate the subtleties of a word or teaching. John Gill, D.D. noted in his book called, *The Antiquity of the Hebrew Language*, "... the Greeks are generally supposed to have their letters, at least most of them, from the Phoenicians, they doubtless had the names of them along with them; and Diodorus Siculus [Bibliothec. Lib. 3.p. 200] expressly says, that as

Cadmus brought the letters from Phoenicia into Greece, so he gave to every one their names, as well as formed their characters; and as the Phoenician, or old Samaritan alphabet consisted of letters of the same name, though of a different character from the Hebrew, it may reasonably be supposed that the names are derived from thence, as the language is but a dialect of the Hebrew, with a little variation and deflexion from it; so that the Hebrews had these names originally; and it cannot be thought otherwise but that when their letters were first invented, and marks made for them, but names were given unto them; and Capellus [Arcanum punctat. Revelat. 1. i. c. 12] himself is quite clear and express in this matter: 'before the age of Cadmus the Phoenician, he says i.e. 1450 years before the birth of Christ, the Hebrew letters had their own names, and indeed the same with those by which they are now called, as is plain by comparing the Greek alphabet with the Hebrew... the same names of Hebrew letters are as they were three thousand years ago..." (*The Antiquity of the Hebrew Language,* Gill; p. 41-42; compare this to the chronology already stated). Dr. Gill then provided the respective significations of the letter-names:

1) Aleph   (א) = "an ox"
2) Beth   (ב) = "a house"
3) Gimel   (ג) = "a camel"
4) Daleth   (ד) = "a door"
5) He   (ה) = "[Dr. Gill was unsure.]"
6) Vau   (ו) = "a hook"
7) Zayin   (ז) = "armor, or spear"
8) Cheth   (ח) = "a beast"

9) Teth   (ט) = "folding or involving"
10) Yod   (י) = "a hand, the finger"
11) Caph   (כ) = "the hollow of the hand"
12) Lamed   (ל) = "a goad"
13) Mem   (מ) = "a spot as impressed upon the hand"
14) Nun   (נ) = "a son, child, or infant"
15) Samech   (ס) = "a support, pedestal, or column"
16) Ayin   (ע) = "an eye"
17) Pe   (פ) = "an open mouth"
18) Tsaddi   (צ) = "a fork"
19) Koph   (ק) = "a revolution, a semicircle, with a descending line, or a monkey"
20) Resh   (ר) = "the head"
21) Shin   (ש) = "a tooth"
22) Tav   (ת) = "a mark, sign, or border, being the boundary of the alphabet"

Gesenius' Hebrew Grammar (Edited and Enlarged by E. Kautzsch) lists the letter-significations this way:

1) Aleph   (א) = "ox"
2) Beth   (ב) = "house"
3) Gimel   (ג) = "camel"
4) Daleth   (ד) = "door"
5) He   (ה) = "air hole (?) lattice-widow (?)"
6) Vau   (ו) = "hook, nail"
7) Zayin   (ז) = "weapon"
8) Cheth   (ח) = "fence, barrier"
9) Teth   (ט) = "a winding (?), a leather bottle, or a snake"

10) Yod   (י) = "hand"
11) Caph   (כ) = "bent hand"
12) Lamed   (ל) = "ox-goad"
13) Mem   (מ) = "water"
14) Nun   (נ) = "fish (perhaps originally נחש snake)"
15) Samech   (ס) = "prop"
16) Ayin   (ע) = "eye"
17) Pe   (פ) = "mouth"
18) Tsaddi   (צ) = "fish hook (?)"
19) Koph   (ק) = "eye of a needle, or back of the head"
20) Resh   (ר) = "head"
21) Shin   (ש) = "tooth"
22) Tav   (ת) = "sign, cross"

Though there seems to be distinctions between the two lists of letter-significations above, it is beneficial to note that their apparent differences are not mutually exclusive.

Dr. Gill's list states that the letter נ signifies a "**son**," while Gesenius' edited list states that this letter signifies a **fish** or a **snake**: Jesus said, "Or what man is there of you, whom if his **son** ask bread, will he give him a stone? Or if he ask a **fish**, will he give him a **serpent**," (Matthew 7:9-10). The "serpent" of Genesis 3 said to Jesus, "If thou be the Son of God, command that these stones be made bread," (Matthew 4:3).

Dr. Gill's list states that the letter ח signifies a "beast," while Gesenius' edited list states that this letter signifies "a fence, barrier" – which is where beasts can be kept. Dr. Gill's list states that the **19**th letter signifies "a semicircle, with a descending line" in agreement with Gesenius' edited list that states that this letter signifies the *"eye of a needle"*

– Dr. Gill described the shape of the entity and Gesenius described the entity itself (regardless of the auxiliary opinions of both men). As we have already understood that the "eye of a needle" can refer to a "womb" (Rubric i.33) it is interesting to note that "Eve" = "חוה" (ref. 2332) = "ה+ו+ח" = 5+6+8 = **19**.

Letter significations are conceptual. Like the ancient star maps, it is the names of the letters that determine their significations just as it is the names of the stars that determine their pictures. Accordingly, the names of Hebrew letters are reminiscent of the names of various stars, and at one point in history, they probably shared the same names. The letter-names listed above have also more meanings than what Dr. Gill listed. For instance, the 9th letter also signifies "sweeping"; **the 18th letter (צ) also signifies a "tree"**; the 21st letter also signifies "fire" (both "tooth" and "fire" in the sense of "consumption"). The pronunciation of a given letter-name is also a Hebrew word (or words) that conveys a concept.

The Lock   197

Dr. Ginsburg listed the names of the letters this way:

א	=	אלף
ב	=	בית
ג	=	גימל
ד	=	דלת
ה	=	הא
ו	=	ויו
ז	=	זין
ח	=	חית
ט	=	טית
י	=	יד
כ	=	כף
ל	=	למד
מ	=	מים
נ	=	נון
ס	=	סמך
ע	=	עין
פ	=	פא
צ	=	צדי
ק	=	קוף
ר	=	ריש
ש	=	שין
ש	=	סין
ת	=	תו

When one says the name of a Hebrew letter aloud, the name is also a word for which the letter stands conceptually. The letter "ב" can signify a "house" because the name of the letter is "בית" (ref. 1004) = "a house." In the same way, the letter "א" can signify and "ox" because the name of letter is "אלף" (ref. 504) = "a family; also (from the sense of yoking or taming) *an ox or cow, kine.*" In the Gematria matrices of the Hebrew and Greek alphabets, the number/letter "א" = "1" is also "1000" (though not often calculated as such), as "1" describes the beginning of a cycle, whereas "1000" describes the end of a cycle (Deuteronomy 32:30: "How could one chase a thousand...?"). Thus, we can observe the various definitions attached to "א" = "אלף" for "אלף" (ref. 505) = "*an ox's head;* the numeral 1,000, a thousand". The words composed of the letters "אלף" are related by similar sounds, but the gematria of these words is identical, as we can see an inherent relationship:

"אלף" (ref. 502) = "to associate with; hence, to learn, to teach, to utter" = "א+ל+ף" = **111**

"אלף" (ref. 503) = "to make a thousandfold:- to bring forth thousands" = "א+ל+ף" = **111**

"אלף" (ref. 504) = "a family; also (from the sense of yoking or taming) an ox or cow, kine" = "א+ל+ף" = **111**

"אלף" (ref. 505) = "an ox's head; the numeral 1,000, a thousand" = "א+ל+ף" = **111**

"אלף" (ref. 506) Chaldee = "a thousand" = "א+ל+ף" = **111**

"אלף" (ref. 507) = "(same as ref. 505) a place in Palestine" (*Eleph* [*Thousand*])" = "א+ל+ף" = **111**

The vowelized Hebrew Scriptures select one of these words over another so that a specific sense is given in order that the readings remain consistent. In other words, there is a distinction between ref. 502, ref. 503, ref. 504, ref 505, and ref. 506 as indicated by the different vowels (points) affixed to these words (not present in the examples above). When Christ *taught* ["אָלַף" (ref. 502)] the *multitudes* ["אֶלֶף" (ref. 503)], He said, "Come to Me, *all* ["אֶלֶף" (ref. 503)] you that are weary and are carrying heavy burdens, and I will give you rest. Take my *yoke* ["אֶלֶף" (ref. 503)]..." (Mathew 11:28-29); to think of this in a mathematical way, then, When Christ *taught* [**111**] the *multitudes* [**111**], He said, "Come to Me, *all* [**111**] you that are weary and are carrying heavy burdens, and I will give you rest. Take my *yoke* [**111**]..." (Mathew 11:28-29). Christ's Oral Law explained the intricacies of the Written Law on a far more intense level than the traditions of the elders, for Christ even accounted for the very conceptual essence of single letters that constitute words, hence His title of being the "Computation" = the "Logos": "...λογος (logos), generally speaking, is taken as meaning a word as made up of letters; and ρημα (rhema), a saying as made up of words," (*How to Enjoy the Bible, Bullinger*, p. 183). Christ, the Logos, explained the Written Law when He said, "Man shall not live by bread alone, but by every rhema proceeds from the mouth of God," (Matthew 4:4 & Deuteronomy 8:3).

Unfortunately, because Gematria has been abused to the point of Satanic degeneration, many Christians have abstained from the wonders it unearths. The inheritance is ours, not the Enemy's! It is only the ridiculous mystical perversions of Gematria that attempt to convert its exactitude into sorcery. The first letter-name of the Hebrew alphabet is "aleph" = "אלף" = "א+ל+ף" = 80+30+1 = **111**. The first letter that Satan spoke in Eden was "א" = "אלף" = "א+ל+ף" = 80+30+1 = **111**, and Satan's first recorded words in Genesis are "אף כי" = "א+ף+כ+י" = 10+20+80+1 = **111**.

[2.26] Holy Scripture was written by very specific formulas. Satan attempts to manipulate the words of God in order to confuse our comprehension of what God has spoken to us, as the battle between good and evil revolves around the Word of God. The words of God are extremely weighted. The letter "ש" signifies both "tooth" and "fire" as connected to the mouth by way of consumption. Fittingly, God asked in Jeremiah 23:29, "Is not My word like fire...?" Hebrews 12:29 says, "for indeed our God is a consuming fire." "Then the Lord spoke to you out of the fire. You heard the sound of words but saw no form; there was only a voice," (Deuteronomy 4:12). Acts 2:3-6 depicts the Pentecost where, "Divided tongues, as of fire, appeared among them, and a tongue rested on each of them. All of them were filled with the Holy Spirit and began to speak in other languages, as the Spirit gave them ability {4}." Now there were devout Jews from every nation under heaven living in Jerusalem. And at this sound the crowd gathered and was bewildered, because each one heard them speaking in the native language of each." The flying *Seraph* (*fiery serpent*) angel of Isaiah 6 put a burning coal on Isaiah's lips so that Isaiah could properly prophesy.

Though the pronunciations of these letter-names are not all now exactly as they were originally, a general sense can be perceived through both Old and New Testaments as they quietly utilize these names within their respective accounts. As the Scriptures often refer to human physicality in terms of pottery, clay, dust, *houses* (II Corinthians 5; Job 4:19) the ninth letter (ט) was probably alluded to by Jesus in Luke 11:24-26: "When the unclean spirit has gone out of a person, it wanders through waterless regions looking for a resting place, but not finding any, it says, 'I will return to my house from which I came.' When it comes, it finds it *swept* and put in order. Then it goes and brings *seven other spirits* more evil than itself, and they enter and live there; and the last state of that person is worse than the first." The eight total spirits within the one person sum to 9, and "ט" is also the number "9"; the signification of this ninth letter is "*sweeping*": "טיט" (ref. 2916) = "to be sticky, from ref. 2894, through the idea of dirt to be swept away; mud or clay; (figuratively) calamity:- clay, dirt, mire." In other words, the teachings of Christ were delivered according to the very letter and computation of the words of Scripture that were first received at Sinai. By discussing the number of "spirits" in connection with the ninth Hebrew letter (which is also the number 9) and the signification of that letter/number, we can understand the constitution of "a word as made up of letters" to the point that Christ was so specific in His correctness that He not only accounted for the explicit standards of the Torah, but He also accounted for the minute aspects of number and letter-significations in order to explain the intricacies of the Torah as He fulfilled all of those intricate standards accordingly.

[2.27] When considering the weight of even the alphabetic system by which the Torah was composed, let us examine a small portion of this alphabet's history. "The labors of the Massorites may be regarded as a later development and continuation of the early work which was carried on by the *Sopherim* (סופרים, γραμματεις) = the doctors and authorized interpreters of the Law soon after the return of the Jews from the Babylonish captivity (comp. Ezra VII 6; Neh. VIII 1&c.). And though it is now impossible to describe the chronological order the precise work which these custodians of Holy Writ undertook in the new Commonwealth, it may safely be stated that the gradual substitution of the square characters for the so-called Phoenician or archaic Hebrew alphabet was one of the first tasks," (*Introduction to the Massaretico-Critical Edition of the Hebrew Bible*, Ginsburg; p. 287).

In his informative and astute book, *Phoenicians* (Copyright 2000, The Trustees of the British Museum; University of California Press, Berkeley, Los Angeles), Glenn E. Markoe elaborated on the origin and development of the Phoenician alphabet:

"There is general agreement among scholars that the modern linear alphabet arose somewhere in the Levant during the second millennium BC. The precise date and point of origin, however, remain highly debated. Where in the Syro-Palestinian realm did the alphabet originate and how was it transmitted to the Phoenicians?
"The Modern story begins in the early twentieth century with the discovery of a series of pictographic inscriptions at Serabit el-Kadem, an Egyptian mining community

of the Middle and early New Kingdoms in the Sinai peninsula... The individual pictographs each marked a discrete sound, the phonetic value of which appears to have been determined by the initial value of the Semitic word represented, according to the acrophonic principle. (The picture of a house, for example, denoted the letter 'b' – from the Semitic word bayt for 'house'.) Proto-Sinaitic's pictographic character, combined with the use of the acrophonic principle, suggest that it may have been inspired by Egyptian writing recorded on hieroglyphic stelae at the site.

"While attempts at decipherment of the script have proved only partially successful, enough of the individual signs have been identified to support the conclusion that the proto-Semitic inscriptions represent a rudimentary form of alphabetic writing... Like their Sinaitic counterparts, these 'proto-Canaanite inscriptions were initially written both vertically and horizontally (the latter in either direction: right-to-left or left-to-right); through time the horizontal orientation prevailed. The characters were gradually simplified and abstracted, setting the stage for the emergence of the Phoenician linear alphabetic script at the close of the second millennium BC.

"Around the mid-fourteenth century or shortly before, the Canaanite linear alphabet was adapted to the prevailing cuneiform writing system of Ugarit in north Syria. Spelling-books of the period reveal that the order of its characters, originally totaling thirty in number, corresponded roughly with that of the Phoenician system. In the course of the succeeding centuries, the Canaanite linear alphabet underwent a process of simplification, leading ultimately to a reduced system of twenty-two characters or graphemes. The latter formed the direct antecedent of the Phoenician alphabet...

"At Byblos itself, a pseudo-hieroglyphic syllabic writing system of about one hundred and twenty signs was employed in the second millennium. Its exact chronology remains unclear... Despite several efforts, the Byblian pseudo-hieroglyphic script remains undeciphered...

"With its twenty-two consonants, the Phoenician alphabet is well documented on early Byblian monuments... Already by this time, the stance and form of its letters had become fixed. So, too, had the horizontal direction of its script, which read uniformly in sinistrograde fashion (i.e. from right to left). In the early Byblian texts, words within sentences were delineated by short vertical strokes; in later Phoenician and Punic texts, however, the words were presented in unbroken sequence, often dividing arbitrarily at the end of lines.

"As the inscriptional evidence reveals, the Phoenician alphabet spread quickly beyond the borders of the homeland. By the ninth century, it had been adopted by a variety of neighboring tongues, including Aramaic, Hebrew, Ammonite, Moabite, and Edomite. In each of these languages, the alphabet soon evolved along its own lines; a clear distinction from the Phoenician may be seen in the use of certain letters ('aleph, waw, yod) to denote vowel sounds. The Phoenician script itself... remained unvocalized.

"Phoenician commercial expansion abroad within the Mediterranean led to the export of the alphabet – at first to Cyprus and the Aegean (Crete)... As ancient classical tradition underscores, the Phoenicians were responsible for the introduction and adoption of the Greek alphabet, a fact confirmed by the names, shapes, values, and order of the letters attested to in early Greek scripts...

"The innovative use of vowels by the Greek initiator (using 'left-over' Phoenician signs such as '*aleph*, he, and 'ayin which had no consonantal equivalent in ancient Greek) lends support to this assumption," (*Phoenicians*, Markoe; p. 110-112).

Greek letters are numeric equivalents to Hebrew letters; this fact is shown by the construction of their respective alphabets, particularly with respect to Gematria, as it is more apparent why the New Testament had to be written in Greek. In the holy languages of the Scriptures, each letter is its own number:

Hebrew

Aleph (א) = 1	Yod (י) = 10	Koph (ק) = 100
Beth (ב) = 2	Kaph (כ) = 20	Resh (ר) = 200
Gimel (ג) = 3	Lamed (ל) = 30	Shin (שׁ) = 300
Daleth (ד) = 4	Mem (מ) = 40	Tau (ת) = 400
He (ה) = 5	Nun (נ) = 50	Kaph (ך) = 500 or 20
Vau (ו) = 6	Samech (ס) = 60	Mem (ם) = 600 or 40
Zayin (ז) = 7	Ayin (ע) = 70	Nun (ן) = 700 or 50
Cheth (ח) = 8	Pe (פ) = 80	Pe (ף) = 800 or 80
Teth (ט) = 9	Tsaddi (צ) = 90	Tsaddi (ץ) = 900 or 90

Greek

Alpha (α) = 1	Iota (ι) = 10	Rho (ρ) = 100
Beta (β) = 2	Kappa (κ) = 20	Sigma (σ) = 200 or 6
Gamma (γ) = 3	Lambda (λ) = 30	Tau (τ) = 300
Delta (δ) = 4	Mu (μ) = 40	Upsilon (υ) = 400
Epsilon (ε) = 5	Nu (ν) = 50	Phi (φ) = 500
Stigma (ς) = 6	Xi (ξ) = 60	Chi (χ) = 600
Zeta (ζ) = 7	Omicron (o) = 70	Psi (ψ) = 700
Eta (η) = 8	Pi (π) = 80	Omega (ω) = 800
Theta (θ) = 9	Koppa = 90	Sampsi (ϡ) = 900

"Βιβλος" is the first word of Matthew's Gospel; the first letter of the New Testament is "B" = 2, and the first letter of the Old Testament is "ב" = 2.

[2.28] "Aramaic was Hebrew, as it was developed during and after the Captivity in Babylon. There were two branches, known roughly as Eastern (which is Chaldee), and Western (Mesopotamian, or Palestinian). This latter was also known as Syriac; and the Greeks used "Syrian" as an abbreviation for Assyrian. This was perpetuated by the early Christians. Syriac flourished till the seventh century A.D. In the eighth and ninth it was overtaken by the Arabic; and by the thirteenth century it had disappeared... certain parts of the O.T. are written in Chaldee (or Eastern Aramaic): viz. Ezra 4:8-6. 18; 7:12-26; Dan. 2.4 – 7.28. Cp. Also 2 Kings 18.26." (*Companion Bible,* Bullinger; Appendix 94 III.3 – page 135).

Consider again that, "As the inscriptional evidence reveals, the Phoenician alphabet spread quickly beyond the borders of the homeland. By the ninth century, it had been adopted by a variety of neighboring tongues, including Aramaic, Hebrew, Ammonite, Moabite, and Edomite. In each of these languages, the alphabet soon evolved along its own lines; a clear distinction from the Phoenician may be seen in the use of certain letters ('aleph, waw, yod) to denote vowel sounds. The Phoenician script itself... remained unvocalized"; compare to, "The Hebrew language probably came into existence during the patriarchal period, about 2,000 B.C. The language was reduced to writing about 1,250 B.C." (*Vine's Expository Dictionary of Old and New Testament Words;* Forward – Introduction), for regarding the Sopherim, "...it may safely be stated that the gradual substitution of the square characters for the so-called Phoenician or archaic Hebrew alphabet was one of the first tasks," (*Introduction to the Massaretico-Critical Edition of the Hebrew Bible,* Ginsburg; p. 287) – however the chronology works out.

[2.29] *National Geographic* reported, "The Phoenicians were the Canaanites – and the ancestors of today's Lebanese," (October 2004; p. 48), a quotation of the American geneticist Spencer Wells, as this assessment agrees with the astronomer G. Schiaparelli who said, "Phoenicians... is equivalent to saying the Canaanites..." (*Astronomy of the Old Testament*, Schiparelli; p. 71). Dr. Lightfoot commented that, "It was the land of the Hebrews before it was the Canaanites... Abraham is called עברי Hebrew, then only when the difference between him and the Elamites was to be decided by war. And the reason of the surname is to be fetched from the thing itself which then was transacted... For my part, I scarcely believe, either that the Canaanites went thither before the confusion of tongues, or that Shem, at that time, was not there: but that he had long and fully inhabited the land of Canaan (as it was afterward called), before the entrance of the Canaanites into it: and that by the privilege of divine grant, which had destined him and his posterity hither: and that afterward the Canaanites crept in here; and were first subjects to the family of Shem, whose first-born was Elam, but a length shook of the yoke... The borders of the Canaanites, saith the Holy Scripture, 'were from Sidon to Gerar, even unto Gaza,' Gen. x. 19. You will say they were from Antioch, and utmost Phoenicia, and a great part of Syria. True, indeed, those countries, as we have seen, were planted by the sons of Canaan, but the Scripture doth not call them Canaanites; but where their coasts end towards the south, there the Canaanites begin." (*Commentary on the New Testament from the Talmud and Hebraica*, Lightfoot; Vol. 1, p. 276-281).

The Holy Bible refers to some of the Canaanite people as "Nephilim" (Numbers 13:33). The Nephilim story is often skimmed over because it sounds so mythic and so near the Greek legends of the demi-gods. The Greek legends of the demi-gods are but the offspring of a historical tradition of a forgotten origin which became little more than mythical fantasy. Sinfully, the sons of God erred by coupling with mortal women (against the design); conversely and by perfect justice, God impregnated Mary that the Son might be birthed into the world through her (within the design). Genesis 6 declares that the Nephilim were the offspring of the angels ("Sons of Elohim"). Offspring speak the language of their parents. It is known that the Hebrew and Greek alphabets are linked to the Phoenician alphabet. Hebrew and Greek letters are partially pictographic, and these letters illustrate concepts. The concepts represented by Biblical letters are preserved in the names of the letters themselves, similar to how the ancient maps drawn around the constellations help preserve the names of the stars they surround; by these facts, it can be reasonably deduced as to how Greek mythology and astrology are so closely related to the account of the Nephilim.

"Phoenician commercial expansion abroad within the Mediterranean led to the export of the alphabet – at first to Cyprus and the Aegean (Crete), by 900 BC... and a century later, to the western Mediterranean (Sardinia and southern Spain)... Its impact was most clearly felt in the Aegean realm. As ancient classical tradition underscores, the Phoenicians were responsible for the introduction and adoption of the Greek alphabet, a fact confirmed by the names, shapes, values, and order of the letters attested in early Greek scripts," (*Phoenicians*, Markoe; p. 112).

The title "Nephilim" is connected to several concepts:

"נפל" (ref. 5303) = "tyrant, giant" = "ל+פ+נ" = **160**
"נפל" (ref. 5307) = "to fall, divide, perish, rot, slay, smite, throw down" = "ל+פ+נ" = **160**
"נפל" (ref. 5308) = "to fall" = "ל+פ+נ" = **160**
"נפל" (ref.5309) = "something fallen, i.e. an abortion:- untimely birth" = "ל+פ+נ" = **160**

We must remember that the punishment for sin perfectly fits the crime of sin, and God's grace perfectly fits the punishment. Genesis 6:1-5 says, "And it came to pass, when men began to multiply on the face of the earth, and daughters were born unto them, that the sons of God saw the daughters of men that they were fair; and they took them wives of all which they chose. And the Lord said, 'My spirit shall not always strive with man, for that he also is flesh: yet his days shall be 120 years.' The Nephilim were in the earth in those days; and also after that, when the sons of God came in unto the daughters of men, and they bare children to them, the same became mighty men which were of old, men of renown. And God saw that the wickedness of man was great in the earth, and that every imagination of the thoughts of his heart was only evil continually." As a result, God flooded the earth.

We must understand the sense of one "untimely born" as it is not confined to an abortive birth only. The fact that the title "*Nephilim*" is also related to "נפל" (ref. 5309) = "something fallen, i.e. an *abortion:- untimely birth*" alludes to the fact that the reign of the Nephilim was to be short-lived and untimely which is a reason why God pronounced a judgment of water to wipe these Nephilim out *before their time* (in a manner of speaking) by a drowning death. Concerning Jewish practice, "Seven relatives of the deceased are required to mourn (father, mother, brother, sister, son, daughter, and spouse). The mourning period, called *aveilus*, begins with the sealing of the grave. Until that time, the mourners are in a state of *aninus*...there is no *aninus* for a *neifel* ["נפל" (ref. 5309) = "something fallen, i.e. an *abortion:- untimely birth*"], i.e. a nonviable infant, and an infant that died within thirty days of its birth is considered a neifel," (*Baal Ha Turim*, Gold,; p. 978). "The first-born was to be redeemed immediately after the thirtieth day from his birth [Numbers 18:16]," (*Commentary on the New Testament from the Talmud and Hebraica*, Lightfoot, Volume 3; p. 38).

The Nephilim were a short-lived race (relatively speaking), and they were considered in the same fashion as nonviable offspring were considered; by such a title, the name "Nephilim" is connected to infant death in the sense that they were doomed to a short reign like a child bound to a brief life extinguished by infant death. The immediacy of judgment that secured the Nephilm's demise pronounced by God in Genesis 6 likened them to a "נפל" (ref. 5309) or a *doomed infancy* as the concept attached to their title specifically indicates. Merely rendering the title "Nephilim" to only indicate "giants" disallows the reader from understanding why the judgment pronounced against them is mentioned in Genesis 6:3 **before** their birth in Genesis 6:4; in other words, the expression of "one untimely born" is taken in a similar sense to an "abortion" in that both "untimely birth" and "abortion" describe a human who is not given the opportunity to live out a full life-span – as the Apostle Paul, the mighty warrior of Christ, referred to himself as such in connection with the prophesy of his own demise from in Acts 21.

The Greek equivalent to this word "נֵפֶל" (ref. 5309)= "abortion; untimely birth" is "εκτρωμα" (ref. *1626*) = "to wound; a miscarriage, abortion, untimely birth," and Paul used this word to describe himself in I Corinthians 15:3-9 where it is written, "For I handed on to you as of the first importance what I in turn had received: that Christ died for our sins in accordance with the Scriptures, and that He was buried, and that He was raised on the third day in accordance with the scriptures... Last of all, as to one *untimely born*, He appeared also to me. For I am least of the apostles..." Paul compared himself to an "untimely born" or "non-viable" infant, because he knew he was destined to die without reaching a ripe old age, as we read of his destiny prophesied in Acts 21:2-14: "When we found a ship bound for *Phoenicia*, we went on board and set sail. We came in sight of Cyprus; and leaving it on our left, we sailed to Syria and landed at Tyre, because the ship was to unload its cargo there. We looked up the disciples and stayed there for *seven* days. Through the Spirit they told Paul not to go to Jerusalem. When our days there were ended, we left and proceeded on our journey; and all of them, with wives and children, escorted us outside the city. There we knelt down on the beach and prayed and said farewell to one another. Then we went on board the ship, and they returned home. When we had finished the voyage from Tyre, we arrived at Ptolemais; and we greeted the believers and stayed with them for one day. The next day we left and came to Caesarea; and we went into the house of *Philip* [*Warrior*] the evangelist, one of the *seven*, and stayed with him. He had four unmarried daughters who had the gift of prophecy. While we were staying there for several days, a prophet named Agabus came down from Judea. He came to us and took Paul's belt, bound his own feet and hands with it, and said, "Thus says the Holy Spirit, 'This is the way the Jews in Jerusalem will bind the man who owns this belt and will hand him over to the Gentiles.'" When we heard this, we and the people there urged him not to go up to Jerusalem. Then Paul answered, '**What are you doing, weeping and breaking my heart**? For I am ready not only to be bound but even to die in Jerusalem for the name of the Lord Jesus.' Since he would not be persuaded, we remained silent except to say, 'The Lord's will be done"; again, "*Seven* relatives of the deceased are required to mourn (father, mother, brother, sister, son, daughter, and spouse). The mourning period, called *aveilus*, begins with the sealing of the grave. Until that time, the mourners are in a state of *aninus*... **there is no aninus for a neifel**...," (*Baal Ha Turim*, Gold,; p. 978).

"See what love the Father has given us, that we should be called sons of God; and that is what we are. The reason the world does not know us is that it did not know Him," (I John 3:1). Paul, the mighty warrior for God, "a son of God," followed Christ even to an untimely demise, and he referred to himself in the sense of a *"neifel,"* in accordance with Agabus' prophesy. Conversely, "The *Nephilim* were in the earth in those days; and also after that, when the sons of God came in unto the daughters of men, and they bare children to them, the same became mighty men which were of old, men of renown," (Genesis 6:4). The tremendous irony of *Agabus [A Grasshopper]* is that when the Israelites went up to take the promised land of Canaan, they "...saw the Nephilim (the Anakites come from the Nephilim); and to ourselves we seemed like *grasshoppers*..." (Numbers 13:33). The Scriptures tell the same story over and over cyclically throughout history (as is true of the arrangement of the solar system), though the background takes on various forms of united meaning as time progresses (similar to the proper motion of the constellation patterns). "What has been is what will be, and what has been done is what will be done; there is nothing new *under the sun*," (Ecclesiastes 1:9), but in the end, "...there will be no more night; they need no lamp or *sun*, for the Lord God will be their light..." (Revelation 22:5).

[2.30] *"naw-khash"* = "נחש" (ref. 5172) = "to hiss, whisper a (magic) spell, to prognosticate, enchanter, diligently observe, learn by experience" = "ש+ח+נ" = 300+8+50 = **358**

"nakh-ash" = "נחש" (ref. 5173) = "an incantation, augury, enchantment" = "ש+ח+נ" = 300+8+50 = **358**

"*naw-khawsh*" (from ref. 5172) ="נחש" (ref. 5175) = "a serpent" = "ש+ח+נ" = 300+8+50 = **358**

"*nekh-awsh*" = "נחש" (ref. 5174) Chaldee = "copper; brass" = "ש+ח+נ" = 300+8+50 = **358**

When we consider that ancient Eastern mirrors were made of polished copper (or brass, or bronze), especially in light of the copper mirrors of the women of Exodus 38:8, we may also notice that the concepts of *defending* and *accusing* are 180-degree opposites of each other. It is ironic that *Hymenaeus* [*Nuptial*] and *Alexander* [*Defender*] the coppersmith were "turned over to *Satan* [*Adversary; Accuser* (ref. 4567)], so that they may learn not to blaspheme," (I Timothy 1:20), for Paul also said that "Alexander the coppersmith did me great harm; the Lord will pay him back for his deeds. You also must be aware of him, for he strongly opposed our message," (II Timothy 4:14-15). When Eve stated that "The serpent *deceived* me" in Genesis 3:13, we read of the first instance in Scripture that relates sin to a lack of chastity [Rubric 1.13]. As Adam's firstborn son was a neifel because both he and Eve made an illegitimate decision to follow Satan, so the Nephilim were the doomed products of an illegitimate union between the angels (who fell) and mortal women that mimicked the agreement between Satan and "the woman" who was later named "Eve."

The Nephilim were great war heroes, and King David was also a great war hero; this fact points us to a reason why King David did not lament his son's death (his firstborn with Bathsheba) as there is no mourning period for a neifel: "But now he is dead; why should I fast? Can I bring him back again? I shall go to him, but he will not return to me," (II Samuel 12:23). "I say, a *miscarriage* ["נפל" (ref. 5309) = **160**] is better than he. For he comes in with vanity, and goes out in darkness; his name shall be covered in darkness," (Ecclesiastes 6:3-4). King David devised and exacted an illegitimate union with Bathsheba, and like the fallen angels ("the sons of God" in Genesis 6), he begat a nonviable child – though the saddest facet of King David's neifel was that his neifel committed no error (like Adam's neifel), whereas the Nephilim (the Neifels) received what they deserved for their child sacrifice practices: "The Phoenicians were both lauded and despised in antiquity. They were celebrated – as learned scribes, who passed on the modern alphabet... [but they also] were despised as cheaters and hucksters, who could not be trusted; as insatiable mongers and *unscrupulous profiteers*, who kidnapped the helpless and traded in human lives; a licentious and morally corrupt race of people, who prostituted their daughters *and butchered their infant children* in honor of their gods," (*Phoenicians*, Markoe; p. 10). "Canaan" means "*Merchant.*"

[2.31] Let us consider the Creator:

Elohim said, "Let **Us** *make* man in **Our** image, according to **Our** likeness," (Genesis 1:26). Elohim "*created*" humanity (Genesis 1:27); Jehovah Elohim "*formed*" Adam (Genesis 2:7). Elohim "*created*" humanity (Genesis 5:1); Jehovah "*made*" man (Genesis 6:6), and Jehovah "*created*" man

(Genesis 6:7). Jehovah "*laid the foundations of the earth,*" (Job 38:4); Christ is the "*head of the corner*" (Matthew 21:42), for "The Stone which the builders rejected, the same is become the head of the corner: this is from Jehovah, it is marvelous in our eyes," (Psalm 118:22-23). Though "Elohim" is plural, God is One: "...**I judge no man. And yet if I judge**, My judgment is true: for **I am not alone**, but **I and the Father** That sent Me," (John 8:15-16). Elohim is the Creator, and Jehovah is the same God Who is usually viewed in covenant relation to His creation (compare to Genesis 6:18...). Compare the work of Elohim in Job 28:23-26 in relation to the work of Jehovah in Job 38:9-10). Jesus said, "I and my Father are One," (John 10:30), thus Jehovah Elohim formed man (Genesis 2:7).

As John 1 tells us, Jesus is the Creator called "Elohim." "The sons of Elohim saw the daughters of men, that they were fair. And they took wives for themselves from all those whom they chose. And Jehovah said, ''My spirit shall not always strive with man, for that he also is flesh: yet his days shall be 120 years,'" (Genesis 6:2-3). The sons of the Son (Elohim) made an illegitimate blunder (Mark 12:25; II Peter 2:4; Jude 1:6), and the Father (Jehovah) disapproved of the Sons of Elohim (Jehovah's grandsons) and therefore prophesied the Nephilim-Phoenician-Canaanite's doom. Concerning the first humans, "Elohim blessed them, and Elohim said to them, 'Be fruitful and multiply and fill the earth..." (Genesis 1:28) – and when Adam and his wife sinned, "they knew that they were naked..." (Genesis 3:7). Concerning the repopulation of the earth after the flood of Noah's day, "Elohim blessed Noah and his sons, and said to them, 'Be fruitful and multiply, and fill the earth,"

(Genesis 9:1). "And Noah began to be a husbandman, and he planted a vineyard: and he drank of the wine, and was drunken; and he was uncovered within his tent. And Ham, the father of *Canaan* [*Merchant*], saw the nakedness of his father... And Noah awoke from his wine, and knew what his younger son had done unto him. And he said, 'Cursed be Canaan!" (Genesis 9:20-25). "Noah lived after the flood **350** years," (Genesis 9:28), just as in Genesis 3:6, "...the tree was to be desired *to make one wise* [from "שכל" = "ל+כ+ש" = 30+20+300 = **350**]..." The ancient Jews had an expression: "O you vinegar, the son of good wine!" which meant "O you wicked son of a good father!" (*Commentary on the New Testament from the Talmud and Hebraica*, Lightfoot, Vol. 3; p. 425).

In Eden, as a result of the woman's confusion of the Names of God, she also confused His commands; the only "fruit" God bound to commands given to humanity in Scripture until the Fall of man was the human "fruit" that humanity was commanded to produce in Genesis 1:28 and the fruit of which they were allowed to eat (Genesis 1:29). Satan wanted the human fruit consumed "...as one dead, who proceeded from the womb of OUR mother, and half of OUR flesh be consumed," (Numbers 12:12) through the human consumption of the forbidden tree (as Satan did not mention "fruit"). Hence, the woman began her reply to Satan by stating what "Elohim" had said concerning "the tree" negatively when in fact Elohim alone gave no command concerning humans in relation to "trees" concerning what they *could not* eat, only that they themselves were to be fruitful and multiply and that they *could* eat of every seed-bearing tree. It was Jehovah Elohim Who gave the command about the "tree" that *could not* be eaten of without sin (Genesis 2:17), and unlike Elohim alone, Jehovah Elohim made no mention of "fruit" at all concerning what was forbidden. The Creator (*Elohim*), Who gave the command (Genesis 1:28) concerning "fruit," also gave His life for the sinning humans by dying on a "ξυλον" (ref. *3586*) = "tree" as the "True Vine" (John 15:1) because they transgressed the law of *Jehovah Elohim* concerning the forbidden "tree" (Genesis 2:17) which was a vine-tree coiled around the Tree of Life. Christ mirrored the events in Eden by being the "Firstborn of the Dead" (Colossians 1:18; Revelation 1:5) and the "True Vine" (John 15:1) on the wicked "ξυλον" (ref. *3586*) = "tree" which is the reflected opposite of the False Vine on the Tree of Life. It is humanity that does not mourn those deaths whose infant names become covered in darkness. However, God was so angry over the first abortion – the very first sin – that the entire earth was punished! The traditions of the elders covered the first sin in the Scriptures, and as a result, we can understand the traditions of today.

[2.32] "It is worthy of observing, that the Holy Bible, reckoning up... the seven nations, which were to be destroyed by the Israelites, names the Perizzites, who were not at all recited among the sons of Canaan, Gen. x., and the Canaanites as a particular nation, when all the seven, indeed, were Canaanites. See Deut. vii. 1, Josh. ix. 1, xi. 3, Judg. iii. 5, &c. The reason of the latter... is to be fetched thence, that Canaan himself inhabited a peculiar part of that (northern) country, with his first-born sons,

Sidon and Heth and thence the name of Canaanites was put upon that particular progeny, distinguished from all his other sons and that country was peculiarly called by the name of 'Canaan,' distinctly from all the rest of the land of Canaan. Hence Jabin, the king of Hazor, is called the 'king of Canaan,' Judg. iv. 2, and the kings of Tyre and Sidon, if I mistake not, are called, 'the kings of the Hittites,' (Kings x. 29)," (*Commentary on the New Testament from the Talmud and Hebraica,* Lightfoot; Vol. 2, p. 229-230). The descendants of Canaan were linked to the Nephilim. Noah's grandson Canaan who somehow deceived Noah into shameful nudity through wine little different than in the case of the "serpent" of Genesis 3 in regards to Adam. The seed of Satan came again through Canaan's line after the flood of Noah's time as it is written, "The Nephilim were in the earth in those days; and also after that..." (Genesis 6:4).

[2.33] Mythology recalls the Nephilim as "demigods" whom the Greeks claimed were the offspring of divine-mortal unions. The fathers of the Nephilim were the fallen angels described in Revelation 12:4 as "stars" which is one reason why the gods of Greek Mythology are often linked to celestial lights. The Nephilim, called "warriors of renown" (Genesis 6:4), were the offspring of the sinning angels' rebellion discussed in II Peter 2:4 and Jude 1:6. We can hardly believe that stars came down and had human relations, but we can certainly understand why angels are likened to the brilliance of stars, lightning, etc. as they are described as having "clothes that gleamed like lightning," (Luke 24:4) and their appearance was usually awe-inspiring. The sinning angels left Heaven rebelliously to copulate with mortal women in order to produce children of their own, and these children, by their very name which also alludes to "abortion," are likened to untimely births; they were as doomed children born partially from above, but children who completely drenched themselves in sin and were products of sin. However, they were more powerful than humans (obviously), and the flood of Noah's time was sent to destroy them, not just people in general. [2.34] The Scribes were like a combination of editors and princes. We can see the type of influence they wielded by their Greek name "γραμματευς" (ref. *1122*) = "C.E.O. of a governmental entity, an expert in matters of divine revelation," translated "Scribe" meaning "specialists in the Law of Moses: experts in the law, scholars versed in the law, scribes; mentioned together with the high priests whom with the elders... formed the Sanhedrin," (*Greek-English Lexicon*, Danker; p. 206). However, as far as being experts in "divine revelation," sometimes what appeared to be divine revelation was not so in reality when we recall some of the hypocritical members of the Sanhedrin during the earthly days of Christ. Let us consider the rule called "born before noon or born after noon," found in the *Talmud: Rosh Hashanah* 20b.

"The precise moment of 'conjunction,' at which the moon completes its revolution of the earth to begin a new revolution, and changes from an 'old' moon to a 'new' moon is called... *birth of the moon*, or מולד, *molad*..." (*Talmud: Rosh Hashanah*, Scottenstein Edition; General Introduction). Regarding the *molad*, it is "...at precisely that instant that the moon begins its movement to its next phase, when it starts to be 'reborn,' or visible again. A number of hours later, as it gradually moves out of alignment with the earth, the moon reaches a point where *some* sunlight is reflected toward the earth. Then, a small part of the moon becomes visible as a very thin crescent, which is known as the *first phase* of the moon... In Rabbinic terminology, this first phase is called... *renewal of the moon* or... *chodesh.* The word *chodesh* means not only 'month' but 'renewal,' in the sense that the moon is 'renewed' after having disappeared," (*Talmud: Rosh Hashanah*, Scottenstein Edition; General Introduction).

The renewal of the moon and its accompanying celebration, Rosh Chodesh, was declared by the Sanhedrin based on the (apparent) testimony of credible witnesses who affirmed that they had seen the first crescent of the new moon; however, most of the commoners and subordinates who were witnesses of the new moon were also unaware that the Sanhedrin (who were "Masters of Sorcery") did not need testimonials to determine when to declare the holiday of Rosh Chodesh as they already knew the astronomical calculations necessary to determine a new moon and therefore its accompanying celebration, and by such calculations they could declare Rosh Chodesh on the nearest whole day without error. Astronomical calculations also served to declare Rosh Chodesh when the moon could not be seen due to cloud-cover, as the festival was (apparently) determined by the sight of the renewed moon and not by the moment of its conjunction. The first crescent of the moon (the "renewal") occurs slightly after the conjunction when the moon was said to be "born," and the Sanhedrin let the people assume that they had more of a part in determining the holiday of Rosh

Chodesh than they actually did, for the Sanhedrin held the "secrets" of astronomy. "The calendrical secrets referred to here are no more than astronomical computations concerning the cycles of the sun and moon which are the basis of the calendrical units of a year and of a month. There is nothing esoteric about these calculations, but they are known as 'secrets' because the sages did not publicize them, but taught them only to a select few... *Yesod Olam* (a work on astronomical matters authored by a disciple of Rosh) maintains that the sages purposely suppressed calendrical knowledge and kept it secret from the masses in order to avoid disparagement of [the court] due to their decisions regarding the calendar. [The court] did not strictly follow the calculated results. For example, intercalating an extra month in the year was practiced for an assortment of reasons (see Sanhedrin 11a-12a...)... Thus, persons knowledgeable of the calculations but ignorant of [the court's] methods might criticize and disparage [the court's] decisions. To avoid such undermining of [the court], calendrical knowledge was suppressed and thus the masses accepted [the court's] decisions without question," (*Talmud: Rosh Hashanah*; Schottenstein Edition; Notation on 20b). Christ called the Scribes and Pharisees "hypocrites" numerous times, and He also called them "snakes" (Matthew 23). A violation of the celebration of the new moon was a violation of the very first law of the Torah that was addressed to the Jews as a nation (Exodus 12:2).

According to Jewish terminology, a 29-day month was considered "deficient" and a 30-day month was considered "full" or "*pregnant*," (*Talmud: Rosh Hashanah*,

Scottenstein Edition; General Introduction). It may be that the total solar eclipse of November 24, 29 A.D. over Israel indicates the year of Christ's death; yet keep in mind that Passover is not in November, and Passover does not occur at new moon as solar eclipses do. The significance of this particular eclipse, if counting backward from it, may indicate a reason that Jesus cursed the fig tree.

[2.35] The constellations (indicating astronomical dating, not astrological nonsense) were of much importance to the ancient Jews as the morning stars (stars that rose above the horizon just prior to being extinguished by the sun) indicated the Jewish agricultural periods and seasonal boundaries (Genesis 3:14). Remember that "... the riches of the earth are for all; the king, himself, is served by cultivating his own field," (Ecclesiastes 5:9), for "...their principle employments were agriculture and the care of *cattle*; they were a nation of husbandmen and shepherds. The lands had been originally parceled out to the different families; the portions of which (by the laws of the country) could not be alienated by sale, and therefore descended to their posterity without diminution. The fruits of the earth, the produce of his land and labor, constituted the *wealth* of each individual," (*Lectures on the Sacred Poetry of the Hebrews*, Lowth; p. 32). "Now the serpent was subtle above any *beast of the field* that the Lord God had made," (Genesis 3:1); when Satan was cursed for his part in the great Fall of humanity, Jehovah Elohim declared "...thou art cursed above all *cattle, and above every beast of the field*; upon thy belly shalt thou go, and dust shalt thou eat all the days of thy life," (Genesis 3:14). It is highly probable that when the constellations were first mapped out, the vernal equinox was in the constellation of Taurus the Bull and the Polar Star was Thuban inside of Leviathan (ref. 3882) = "the constellation of the dragon; mourning" that we call "Draco" (as the various serpentine constellations discuss the same being); however, considering that these celestial maps were probably first devised when the vernal equinox was in Taurus says nothing as to where the pattern actually begins. Knowing that the vernal equinox was in the constellation of Taurus the Bull at such a time under our *thematic* discussion, we can understand that the equinoxes and soltices were within the constellations paralleled by the faces of the creatures described Ezekiel 1:10, Revelation 4:6-7, in connection with the Cherubs of Genesis 3:24. However, the autumnal equinox is paralleled by the constellation Aquilla the Eagle in Ezekiel 1:10 and Revelation 4:6-7 even though the actual autumnal equinox oriented to the Age of Taurus was near the foot of the Ophiuchus the Serpent Holder who crushes Scorpio's head (despite astrology's false connections). By describing the autumnal equinox through the constellation of Aquila the Eagle (which that equinox was not in; Aquilla is not Zodiacal), we can observe the conceptual melding of wings, a man, and a serpent – like the angelic Seraphs of Isaiah 6 (see Rubric i.4), i.e. dragons.

Genesis 3:1, is oriented (thematically) to the astronomical period or "Age" of Taurus (when the vernal equinox was in the constellation of Taurus, the bull) – as this fact is explicit when regarding the serpentine constellations that describe Satan or "Leviathan" (for Cetus is not the only constellation that describes the Leviathan). When the earth was in the Age of Taurus, "The lower part of the autumnal colure was marked by the Scorpion, and the foot of the Serpent-holder pressed down the creature's head, just where the colure, the equator, and the ecliptic intersected... **the equator [1], the colure [2], the zenith [3] and the poles [4]** were all marked out by these **serpentine or draconic forms**..." (*Astronomy of the Bible*, Maunder, p. 159-160); "Then I saw an angel coming down from heaven, holding in his hand the key to the bottomless pit and a great chain. He seized **the dragon [1], that ancient serpent [2], who is the Devil [3] and Satan [4]** and bound him for a thousand years, and threw him into the pit, and locked and sealed it over him, so that he would deceive the nations no more, until the thousand years were ended. After that he must be let out for a little while," (Revelation 20:1-3). Simply put, when the beginning of the Spring season aligned with the center of the constellation of the *Bull*, the *serpent*-figure was the most prominently pronounced figure in the night sky; when Satan (the "*serpent*") was cursed, Jehovah Elohim said, "... thou art cursed above all *cattle*..." (Genesis 3:14).

The celestial beings are not stars, but physical nature illustrates spiritual reality, as it is written, "But someone will ask, 'How are the dead raised? With what kind of body do they come?' Fool! What you sow does not come to life unless it dies. And as for what you sow, you do not sow the body that is to be, but a bare seed, perhaps of wheat or of some other grain. But God gives it a body as He has chosen, and to each kind of seed its own body. Not all flesh is alike, but there is one flesh for human beings, another for animals, another for birds, and another for fish. There are both heavenly bodies and earthly bodies, but the glory of the heavenly is one thing, and that of the earthly is another. There is one glory of the sun, and another glory of the moon, and another glory of the stars; indeed, star differs from star in glory. So it is with the resurrection of the dead. What is sown is perishable, what is raised is imperishable. It is sown in dishonor, it is raised in glory. It is sown in weakness, it is raised in power. It is sown a physical body, it is raised a spiritual body. If there is a physical body, there is also a spiritual body. Thus it is written, 'The first man, Adam, became a living being'; the last Adam became a life-giving spirit," (I Corinthians 15:35-45). Paul used agriculture along with the stars to illustrate the resurrection in accordance with the fact that agricultural periods were indicated by the stars (thus the turning seasons: Genesis 3:14), though it was the lunar cycle (the synodic month, not the sidereal month) that ordered the Jewish festivals.

[2.36] The patterns of time (sun, moon, stars, etc.) are cyclic. The sun, moon, and stars were made "for signs and for seasons and for days and years" (four attributes for Day Fourth in Genesis 1:14). Earth's North Celestial Pole traces a full circle in the night sky once fully in about 25,800 years in a process called "Precession of the Equinoxes": "...Earth's axis wobbles and the equinoxes precess largely because of the gravitational influence of the Moon. Earth's relatively rapid 24-hour spin causes the Earth to bulge at its equator. Earth's equatorial diameter is 21 kilometers (13 miles) greater than its polar diameter. The Moon – and to a lesser extent the Sun and to a far lesser extent the planets – pull on this slight bulge. The bulge is oriented along Earth's equator, but the Moon and

Sun pull from a different direction – from the ecliptic. The effect is to try to pull Earth into a more upright orientation. But Earth is spinning like a gyroscope, and it resists being pulled over. Instead, it precesses, or wobbles; the amount of tilt (in this case, 23 1/2°) remains constant while the direction of the tilt changes. Earth's axis traces a huge circle in the sky with a radius of 23 1/2° in a time span of 25,800 years... The celestial equator, which is always 90° from the poles, wobbles at the same time and at the same rate as the poles," (*Starry Night Companion*, Mosley; p. 77).

We must continually distinguish between the dating of astronomy and absurdity of astrology. "Precession has an interesting effect on astrology, and especially on *birth signs* or *astrological signs*. The signs – such as 'Scorpio' – are each a uniform section of the sky 30° wide [in astrological conceptual thought, but not in reality]... When this system was first set up around 600 BC [long after the Torah was written down], the zero point was in Aries and was called the 'first point of Aries.' The constellation Aries encompassed the first 30° of the ecliptic [the apparent path of the sun across the sky]; from 30° to 60° was Taurus... This ignored actual stars, but uniformity was more important than fussing about star positions... Your birth sign in your morning newspaper horoscope ignores precession. What your horoscope calls 'Aries' is the 30° segment along the ecliptic that is east of the current location of the vernal equinox – but most of it is in Pisces!" (*Starry Night Companion*, Mosley; p. 80). We can see that astrology is a geometrically uniform system of falsehood that ignores the facts. Many people eagerly anticipate the

Age of Aquarius without realizing that this astronomical age does not begin for nearly another six centuries.

The boundary-lines of the current celestial maps are agreed-upon approximations that provide a standard reckoning of where one constellation ends and another begins. However, since the people of Jesus' earthly days viewed the heavens with the naked eye, those people's specific constellation boundaries (which were not universal) were drawn within the spaces that separate the stars of one constellation and the stars of another – spaces that were larger (apparently speaking) than ours today. In other words, the precise end of one constellation was a larger approximation to the ancients. With respect to Precession of the Equinoxes, the fixed boundaries we have now were not fixed precisely as such during the earthly days of Christ (from man's perspective). We can therefore see that Christ came to earth near the transition from the astronomical Age of *Aries* [*the Ram/Lamb*] to the astronomical Age of *Pisces* [*the Fish*]; the age of animal sacrifice had ended, and the age of the Christian Church began (compare to Matthew 27:20 and Acts 2:2-3). The Christian *Fish* [*Icthus*] originated from the divinely directed recognition of astronomical knowledge as a mark of distinction for the Church, for the Sanhedrin (who were largely astrologers, not astronomers) endeavored their utmost to suppress astronomical knowledge in order that they themselves would be the sole masters of it (or something like it) among the masses. However, Precession is a much more difficult pattern to observe and calculate than the cycles of months, and the Church's knowledge was unstoppably superior to those who headed the Sanhederin – despite the fact that many of the Church leaders were commoners: "Consider your own call, brothers and sisters: not many of you were wise by human standards, not many were powerful, not many were of noble birth. But God chose what is foolish in the world to shame the wise; God chose what is weak in the world to shame the strong; God chose what is low and despised in the world, things that are not, to reduce to nothing things that are, so that no one might boast in the presence of God. He is the source of your life in Christ Jesus, Who became for us wisdom from God, and righteousness and **sanctification** and redemption, in order that, as it is written, 'Let the one who boasts, boast in the Lord,'" (I Corinthians 1:26-31). The Sanhedrin suppressed the knowledge of astronomy (a knowledge that marked the Wise men who sought the Christ Child) so that they could declare festivals for their own reasons without being challenged. "'This month shall be for you the first of the months,' (Exodus 12:2). This verse contains the positive commandment... incumbent upon [the court] to perform the mitzvah of... *sanctifying the renewal*, by **sanctifying** and declaring which day is to be Rosh Chodesh, based on certain criteria..." (*Talmud: Rosh Hashanah*, Scottenstein Edition; General Introduction). The knowledge of the moon cycles that the Sanhedrin suppressed involved calculating the synodic month of about 29 days; the knowledge of Precession that the Church displayed as its insignia involved calculating the cycle of about 25,800 years. The Sanhedrin jealously despised the commoners who were educated by Jesus above the teachings of the Pharisees: "But this crowd, which does not know the law – they are accursed," (John 7:49). The followers of Christ are not to remain in the darkness of ignorance, particularly under the ignorance that the Sanhedrin devised to enshroud them – which is explicitly why I Corinthians 1:26-31 allows us to understand that even though many were formerly of low esteem and were deemed inferior, God can take such people and make them sages above those "sages" who looked down on them before. God causes His followers to prosper, so long as they are willing to let their prosperity to be defined by Him: "But He gives all the more grace; therefore it says, 'God opposes the proud, but gives grace to the humble,' [Proverbs 3:34]. Submit yourselves therefore to God. Resist the devil, and he will flee from you. Draw near to God, and He will draw near to you..." (James 4:6-8).

The constellations are used to mark time (Genesis 1:14), and as "clocks" as we know them were not in the hands of the ancients, the giant sky-clock (Zodiac) served to indicate time as its 12 markers are represented uniformly on our analog clocks today. In essence, the maps drawn around the 12 constellations of the Zodiac were viewed in a somewhat similar fashion to the way we look at clock and say "It is seven o'clock." Pisces is the true Seventh Sign although it is not commonly reckoned as such today. The 12 classical constellations of the Zodiac are not uniformly separated into 12 equal portions of 30 degrees along the ecliptic. Today, 13 constellations are officially counted as Zodiacal because constellation boundaries were often left to the discretion (or lack thereof) of celestial map-makers so that "...each astronomer (and astrologer) was free to place the boundary lines where he saw fit. This caused endless confusion until 1930, when the constellation boundaries were fixed – among astronomers at least – by international agreement... One effect of this tidying-up was to draw the huge and ancient constellation Ophiuchus so that it intersected the ecliptic," (*Starry Night Companion,* Mosley; p. 26).

[2.37] The "scroll" of the heavens, commonly referred to as the "Zodiac" (that the Bible calls the "Mazzaroth": Job 38:32) serves as the partial origin of the various tales of mythology, as one cannot help but notice a striking similarity between many mythological fancies and factual Scripture. In the Scriptures, the prophets or main personalities of stories (Job, for instance) are, strangely and beautifully, able to see the constellations through torrid storms (Job 41; Ezekiel 1; Revelation 4), hence the supernatural aspects of the matter; linguistically, this can be seen in the word "מזלה" (ref. 4208) = "from ref. 5140 (נזל) in the sense of *raining,* a *constellation,* i.e. Zodiacal sign (*as affecting weather*)." As the year is sifted through the Zodiac, the constellations mark out seasons (Genesis 1:14). Job, Ezekiel and John (to name a few) were allowed to see the spiritual significance behind the ancient star groupings as they viewed the constellations through the clouds of storms. The manner in which the prophets and others of the Bible saw these constellations turn in the sky was faster than they actually turn physically in front of our eyes, for this swift turning is a gorgeous description of time that is sped up. Yet, though time was sped up (or turned back swiftly) in the sight of the prophets and other Biblical people, the constellations that they beheld were often displayed to them in a manner that depicted an orientation according to a time before them – in the

Age of Taurus, and the Age of Taurus is cyclic like all of the other Ages of Precession. It is uncertain as to which Age of Taurus the constellations were first mapped in (if, in fact, they were originally mapped in an Age of Taurus), as it is impossible to believe that Adam was caused to comprehend the constellations according to the most recent Biblical alignment of the Age of Taurus which was in about 2,700 B.C. (as the Age of Taurus began near 4,500 B.C. and ended near 2,000 B.C., according to today's official constellation boundaries). It is quite likely that the constellations were first marked out in an Age of Taurus. However, if, in fact, the constellations were not first marked out in an Age of Taurus, it is reasonable to ponder the possibility that the constellations were first marked out so that the Age of Taurus would be defined by serpentine depictions, keeping in mind that the star pictures were drawn to preserve the names of the stars (as the preceding star names serve as a control for the star pictures, not ignoring the slight variances and inventions between cultures; for instance, the Little Bear and the Lesser Winnowing Fan are two different indifications of the same constellation, not two different names for two different constellations). It may be that the age of Taurus is so often reflected upon by the Scriptures – with reference to the fall in Eden – because the serpent is the most prominent symbol of this time-period, besides the bull.

By knowing the pattern of the Zodiac, one can describe a former or future orientation of time with precision and yet not live during the time of such an orientation. One could describe the facets of a particular Age of

Precession without living to witness it personally, and because of this fact, it is easier to grasp why Genesis 3:1 is specifically aligned with an Age of Taurus and why Genesis 3:15 is aligned with an Age of Virgo, for these two respective Ages are separated by thousands of years. Thus, the specific alignement of time near 2,700 B.C. during the Age of Taurus could have possibly been planned prior to the beginning of that Age (though this is unlikely). Considering the striking consistency of the Age of Taurus in the Scriptures along with the orientation of various constellations located at critical points on the conceptual celestial sphere, it is more than likely that the constellations were first marked out in an Age of Taurus. Since human sin ushered death into human existence whereby time became of dire importance to humanity, it would make much sense for the constellations to have been first mapped out according to the names God gave them during (or aligned with) the Age of Taurus as this Age displays serpent imagery as its most consistent theme with particular respect to Autumn (the season of death).

The themes of Scripture are aligned with the Precession of the Equinoxes. Regarding Precession, the importance of the Christian Fish symbol cannot be ignored – for the Age of Pisces began near the time of the Christian Church's historical origin when the Age of Aries the Ram/*Lamb* had recently passed away (relatively speaking), just as Christ was the *final* sacrifice, our Passover (I Corinthians 5:7), the "*Lamb* that was slaughtered" (Revelation 5:12). Near the time (relatively speaking) of the origin of the Christian Church, the Age of Aries had ended and had given way to the Age of Pisces: simply put, the vernal equinox left the constellation of the Lamb and entered into the constellation of the Fishes; thus, the era of animal sacrifice ended, and the Christian Church began (with Jews and by Jews), for Pisces was "...considered the national constellation of the Jews..." (*Star Names*, Allen; p. 341); "The Hebrew idiom for 'grow' is Let them increase *as fishes do increase*..." (*Great Cloud of Witnesses*, Bullinger; p. 205) – "All authority *in heaven* and on earth has been given to Me. Go therefore and *make disciples of all nations, baptizing* them in the name of the Father and of the Son and of the Holy Spirit," (Matthew 28:18-19) – thus the importance of a water-animal signification in the heavens and on the earth to define Christians, as Christians battle against the powers of the Leviathan who is also signified as a water-animal.

Confusion regarding the relation of Biblical chronology with respect to the Precession of the Equinoxes has occurred in part because many Jewish and Christian Bible Scholars assumed the 12 classical constellations of the Zodiac to be set uniformly along the ecliptic, when the constellations of the Zodiac each have their own respective times and are not set uniformly like an analog clock where the markers each occupy 30 degrees of the circuit; as Taurus began near 4,500 B.C. and ended near 2,000 B.C., we can see that this interval is greater than a 30 degree segment of the roughly 25,800-year precession cycle. Assuming a uniform occupancy of 30 degrees per Zodiacal constellation also assumes Taurus to be smaller than it is in reality.

The language in the heavens was supposed to be recounted on earth without alteration, and the transmission of the "scroll" of the heavens was corrupted by reckoning from a false point of origin; that is, the point of origin is Virgo, not Aries or Taurus, and this is part of the reason that Genesis 3:1 discusses Satan as the "serpent" in relation to the "beast of the field" (Taurus), for Taurus was regarded as the first marker in the Zodiac by many of the ancients when it is not in reality. The lesson to be learned is that arguing from a false premise produces tainted results, as the reader will notice that Satan merely asked a question in Genesis 3:1, but his question was deliberately oriented around the false premise that Elohim had given a prohibition against certain food (Genesis 1:29-30) when it was instead Jehovah Elohim Who gave the prohibition against certain food (Genesis 2:17); this first deceptive question concerned God's Word as is the nature of the battle between good and evil. Mythology and astrology are largely the result of corrupted transmissions of the celestial "scroll," the same scroll "eaten" and digested by Ezekiel, and John, as it was represented by the 12 pillars that Moses erected in Exodus 24:4. "...Moses, when he was about to erect the **tabernacle**, was warned, 'See that you make everything according to the pattern that was shown you on the mountain,'" (Hebrews 8:5). "Have ye not known: have ye not heard? Hath it not been told you from the beginning? Have ye not understood from the foundations of the earth? It is He That sitteth upon the circle of the earth, and the inhabitants thereof are as grasshoppers; That stretcheth out the heavens as a curtain, and spreadeth them out as a **tent** to dwell in," (Isaiah 40:21-22).

Numbers 2:2 states, "Every man of the children of Israel shall pitch by his own standard, with the ensign of their father's house..." "There can be no doubt... that these signs [of the Zodiac] were afterwards identified with the twelve sons of Jacob. Joseph sees the sun and moon and eleven stars bowing down to him, he himself being the twelfth (Gen. xxxvii. 9)," (*Witness of the Stars*, Bullinger; p. 17); this information may be new to Christians, but is standard to Jews. Concerning the 12 classical constellations of the Zodiac, we have no difficulty in observing the fact that the 12 Tribes of Israel have a relationship with the 12 constellations of the Zodiac.

Concerning the time of Noah, "The flood would therefore have lasted for twelve moons and eleven extra days. It is hard not to recognize here the intention of making the flood last for an exact solar year; for if 354 days be assumed for the duration of twelve moons... the total duration of the flood comes to 365 days," (*Astronomy in the Old Testament*, Schiaparelli; p. 127). The solar year can be rounded to the nearest whole number of 365 days. Classically speaking, the sun passes through the 12 constellations of the Zodiac every year. Let us note the first letters of the words that immediately follow the names of Jacob's sons in Genesis 49:3-27:

(verse 3)	Reuben:	ב = 2
(verse 5)	Simeon & Levi:	א = 1
(verse 8)	Judah:	א = 1
(verse 13)	Zebulun:	ל = 30
(verse 14)	Issachar:	ח = 8
(verse 16)	Dan:	י = 10
(verse 19)	Gad:	ג = 3

(verse 20)	Asher:	ש = 300
(verse 21)	Naphtali:	א = 1
(verse 22)	Joseph:	ב = 2
(verse 27)	Benjamin:	ז = 7
		365

The initial letters of the words that immediately follow the names of Jacob's sons have a combined gematria of **365**, the number of full days in the solar year. Concerning Jesus, Matthew 10:1 says, "And having called His 12 *disciples* ["μαθητας" (ref. *3101*)]..." the word "*disciples*" is "μαθητας" = "μ+α+θ+η+τ+α+ς" = 40+1+9+8+300+1+6 = **365**. The word "disciples" in the lexicon is "μαθητης" (ref. *3101*) which is not 365; the point is that when the word "disciples" was used in the context of Matthew 10:1 to describe the 12 (like the Zodiac), the spelling within the context computes to **365** in congruence with the 12 Tribes of Israel in the war against Satan, *the Accuser* = "Σατανας" (ref. *4567*) = "Σ+α+τ+α+ν+α+ς" = 6+1+300+1+50+1+6 = **365**. Satan *the Accuser* is also marked out by the number **365** in conjunction with another of his names: "Leviathan" or what we call the constellation of "Draco," or The Dragon. Leviathan occupied the very crown of the heavens when the ancient constellation pictures were, most likely, first mapped out, as this date can be calculated to be near 2,700 B.C. (*The Astronomy of the Bible*, Maunder; 149-161) or about 25,800 years before that (acknowledging the proper motion of the constellations, if one can entertain the notion of Biblical chronology being figuratively formulaic). Evil is parasitic, for the 12 gates and the 12 angels at the gates of the New Jerusalem are for righteousness (Revelation 21:12).

The angels discussed in Scripture are not stars. However, the stars were marked out to identify the Savior (Genesis 3:15), and from the prophet Daniel, the Magi who we call "Wise Men" were able to calculate the location of the Messiah, and they followed "His *star*" (Matthew 2:3) in order to find Him and pay Him due honor just as the *angels* spoke to the shepherds about the same event. Scripture uses visible nature as an illustration of the spiritual world. When false "Wise Men" began connecting dots on the celestial "scroll" and drawing their own pictures, astrology and mythology reared their blasphemous heads. When those who were wise began foolishly worshipping the stars, astrology and mythology reared their blasphemous heads. Consider Romans 1:18-23: "For the wrath of God is revealed from heaven against all ungodliness and wickedness of those who by their wickedness suppress truth. For what can be known about God is plain to them, because God has shown it to them [*as it was shown to the Magi*]. Ever since the creation of the world His eternal power and divine nature, invisible though they are, have been understood and seen through the things He has made. So they are without excuse; for though they knew God, they did not honor Him [*as the Magi did honor Him*], but they became futile in their thinking, and their senseless minds were darkened. Claiming to be wise [*like the false Magi, i.e. sorcerers*], they became fools; and they exchanged the glory of the immortal God for images resembling a mortal being or birds or four-footed creatures or reptiles [*like the pictures drawn around the stars that were worshipped in idolatry*]." The star pictures referred to in Romans 1:23 were once the four corners of the sky,

marked out specifically by Ezekiel and John, and are listed according to the order of Creation in Genesis 1:14:
"...for signs [1] and for seasons [2] and for days [3] and years [4]," (Genesis 1:14)
"a mortal being [1] or birds [2] or four-footed creatures [3] or reptiles [4]," (Romans 1:23)

The link between "years" [4] and "reptiles" [4] is that Leviathan = Satan [*the Accuser*] = "Σατανας" (ref. *4567*) = "Σ+α+τ+α+ν+α+ς" = 6+1+300+1+50+1+6 = **365**. Satan used astrology in an attempt to cover the astronomical aspects of the Scriptures, particularly in relation to the Savior, as both Christ and Satan are marked out in Genesis 3:15 to Satan's ultimate demise – and thus it is written that "...the wrath of God is revealed from heaven against all ungodliness and wickedness of those who by their wickedness suppress truth," (Romans 1:18); "...Thus, persons knowledgeable of the calculations but ignorant of [the court's] methods might criticize and disparage [the court's] decisions. To avoid such undermining of [the court], calendrical knowledge was suppressed and thus the masses accepted [the court's] decisions without question," (*Talmud: Rosh Hashanah*; Schottenstein Edition; Notation on 20b) – Satan took such a line of reasoning and made it appear that God was suppressing beneficial knowledge in Genesis 3, as the humans were to obey God without question, which is why Satan began his attack with a question. Confusion concerning the intentions of God sparked a curiosity in humanity, and such a curiosity (being misdirected) led to a faulty assumption as to Who was righteous and who was not.

"Messiah" = (ref.4899) = "משיה" = "ה+י+ש+מ"
=8+10+300+40 = **358**

"Serpent" = (ref. 5175) = "נחש" = "ש+ח+נ" = 300+8+50 = **358**

"Satan" = (ref. *4566*) = "Σ+α+τ+α+ν" = 6+1+300+1+50 = **358**

As the first humans reckoned the message falsely after being prompted by Satan, Genesis 3:15 specifically marks out the constellations of Hercules and Draco when it is written, "...He will crush your head, and you will strike His heel" – which are the very pictures of those celestial maps; that is, since Virgo is actually the first in the order of the Zodiac, the Age of Virgo (i.e. when the vernal equinox was in the constellation of Virgo) was the time-period when Earth's North Celestial Pole was housed in the foot of the constellation we now call "Hercules." Simply put, God realigned what humanity miscalculated by restating the origin of His creation's design.

[2.38] The principle direction of the ancient Jews was East: "And those who encamp to the front, at the east, shall be the division of the camp of Judah..." (Numbers 2:3). East was the principle direction of the Jews because the sun rises in the East and identifies the passage of the morning stars. "The Lord God planted a garden in Eden, in the east..." (Genesis 2:8). Concerning Leviticus 23:7, "The word קדם means before or in front of, either in space or in time. In the Holy Tongue, directions are often expressed from the vantage point of a person facing east. Accordingly, the direction before him, i.e., east, is called קדם (Genesis 2:8, 10:30, 29:1); the direction to his rear, i.e., west, is called אחור, literally behind or in the back of (e.g., Isaiah 9:11); the south is to his right side and is called ימין, literally right (e.g., Psalms 89:13); and the north, to his left, is called שמאל, literally, left (e.g., Genesis 14:15)," (*Baal Ha Turim*, Gold; p. 1643). (Note Ezekiel's orientation in Ezekiel 1:10.)

[2.39] The Egyptians called Leviathan "Typhon," and they had a sacrificial furnace on which to incinerate humans in the worship of Typhon (Exodus 9:8). Draco or Typhon or *Leviathan* [*A Water Monster; A Coiled Animal; Crocodile; the constellation of the Dragon; Mourning*] was thought to swallow the sun to produce solar eclipses, as Job 3:5-6 depicts Job exclaiming figuratively, "Let darkness and the shadow of death stain it; let a cloud dwell upon it; let all that **blackens** the day terrify it. As for that night, let darkness seize upon it; let it not be joined unto the days of the year, let it not come into the number of the months." The sense of what **blackens** the day is given by "כמריר" (ref. 3650) = "from ref. 3648; an obscuration (as if from shrinkage of light, i.e. an **eclipse**:- blackness." Typhon was also linked to intense storms that blackened the sky.

As the sun, moon, and stars are set to keep time (for we could not gauge time without them), the fact that the prophets saw these constellations move so quickly (Ezekiel 1) illustrates also how these prophets were able to see time at a different rate than ordinary people; it is similar to increasing the rate at which a clock's hands turn. Consider the Cherubs – the Cherubs are described as guardians or watchmen in Genesis 3:24 set at the "east of the Garden of Eden... to guard the way to [or '*of*' as J.P. Green translates] the Tree of Life," for Adam had failed to "guard" (Genesis 2:15) the garden from the "serpent." Adam was to be fruitful and multiply. *Ezekiel* [*Strength of God*] is described as, "the son of *Buzi* [*Contemned of Jehovah*] in the land of the *Chaldeans* [*Astrologers; Wanderers*] by the river *Chebar* [*Vehement* (root = to *multiply*]..." (Ezekiel 1:3) as he was prepared to prophesy rightly by way of spiritual enlightenment from God illustrated with (and/or by) righteous astronomical information.

Dr. Bullinger stated that the Greek "Ζωδιακος" [*Zodiac*] comes from the Hebrew "Sodi" which in Sanscrit means "a way" or "a step" (*Witness of the Stars*, Bullinger; p. 15). The Book of Revelation discusses the celestial "living creatures" or "beasts" in this manner: "...in front of the throne there is something like a sea of glass, like crystal. Around the throne, on each side of the throne, are four living creatures, full of eyes in front and behind: the first living creature like a lion the second living creature like an ox, the third living creature with a face like a human face, and the fourth living creature like a flying eagle. And the four living creatures, each of them with six wings, are full of eyes all around and inside..." (Revelation 4:6-8). Ezekiel 1:10 states that the four "living creatures" had "the face of a human being, the face of a lion on the right side, the face of an ox on the left side, and the face of an eagle." The four faces of the "living creatures" are related to the *Cherubs* [*Celestial; as if Contending*] of Genesis 3:24, and the six wings remind us of the *Seraphs* [*Fiery Serpents*] of Isaiah 6. Whatever the various heavenly beings actually are is presently unknown, but it is certain as to why they are, celestially speaking, described as such, "For the constellations were originally so designed that the sun at the time of the summer solstice was in the middle of the constellation *Leo*, the Lion; at the time of the spring equinox in the middle of *Taurus*, the Bull; and at the time of the winter solstice, in the middle of *Aquarius*, the Man bearing the waterpot. The fourth point, that held by the sun at the autumnal equinox, would appear to have been already assigned to the foot of the Serpent-holder as he crushes down the Scorpion's head; but a flying eagle, *Aquila*, is placed as near the equinoctial point as seems to have been consistent with the ample space that it was desired to give the emblems of the great conflict between the Deliverer and the Serpent. Thus, as in the vision of Ezekiel, so in the constellation figures, the Lion, the Ox, the Man, and the Eagle, stood as the upholders of the firmament, as the 'pillars of heaven.' They looked down like watchers upon all creation; they seemed to guard the four quarters of the sky," (*The Astronomy of the Bible*, Maunder; p. 167). The Cherubs can be understood similarly as they guarded the way to (or of) the Tree of Life "with its 12 kinds of fruit, producing its fruit each month..." (Revelation 22:2) as there are 12 months in the year and therefore 12 classical Zodiac markers that sift the year. As the 12 kinds of "fruit" are illustrated by the 12 constellations of the Zodiac, the beasts that John describes in Revelation 4:8 are "full of eyes all around and inside," for the constellations he describes are groupings of glittering stars. Ezekiel said that, "As I looked at the living creatures, I saw a *wheel* on the earth beside the living creatures," (Ezekiel 1:15), for the word "star" = "כוכב" (ref. 3556) = "...(in the sense of *rolling*)... or (in the sense of *blazing*); a star." [2.40] The visions of the prophets are not mere stars; the stars simply served as illustrations for their visions: "...as I was among the exiles by the river *Chebar*, the heavens were opened, and I saw visions of Elohim," (Ezekiel 3:1), for Elohim gave the positive commands regarding fruit and trees (Genesis 1:28) and Jehovah Elohim gave the negative command concerning the forbidden tree (Genesis 2:17). Thus, "The word of Jehovah came to the priest *Ezekiel* [*Strength of God*] son of *Buzi* [*Contemned of Jehovah*] in the land of the *Chaldeans* [*Astrologers; Wanderers*] by the river *Chebar* [*Vehement* (root = to *Multiply*]..." Elohim is connected to the production of fruit as Jehovah is connected to husbandry: "I am the true vine, and My Father is the vinegrower. He removes every branch in me that bears no fruit. Every branch that bears fruit He prunes to make it bear more fruit," (John 15:1-3).

The sons (or fruit) of Elohim are distinguished from the Triune God as in Job 1:6: "And a day came when the sons of Elohim came to present themselves before Jehovah. And Satan also came among them." The stars are also paralleled to "fruit" by way of illustration in visions as we read of God's blessing to Abram: "...the word of Jehovah came to Abram in a vision, 'Do not be afraid, Abram, I am your shield; your reward shall be very great.' But Abram said, 'O Lord Jehovah, what will you give me, for I continue childless...You have given me no offspring...'" (Genesis 15:1-3), so God, "...brought him outside and said, 'Look toward heaven and count the *stars*, if you are able to count them... So shall your *descendant*s be," (Genesis 15:5).

The illustrative words "eyes" and "fruit" used to describe the stars have a very deliberate and intimate connection. When Elohim (the One Who commanded humanity concerning "fruit") created the sun, moon, and stars in Genesis 1:14, He said, "...Let *luminaries* be in the expanse of the heavens, to divide between day and night..."; the word "*luminaries*" = "מארה" (ref. 3974) = "a chandelier; bright, light," and is similar to the next word in order "מאורה" (ref. 3975) = "something *lighted*, i.e. an *aperture*; by implication, *a crevice or hole of a serpent*:-den." There is a connection between "eyes," "fruit," and a "serpent," for when the constellations were first mapped out, the highest of them all, the pinnacle of the firmament that separated the "waters" below it from the waters above it (Genesis 1:7), the one which all the others revolved around, was *Leviathan* [*A Water Monster, A Coiled Animal; Mourning*] who "surveys everything that is lofty," (Job 41:34). "Yes, let that night be *barren*; let no joyful cry be heard in it. Let those who curse it curse the Sea, those who are skilled to rouse up Leviathan. Let the stars be dark; let it hope for light but have none; may it not see the eyelids of the morning – because it did not shut the doors of my mother's womb and hide trouble from my *eyes*," (Job 3:7-10). "How you are fallen from heaven, O Day Star, son of Dawn! How you are cut down [*like a tree*] to the ground, you who laid the nations low! You said in your heart, I will ascend to heaven; I will raise my throne above the stars of God; I will sit on the mount of assembly on the heights of *Zaphon* [*North; a place exposed to the north wind*]; I will ascend to the tops of the clouds, I will make myself like the Most High,'" (Isaiah 14:12-14). Because of the sin in Eden, out of mercy for us, Christ crushed the head of this evil "serpent," as constellation we now call Hercules is depicted by a kneeler (kneeling because of a wounded heel) who holds a vine and a serpent in one hand, and a club in the other (to smash the head of the serpent amongst the vines) while his foot stomps the head of Draco (Leviathan) beneath him. "...He will bruise your head, and you will bruise his heel," (Genesis 3:15), and the autumnal equinox during the Age of Taurus when the constellations were, most likely, first mapped out is actually near to foot of Ophiuchus the Serpent Holder who wrestles the serpent while crushing the head of the Scorpion. The silly mythological adventures of Hercules are merely reflections of traditions that forgot and corrupted the transmission of the message of the stars around the constellation (that was not always known as Hercules) that prophesied the coming Savior. Myth is but oral tradition that has been eroded to the point that it becomes its own entity. Astrology and mythology mingled, and such a mixture obscured the science of God's Word from our eyes: "...the wrath of God is revealed from heaven against all ungodliness and wickedness of those who by their wickedness suppress truth," (Romans 1:18).

[2.41]   Let us ponder the considerable emphasis placed on the signification of the "head" in the Gospel accounts: "And they... platted a crown of thorns, and put it about His *head*," (Mark 15:17); "And they smote Him on the *head*..." (Mark 15:19); "And they that passed by railed on Him, *shaking their heads*..." (Mark 15:29); "Over *His head* they put the charge against Him, which read, 'This is Jesus of Nazareth, the King of the Jews," (Matthew 27:37); "...Then

He bowed His *head* and gave up His Spirit," (John 19:30). As we recall from Rubric 2.25, each Hebrew letter also has a signification that is apparent when one articulates each letter's name. Let us consider the letter "ר"; this letter is pronounced "Resh" today, but the fact that it signifies a "head" reflects the fact that "head" is pronounced "rosh," not "resh."

Signification: ר = *a head*

"ראש" (ref. 7217) corresponds to ref. 7218; Chaldee = "*the head;* (figuratively) the sum:- chief" = "ש+א+ר" = 300+1+200 = **501**

"ראש" (ref. 7218) = "from an unused root apparently meaning to *shake:* the *head (as most easily shaken),* whether literally or figuratively (in many applications, of place, time, rank, etc.):- band, beginning, captain, chapter, chief, excellent, first, forefront, height, (on) high, ruler, sum, top" = "ש+א+ר" = 300+1+200 = **501**

"ראש" or "רוש" (ref. 7219) = "a poisonous plant; poison (even of *serpents*):- *gall.*"
= "ש+א+ר" = 300+1+200 = **501**

The "poison (even of serpents)" that Christ drank as He hung on the tree in John 19:30 = "ראש" (ref. 7219) = "ש+א+ר" = 300+1+200 = **501** which shows how this word is also linked to the letter ר (Resh) which signifies "the *head*" as well. "[Christ] is the *head* [ר] of the body, the church; He is the beginning, the *firstborn from the dead,* so that He might come to have first place in everything." The description of "firstborn from the dead" cannot mean that Christ was first to be raised from the dead, for He Himself raised others from the dead prior to His own death and resurrection. Since Christ is the "True Vine" (John 15:1), there must also be a false vine. Furthermore, when we consider our True Vine's death on the tree, we can better understand the Greek definition of "vineyard" that Christ used in Mark 12:1 for His parable: "vineyard" = "αμπελον" (ref. *290*) and is from the word "αμπελος" (ref. *288*) which means "a vine (as *coiling* about a support)." Consider the Hebrew word "גפן" (ref. 1612) = "a vine (as *twining*), esp. the grape:- vine, tree" in comparison to the word "עכשוב" (ref. 5919) means "an asp (from *lurking coiled up*):- adder." Jesus described Himself as a serpent in John 3:14; Satan is referred to as a "serpent" in Genesis 3:1. Since a solar eclipse would indicate when the Head of the Month (Rosh Chodesh) should be celebrated, it may be that the total solar eclipse of November 24, 29 A.D. indicates something as to the year of Christ's death and resurrection.

[2.42] The Hebrew "Leviathan" is as the Egyptian deity called "Typhon," and "Leviathan" is the name used to discuss the constellation we call "Draco" the Dragon. The other serpentine pictures drawn around the stars discuss this "dragon" also, as is evident by the depictions of Revelation 12:15-16: "Then from his mouth the serpent poured water like a river after the woman, to sweep her away with the flood. But the earth came to the help of the woman; it opened its mouth and swallowed the river that the dragon poured from his mouth," and this is an overt description of the ancient star maps drawn around Andromeda the Chained Woman, Cetus the Sea Monster, and Eridanus the River that is "swallowed" by the earth, i.e. it disappears into the horizon because of the latitude of the observer.

Earth's North Celestial Pole was housed in the constellation Draco (Leviathan) during the Age of Taurus the Bull.

"בקר" (ref. 1241) = "an animal of the ox kind of either gender (as used for plowing)" = "ר+ק+ב" = 200+100+2 = **302**

"בקר" (ref. 1242) = "dawn (as the break of day), morning")" = "ר+ק+ב" = 200+100+2 = **302**

Precession of the Equinoxes requires about 25,800 years in order to reach its completion, as each of its 12 periods (or ages; 13 today) holds the vernal equinox for an uneven amount of time. When the "age of Taurus" is discussed, it means time period when the vernal equinox is in Taurus. "The North Star at the time of the construction of the Great Pyramid was Thuban, an unassuming 4th magnitude star in Draco the Dragon... In 2,700 BC Earth's axis pointed near Thuban, and the star held special significance to the Egyptians, who associated it, and the 'undying' stars that were circumpolar and that never set, with the Pharaoh. The northernmost 'air shaft' leading upward from the King's Chamber in the Great Pyramid pointed to Thuban, symbolically connecting the dead pharaoh with the central undying star. Thuban is corrupted Arabic for 'serpent's head,'" (*Starry Night Companion*, Mosley; p.

78). "Now the serpent was *subtle* above every beast of the field that the Lord God had made," (Genesis 3:1); the star named "*Thuban*" means "*Subtle*" in Hebrew (*Witness of the Stars*, Bullinger; p. 72). Since Thuban was the polar star during the Age of Taurus the Bull, we can understand that "Now the *serpent* [*Draco*] was *subtle* [*Thuban*] above every *beast of the field* [*Taurus*] that the Lord God had made," (Genesis 3:1) because of the Precession of the Equinoxes; in other words, Genesis 3:1 provides the reader with the constellation that held the polar star, the polar star itself, and the vernal equinox in order to understand the nature of the first human sin. The Scriptures provide three distinctly mapped markers (when only one of these is necessary for a round reckoning of Precession ages) so that we might be made explicitly aware of exactly what celestial orientation is being discussed and for what purpose: many of the ancients regarded Taurus (the golden calf) as being the first constellation in order of the Zodiac when, in fact, Virgo is the first in order; this manner of imagery allows us to comprehend that the first woman was deceived into reasoning from a false point of origin regarding the forbidden tree. "How you are fallen from heaven, O Day Star, son of Dawn! How you are cut down [*like a tree*] to the ground, you who laid the nations low! You said in your heart, I will ascend to heaven; I will raise my throne above the stars of God; I will sit on the mount of assembly on the heights of *Zaphon* [*North; a place exposed to the north wind*]; I will ascend to the tops of the clouds, I will make myself like the Most High,'" (Isaiah 14:12-14). The false assumption of Taurus being the first in the order of the Zodiacal constellations also falsely assumes

Leviathan (Draco) to be their presiding king seated on the Earth's North Celestial Pole. Many ancients assumed that the North Celestial Pole would always remain in Draco, when, in fact, time shifts this pole out of the Serpent's grasp. Earth's North Celestial Pole traces a giant circle in the heavens because of Precession, and this circle is traced around the North Ecliptic Pole completely in about 25,800 years. In a manner of speaking, the Serpent is not allowed to retain possession of the North Celestial Pole indefinitely, for he possesses the North Ecliptic Pole. Earth's tilted North Celestial pole allows for seasons, for if it were not tilted, we would not have seasons. The ecliptic is the sun's apparent annual path through the apparently fixed stars – it is Earth's orbit (if it could be seen in the sky). The North Ecliptic Pole is in Draco (Leviathan/Typhon) and is indicated by the *Serpent*: "the Accuser" = "Σατανας" (ref. *4567*) = "Σ+α+τ+α+ν+α+ς" = 6+1+300+1+50+1+6 = **365** = the solar year. As such, we can understand why, "...there is nothing new *under the sun*," (Ecclesiastes 1:9) as the North Ecliptic Pole remains in Draco. However, in the end, "...there will be no more night; they need no lamp or *sun*, for the Lord God will be their light..." (Revelation 22:5) when Satan is ultimately defeated.

Regarding the unmapped regions of the ancient starcharts that the Astronomer E.W. Maunder studied, he deduced that such unmapped portions of the sky must have corresponded roughly to the horizon of the first people who mapped the heavens: "From this we learn that the constellations were designed by people living not very far from the 40th parallel of north latitude, not further south than the 37th or 36th. This is important, as it shows that they did not originate in ancient Egypt or India, nor even in the city of Babylon, which is in latitude 32 ½°," (*The Astronomy of the Bible*, Maunder; p. 157) – the "people" who "designed" the constellations should probably be more regarded as those who mapped the stars named by God (names that were passed down through antiquity) as, "He determines the number of the stars; He gives to all of them their names," (Psalm 147:4). Also, the era referred to by Maunder is near 2,700 B.C. which is in but the most recent Age of Taurus, for it cannot be assumed that Adam lived at this time, but rather that Taurus was regarded as the beginning of the Zodiac by many of the ancients. The Age of Taurus falsely reckoned only originates from (or is illustrated by) the beginning of human sin (Genesis 3:1), not the beginning of Creation (Genesis 1:1) which is illustrated by the orientation of the Age of Virgo.

The true leader of the Zodiac is in fact Virgo (not Aries or Taurus) as is also indicated by the signs of Virgo and Leo on the ceiling of the Portico of the Temple of Esneh that shows a sphinx uniting Virgo (1) and Leo (12) through the face of a woman and the body of a lion; the Biblical parallel can be seen in the fact that Christ was born of a virgin (Luke 1:34) and that He is called the "Lion of the tribe of Judah" (Revelation 5:5), thus He is "...the first and the last, the beginning and the end," (Revelation 22:13). Regarding sphinxes adds more clarity to the passages that state, "Out of Egypt have I called My Son," (Matthew 2:15 & Hosea 11:1), though the Egyptians were not the first to identify the constellations, yet they were linked to golden calf idolatry as the golden calf signified the shining sun in the vernal equinox in the Age of Taurus, and it was mistakenly thought by many ancients that Taurus led the Zodiac when Taurus is 9th in order of the pattern, which is a reason why Genesis 3:1 is oriented around the Age of Taurus in relation to various human mistakes in connection with the months of a full term pregnancy. **In other words, Taurus is linked to idolatry (Exodus 32) and the anointed priesthood (Leviticus 4:3) as an indicator of sin because the polar star during the Age of Taurus was Thuban inside of the Leviathan, and these facts extend from the 9th Age (like a full-term pregnancy) when the Dragon (like the "serpent" of Genesis 3) who was subtle (like Thuban, the polar star at that time) above every beast of the field (like a bull, or Taurus) coaxed the woman into mistakenly destroying her fruit (like an agricultural product) as humans were made from the dust of the ground (like vegetation).** In a related way, Dr. Bullinger noted that when John 1:14 states, "The Word became flesh and *tabernacled* with us," the allusion here is probably linked to the Feast of *Tabernacles* (*Companion Bible*, Bullinger; Appendix 179) as this month's sun was in the constellation of Virgo, the Virgin.

[2.43] Earth's axis precesses, and so the North Celestial Pole traces a circle around the North Ecliptic Pole once about every 25,800 years – and the North Ecliptic Pole is in Draco, the Leviathan. During the Age of Taurus, the North Celestial Pole (Earth's Axis) shared its home in the same constellation with the North Ecliptic Pole (in Leviathan) so that these two important axes of time became one with this serpentine constellation. Genesis 2:24-25 states, "Therefore shall a man leave his father and his mother, and shall cleave to his wife: and they shall be one flesh.

And they were both naked, the man and his wife, and were not ashamed" – and the very next passage in Scripture states, "Now the *serpent* [*Leviathan*] was *subtle* [*Thuban*] above every *beast of the field* [*Taurus*] that the Lord God had made," (Genesis 3:1). The two humans became one flesh for righteousness, and the natural illustration of evil working against this pure human unity is depicted by the North Ecliptic Pole and the North Celestial Pole uniting in the one flesh of Leviathan.

Precession of the Equinoxes was not known by the common man in the ancient world. "A mysterious religion, now extinct, once incorporated secret knowledge of the precession of the equinoxes. This knowledge was kept so private that only in the last few decades was it rediscovered. Yet at one time its followers were spread through the Roman Empire from England to Palestine and their religion was a rival to young Christianity. Worshippers of Mithras portrayed their hero slaying a bull in the presence of figures of the zodiac. Taurus, the celestial bull, died in the sense that precession had moved the location of the vernal equinox from Taurus into Aries, ending the Age of Taurus. A force that could move the equinox was stronger than any other yet known, for it moved the entire cosmos. Such a force must come from beyond the cosmos, and it was worshipped by the followers of Mithraism – who kept this knowledge a secret. They certainly would have been shocked to learn that the force originates with the pull of the Sun and the Moon on Earth's equatorial bulge!" (*Starry Night Companion*, Mosley; p. 76). Worshipping the stars is ridiculous. However, worshipping the One Who made the stars is our privilege. The stars tell us time, and as such, they were marked out in the Scriptures accordingly in order to leave behind a specific witness of the events inscribed therein.

Consider the sin offering of the bull regarding the Anointed Priest (Leviticus 4) and the red cow in connection with a dead body (Numbers 19) in relation to the fact that the name "Adam" = "אדם" (ref. 121) is composed of the concepts of an "ox" and "blood":

"Adam" = "א+דם":

"א" = "אלף" (ref. 504) = "a family; also (from the sense of yoking or taming) *an ox or cow, kine.*"
"דם" = "דם" (ref. 1818) = "*blood* (as that which when shed causes death) of a man or animal; by analogy, *the juice of the grape*; figuratively bloodshed (i.e. drops of blood)."

The name "Adam" is connected to the origin of the sin-offering of a bull regarding the Anointed Priest (Priest Messiah) in connection with a dead body, as we read of the prophesied crucifixion in Psalm 22 that begins with some of Jesus' words on the cross and contains the statement, "Many bulls encircle me..." (Psalm 22:12) as is connected to the construction of the Molten Sea that was supported by 12 oxen (I Kings 7 & II Chronicles 4), for reflection pools were sometimes used by the ancients to study the stars (note also the ten movable stands, that had wheels, in I Kings 7:27-29 which displayed lions, bulls, and cherubs). In a similar way, the "lake of fire" (Revelation 20:14) is antithetically paralleled to "Heaven" = "שמים" (ref. 8064), for the word "Heaven" is composed of the concepts of "fire" and "water":

"Heaven" = "שׁ+מים"

"שׁ" = "fire"

"מים" = "מים" (ref. 4325) = "water."
As such, we can understand a baptism as with "fire" (Matthew 3:11).

The concepts of a "cow/ox" + "blood/ juice of the grape" are all linked to Adam. The Polar Star was in Leviathan during the Age of Taurus the *bull*. "The Lord God said unto the serpent, 'Because thou hast done this, thou art cursed above all *cattle* and above every beast of the field..." (Genesis 3:14). "He [God] drove out the man; and at the **east** of the garden of Eden He placed the cherubs, and a sword flaming and turning to guard the way to the tree of life," (Genesis 3:24).

[2.44] It is a common, and false, notion that the Hebrew Scriptures arose from an amalgamation of previous myths, for such a stance neglects the fact that most of the Biblical accounts of prophets depict the prophets as placed in the midst of moral decay whereby the prophet is instrumental in realigning what has been made crooked by humanity's own selfish hand. The fact that so much ancient myth exhibits such unavoidable similarities admits a common source – an admittance that is heightened by regarding the oral transmission that led to the fully formed myth.

It was found necessary to solidify, on page, the true meaning of the original truths from which myth ramified and mutated in order to inhibit the further inventive influx of defective thought and deficient practice concerning the pristine truths of antiquity. Disregarding the consistent and precise prophetic formula explicitly provided by the Scriptures forces one into the faulty position of assuming written chronological seniority to be definite historical superiority. A child is not disciplined until after a child misbehaves. A child is instructed secondarily after a child transgresses an initial command: "And your have forgotten the exhortation that addresses you as children – 'My child, do not regard lightly the discipline of the Lord, or lose heart when you are punished by Him; for the Lord disciplines those whom He loves, and chastises every child whom He accepts,' [Proverbs 3:11-12]. Endure trials for the sake of discipline. Gods treating you as children; for what child is there whom a parent does not discipline? If you do not have that discipline which all children share, then you are illegitimate and not His children," (Hebrews 12:5-8). "Whom shall He teach knowledge? And whom shall He make to understand doctrine? Them that are weaned from the milk, and drawn from the breasts," (Isaiah 28:9). "Brothers and sisters, do not be children in your thinking. In regard to evil be infants, but in your thinking be adults," (I Corinthians 14:20).

Scriptural ink serves to correct human memory erosion and intentional transgression as is observed in the unavoidable parallels Scripture shares with the illegitimacy of myth. Based on faulty tradition, it is assumed that the Bible contains a story about a talking snake much like the myth of Hercules who wore a cloak of lion's skin and who traveled to a garden to battle the serpent for the

The Lock   259

Golden Apples of Immortality that hung on the Tree of Life. However, such a tradition was formed errantly from a concise teaching tool that was designed to absorb the basic tenets of Scripture and to place those rudiments in the storehouses of our memory so that we could eventually feed on the wholeness of what was given to us for the cultivation of our minds regarding the knowledge of Salvation. Instead, many have been often drawn to the contradictory complacency of consuming children's milk in expectation of Herculean strength against the original design marked out for fruitful production, savored enjoyment, rapt thankfulness, and resplendent unity.

[2.45] "So they read in the book in the law of God distinctly, and gave the sense, and caused them to understand the reading," (Nehemiah 8:8). "The Talmud explains that 'the book' meant the original text; 'distinctly' means explaining it by giving the Chaldee paraphrase; 'gave the sense' means the division of words, &c. according to the sense; and 'caused them to understand the reading' means to give the traditional pronunciation of the words (which were then without the vowel points)," (*Companion Bible, Bullinger*, Appendix 30).

[2.46] Deuteronomy 29:29 in our English Bibles says, "The secret things belong unto the Lord our God; but those things which are revealed belong unto us and to our children forever, that we may do all the words of this law." However, the ancient Scribes inserted peculiar vowels into Deuteronomy 29:29 referred to as one of the "15 Extraordinary Points of the Sopherim" and as one of the "Ten Nequdoth of the Torah." It is agreed upon by some of the greatest scholars that Deuteronomy 29:29 is better translated to say that when you shall perform the things which are revealed, God will also reveal to you things which are concealed. This translation arises because of the stance that, "The words rendered, 'unto the Lord our God,' have the extraordinary points... to show that they form no part of the text, and should come out. The reading then is: 'The secret things, even the revealed things, [belong] to us and our children forever, that we may do all the words of this Law,'" (*Companion Bible*, Bullinger; p. 279). Dr. Butin concludes his book on the Extraordinary Points of the Torah this way: "... the Nequdoth or Extraordinary Points of the Pentateuch were devised by their author or authors, to condemn, as spurious, the words or letters over which they were placed," (*The Ten Nequdoth of the Torah*, Butin; p. 117). Thus, an attractive gift is offered to all those who adhere to the words of Scripture, especially considering that Christ fulfilled the Torah so that we may embrace the "law of liberty" (James 2:12) and have our eyes opened to the secret things of positively enduring truth.

[2.47] Jesus said to the Scribes and the Pharisees, "You abandon the commandment of God and hold to the tradition of men," (Mark, 7:8) after quoting Isaiah 29:13 where it is written, "... in vain do they worship Me, teaching human precepts as doctrines." Tradition is a place to start (at best), but it is not a beneficial place to finish. The Massorah provides one of the most wonderful and extensive glimpses into the struggle over God's Word. Without the amazing work of the Sopherim and Massorites, the task that took them centuries to complete would be ours, for without the work of these Scribes, the sentence you are reading right now would look something like this: wthtthwrkfthsscrbsthsntncyrrdngrghtnwldlksmthnglkths.

As the ancient Scribes were given such a monumental task, it becomes difficult to criticize their labors, especially when (excepting the Holy Bible) every book out of every human mind is speckled with errors, whether of judgment and/or of printing; thank God that He gave us a flawless Book out of His mind. At the same time, some of the Scribes were "hypocrites," (Matthew 23:23) who were criticized by Christ: "Woe to you, Scribes and Pharisees, hypocrites! For you clean the outside of the cup and of the plate, but inside they are full of greed and self-indulgence. You blind Pharisee! First clean the inside of the cup, so that the outside also may become clean," (Matthew 23:25-26). Christ called the Scribes and Pharisees a "brood of vipers" in Matthew 23:33. With hypocritical Scribes transmitting the Scriptures, it can be seen how, "Dead flies make the perfumer's ointment give off a foul odor; so a little folly outweighs wisdom and honor," (Ecclesiastes 10:1). "How can you say, 'We are wise, and the law of the Lord is with us,' when, in fact, the false pen of the Scribes has made it into a lie?"(Jeremiah 8:8).

[2.48] The manuscripts of the Greek New Testament can be divided into two major classes: 1) *Unical* manuscripts: those written in capital letters, and 2) *Cursives*: those written in the running-hand style. The Unical manuscripts are often considered to be more ancient, "although it is obvious and undeniable that some cursives may be transcripts of uncial MSS. more ancient than any existing unical MS [manuscript]. This will show that we cannot depend altogether upon textual criticism," (*Companion Bible*, Bullinger; Appendix 94.1-2, p. 136). Dr. Bullinger continued by reminding us, concerning the Greek New Testament, that, "Punctuation also, as we have it today, is entirely absent. The earliest two MSS. (known as B, the MS. in the Vatican and א in the Sinaitic MS., now at St. Petersburg) have only an occasional dot and this on a level with the top of the letters. The text reads without any divisions between letters or words until MSS. of the ninth century, when (in Cod. Augiensis, now in Cambridge) there is seen for the first time a single point which separates each word. This dot is placed in the middle of the line, but is often omitted. None of our modern marks of punctuation are found until the ninth century, and then only in Latin versions and some cursives," (*Companion Bible*, Bullinger; Appendix 94.3, p. 136). To this point, English versions of Luke 23:43 display misplaced punctuation that is an invention of an editor of a translation (in an honest attempt), not the work of the inspired writer. That is, according to the common English rendering of Luke

23:43, Jesus said to the criminal: "... Truly I tell you **,** today you will be with me in Paradise"; the comma so inserted severs the Hebrew idiom found 42 times in Deuteronomy

which is, "I tell you today **,** ..."

The Hebrew idiom rendered, "I tell you today" or "I tell you this day" is a solemn declaration of the utmost sincerity, and was a deliberate mode of speech as is exhibited in the vast number of times it is used in Scripture; hence we comprehend why Christ selected such a striking phrase to make His point known to the dying criminal who put his faith in the Savior of the world amidst execrable public execution. The emphasis of Christ's words here in Luke 23:43 is placed in the solemn certainty of their specific sense, not on the chronology of events – especially considering that Christ did not resurrect until three days after this statement and could not have been in the Heavenly Paradise between His death and resurrection lest it be said that the Heavenly Paradise was somehow beneath the ground.

When attempting to decipher Biblical chronology, it is helpful to keep in mind that the Scriptures not written chronologically as we count chronology, nor are the Books of Scripture ordered chronologically as we count chronology. The events and Books of Scripture are ordered thematically as is observable in the fact that Joshua's death is described in Judges 1:1, for he is recounted again, alive, in Judges 2:6-8. Biblical chronology often moves in a circuit, not always within in a line segment. Consider the creation of humanity in relation to the specificity of Adam's creation:

Genesis 1:27: "So God created man in His Image, in the Image of God He created him; male and female He created them."

Genesis 2:7: "- then the Lord God formed man from the dust of the ground, and breathed into his nostrils the breath of life; and the man [Adam] became a living being."
Genesis 5:1-2 "... When God created man, He made him

in the likeness of God. Male and female He created them, and He blessed them and named them 'Adam' when they were created."

Should we judge the Bible by our own systems in stead of by its own systems, we could easily state that there were three creations of human beings in linear succession based on the sequence of Biblical narrative expressed between Genesis 1:27 and Genesis 5:1-2.

[2.49] In order to keep the Scriptures uniform, the Scribes counted every letter of the Scriptures. They reckoned the following:

א *Aleph*, occurs 42,377 times in the Hebrew Scriptures. Concerning Nehemiah 7:66 and Numbers, 7:17: in the former the number 42,360 occurs, and in the latter 17; thus yielding together 42,377.

The same manner of listing was reckoned for the remainder of the Hebrew alphabet as it occurs in Scripture; these Scribes exhibited a rare devotion, to say the least. Significant letters within the catalogued Hebrew Scriptures were emboldened systematically in larger and darker print than most other letters in order to communicate various aspects of Scriptural phenomena, and this method of reckoning could have been used by the Apostle Paul when he wrote, "See what large letters I make when I am writing in my own hand!" (Galatians 6:11).

[2.50] In accordance with God's prophetic pronouncement of judgment and death on Adam in Genesis 2:7 before the consumption of the rosh in Eden, it should be noted that when God judged Satan in Genesis 3:15, He extended grace to humanity (but none to Satan) by prophesying the coming Savior *before* He punished the humans (Genesis 3:16). It is therefore apparent that the Old Testament Law is not devoid of grace when the very first story of sin provides the remedy to sin prior to any judgment that was pronounced on humanity. The Old Testament Law instills fear as a major motivation for upholding the standard, whereas the New Testament Grace depicts love as the main motivation for upholding the standard – for Christ summed all of the Old Testament Law into two main categories: "'You shall love the Lord your God with all your heart, and with all your soul, and with all your mind [as in Deuteronomy 6:5].' This is the greatest and first commandment. And a second is like it: 'You shall love your neighbor as yourself [as in Leviticus 19:18].' On these two commandments hang all the law and the prophets," (Matthew 22:37-39). We see that the initial standard in Eden was one of love, and once sin was chosen against the love of God, fear became a major motivation entwined with love. It can therefore be understood that when it is written that, "...perfect love casts out fear..." (I John 4:18), a new rule was not instated, but the original design in Eden was reinstated. When Jesus summarized all 613 Torah Laws into two categories, He summarized them by two Torah Laws themselves, not additions to the Torah Laws; as this summary was the rule of the New Testament, it can also be understood that it was mostly the impetus by which people followed God that was realigned and renewed from what had resulted on account of human rebellion. The traditional presumption that the Law was thrown out rather than fulfilled has kept Christians from reading the foundation of their New Testaments, and it seems fitting to credit this misconception to the Enemy when it was he who was the only being in Eden personally cursed. By rejecting Torah study, Christians are kept from the foundational precepts of Scripture, as has been the intention of the Enemy from the beginning. The main conflict between good and evil revolves around God's Word, the recognition of it, and the adherence to it and its purposes.

[2.51] When human reasoning is assumed to be somehow able to improve the Scriptures, error is unavoidable. The Scribes thought that certain Scriptures were indecent. There is no place of indecency in the Scriptures that can be credited to God, and by assuming there to be such indecent places, the Scribes sought to eliminate their concept of indecency from the official reading of the Text. The Scribes, out of reverence, removed various words and inserted others so that the Masters of Assembly directed a euphemized version of the Scriptures to please the ears of the congregation, and to keep both the tradition and the people hedged in – a tactic that shows dedication, but also a tactic that evinces hidden motives at times. Deuteronomy 4:2 commands, "You must neither add anything to what I command you nor take away anything from it, but keep the commandments of the Lord your God"; this direction is echoed by Revelation 20:18-19: "I warn everyone who hears the words of the prophecy of this book: if anyone adds to them, God will add to that person the plagues described in this book; if anyone takes away from the words of the book of this prophecy, God will take away that person's share in the tree of life and in the holy city, which are described in this book."

The attempt to euphemize "indecent" or "displeasing" passages of Scripture reveals the fact that what is considered indecent or displeasing is left to the discretion of those who hold the power to edit. Indeed, those in power certainly could have buried Biblical treasures for themselves and then claimed to do so for the good of the people. Again, it is rash to assume that all the Scribes were somehow members of a giant conspiracy, but it is more than evident that a conspiracy did exist concerning the Scriptures as is made plain by the New Testament accounts of the Sanhedrin, for Christ was given an illegal trial under false circumstances by the group that feigned the utmost piety.

The Scribes inserted vowels into the Scriptures partially to preserve them from human ruin, and so they catalogued their work in hopes that the original and full message (or what they could grasp from it) might also remain unaltered. However, because the oral law was relied on so heavily, the intricacies of the oral law became remembered while the intricacies of the Written Law faded. As such, the oral law became upheld to a greater extent than the Written Law, and the oral law became a written law.

[2.52] The Massorah is one of the most amazing Biblical tools ever constructed. The Massorah is a lock. In the opinion of this author, the Massorah is the most intricate labyrinth ever invented by humanity. The Massorah records the enigmatic phenomena of the Hebrew Scriptures, and it offers these patterns in numeric form. The Massorah records the number of times various letters, words, and groupings of words occur in the Scriptures; it is a massive cipher far beyond ordinary Biblical study. The Massorites realized that, by counting the letters and words of the Scriptures, they could find a deeper meaning that helped to explain the ceaseless, silent (yet speaking) patterns one begins to notice when reading the Scriptures regularly.

[2.53] "Since the circumstances of any given eclipse are reproduced almost exactly 18 years and 11 days later, this period is called an *Eclipse Cycle*, to which the ancient astronomers gave the name of *Saros*; and eclipses separated from each other by an exact cycle, and, therefore, corresponding closely in their conditions, are spoken of as being one and the same eclipse. Each Saros contains, on the average, 70 +/- eclipses," (*Witness of the Stars*, Bullinger; p. 179). "Now the important point is this, that if we take the prophetic reckoning of 360 days to the year, we have the following significant Biblical numbers:- In the first place, we already have the 70 +/- *Sari* divided into two portions of 33+37. A perfect cycle is accomplished in 33 *Sari*, or 595 years, when the eclipse, by a series of unbroken *Sari*, has accomplished a passage through the year of 360 days; or, if we reckon only the whole numbers, i.e., the 18 completed years, we have for the 33 *Sari* the period of 594 years, while the remaining portion of 37 *Sari* makes **666** years (37x18); and the whole 70 +/- *Sari* makes **1,260** years (594+666)," (*Witness of the Stars*, Bullinger; p. 180-181).

The Scriptures count the same essential time interval in four ways: "a time, and times, and half a time," 3.5, 42, and 1,260, and these four are in accordance with Day 4th of Genesis 1 which is when the sun, moon, and stars were created, "for signs [1] and for seasons [2] and for days [3] and years [4]," (Genesis 1:14). The Scriptures often count in what is called the "prophetic year" which is 360 days. Thus, 1,260 "days" on a 360-day "year" equals 42 "months" which equals 3.5 "years." The "time, and times, and half a time" (Revelation 12:14 & Daniel 7:25) description uses the word "time" in the sense of the prophetic year of 360 days; so, 360 x 3.5 = **1,260**.

"In the Roman World it was the common opinion, that, in very ancient times, magic originated with the priests of the Persians; and in the Roman World, those who practiced magic assumed the name of Magi; the adepts in the black arts shrewdly seeking to impress the popular imagination by taking to themselves the countenance of the name of an order, that, at the height of its glory, but in a time long past, had been widely honored. Thus in the two prevailing languages of the Roman Empire, in the Greek, the language of letters, and in the Latin, the language of laws, the word Magi came into common use in a sense that was related to the distinctive name of the Persian priest-hood, much as the English word magician is. The new sense of the word differed, in all important respects, from its original meaning. It indicated no priestly function, no sacredness of character, little or nothing as to nationality; and the term that best represents it is sorcerer," (*The Wise Men*, Upham; p. 5-6). Concerning the Magi who paid homage to the Christ Child, "... the motive of their pilgrimage was a prophecy of Daniel, who, though a Hebrew, was a Magian, held in honor by their renowned sovereigns of old, and whose bones were in the land of the Medes. This was what the form of their inquiry meant [regarding the 'king' of Matthew 2:2]. This the Evangelist [Matthew] meant to indicate by preserving that form. And this would ever have been clear to the readers of the English version had it rendered the words in the prophecy of Daniel, as the ancient Syriac version did render them, 'the anointed one, THE KING,'" (*The Wise Men*, Upham; p. 137). As a king, the years that Christ lived on the earth are most likely reckoned accurately by counting from the New Year for Kings. The *Talmud: Rash Hashanah 2a* states, "There are four New Years: On the first of Nissan is the New Year for Kings"; the *Schottenstein Edition's* notation explains this by stating, "The Rabbis established that a king's reign begins on the first of Nissan, e.g. in Shevat or Adar... his first year ends when Nissan arrives, and from that day on we start counting his second year," (*Talmud: Rosh Hashanah 2a*; Notation 1).

[2.54] "Paradise" = "Παραδεισος" (ref. *3857*), "is an Oriental word, first used by the historian Xenophon, denoting 'the parks of Persian kings and nobles.' It is of Persian origin (Old Pers. pairidaeza, akin to Gk. peri, 'around,' and teichos, 'a wall') whence it passed into Greek," (*Vine's Expository Dictionary*, p. 457). The word "paradise" is an "old Persian word," (*Commentary: Song of Songs*, Keil & Delitzsch, p. 559) that denoted an enclosing, a manner of fortification by walls (similar to those erected by a military), a circumvallation, and something defended. The word "garden," = "גַן" (ref. 1588) = "garden (as fenced)"; from "גָנַן" (ref. 1598) = "to hedge about; protect; defend"; a "vineyard" = "כרם" (ref. 3754) is also considered a "garden," as Keil and Delitzsch render "vineyard" as "vine-garden" (*Commentary on the Old Testament: Song of Songs*, Keil & Delitzsch; p. 518).

Confusion is one of Satan's most effective tools. As it is written, "...neither shall ye use enchantment, nor observe times," (Leviticus 19:26) as in sorcery. The Magi followed the "the star" to find the young Christ. "In the time of King Herod, after Jesus was born in Bethlehem, *wise men from the east*, came to Jerusalem, asking, 'Where is the child who has been born king of the Jews? For we observed his star in the east, and have come to pay homage," (Matthew 2:1-2), just as, "...Jehovah Elohim planted a garden in *Eden, in the east*...," (Genesis 2:8). Consider:

"...wise men, from the east..."
"...Eden, in the east..."

"...wise men ["μαγοι" (ref. *3097*)], from the east..."
"...Eden ["עדן" (ref. 5731)], in the east..."

Both "wise men" and "Eden" have the same gematria, hence the similarity of description between them concerning the "east":

wise men = "μαγοι" (ref. 3097) = "μ+α+γ+ο+ι" = 40+1+3+70+10 = **124**
Eden = "עדן" (ref. 5731) = "ן+ד+ע" = 50+4+70 = **124**

Deuteronomy 18: 9-14 states: "When thou shalt have entered into the land which the Lord thy God giveth thee, thou shalt not learn to do according to the abominations of those nations. There shall not be found in thee one... who uses divination, who deals with omens, and augury; one who has in him a divining spirit, an observer of signs, questioning the dead. For every one that does these things is an abomination to the Lord thy God; for because of these abominations the Lord will destroy them from before thy face." The abominable diviners were probably similar to those degenerate "Magi" who were not part of (or were no longer part of) the original Persian priesthood, for: "Ye shall not save the lives of sorcerers," (Exodus 22:18); "Ye shall keep My Sabbath, and reverence My sanctuaries; I am the Lord. Ye shall not attend to those who have in them divining spirits, nor attach yourselves to enchanters, to pollute yourselves with them; I am the Lord your God," (Leviticus 19: 30-31). "The soul that shall follow those who have in them divining spirits, or enchanters, I will set my face against that soul, and will destroy it from among the people," (Leviticus 20:6).

"As for a man or woman, whosoever of them shall have in them a diving spirit, or be an enchanter, let them both die the death. Ye shall stone them with stones; they are guilty," (Leviticus 20:27); Dr. Ginsburg noted that, "The woman is here expressly added, both because this art seems to have been principally followed by women (Exod. xxii. 28; I Sam. xxviii. 7; Acts xvi. 16), and because men would naturally be inclined to treat women more mercifully," (*Leviticus*, Ginsburg; p. 207). As there were many female Pharisees, the following is recounted:

"'Joanna the daughter of Retib... was a certain sorceress widow, who, when the time of any child's birth drew near, shut up the womb of the child-bearing woman with magic arts, that she could not be delivered. And when the poor woman had endured long and great torments, she would say, I will go and pray for you; perhaps my prayers will be heard: when she was gone, she would dissolve the enchantments, and presently the infant would be born... she [the female Pharisee being discussed] was a witch. I have therefore cited these passages, not only that it may be shown that there were women-Pharisees, and so that the name is not taken from interpreting or expounding, but that it may be observed also what kind of women, for the most part, embrace Pharisaism; namely, widows and maids, under the veil of sanctity and devotion, hiding and practicing all manner of wickedness. And so much we gain of the history of the Pharisees..." (*Commentary on the New Testament from the Talmud and Hebraica*, Lightfoot; Vol. 2, p. 68-69).

"Members of the Sanhedrin had to be 'masters of sorcery' in order to be able to carry out the death sentence against sorcerers who might otherwise have been able to use their sorcery to protect themselves from capital punishment," (*Baal Ha Turim*; p. 2009). "Members of the Sanhedrin had to be 'masters of sorcery'..." as the term, "...'masters of sorcery'... referred to Torah scholars who had studied the black arts..." (*Baal Ha Turim*, Gold; p. 2009): "Moreover I saw under the sun that in the place of justice, wickedness is there, and in the place of righteousness, wickedness is there also," (Ecclesiastes 3:16). The members of the Sanhedrin who accused Christ of enchantment were known as "Masters of Sorcery" themselves, though they had a convenient excuse for being such masters, and they accused Christ falsely on account of their own guilt. Yet, in a good sense, "...just as Moses lifted up the serpent in the wilderness, so must the Son of Man be lifted up, that whoever believes in Him may have eternal life," (John 3:14). The concept of the "serpent" carried the possibility of either positive or negative applications. Consider these two closely related but opposing ideas:

1)   "לחשׁ" (ref. 3907) = "whisper, charmer; to mumble a spell (as a magician) [possibly originally serpent charming]," (*Brown-Driver Briggs Hebrew & English Lexicon*)" = "שׁ+ח+ל" = 300+8+30 = **338**.

2)   "לחשׁ" (ref. 3908) = "a whisper, (in a good sense) a private prayer," = "שׁ+ח+ל" = 300+8+30 = **338**.

In a similar way, the word "magic" was positively (though not altogether accurately) applied to the study of disciplines of intense observation and study outside of common knowledge: astronomy, meteorology, medicine, etc.

Matthew 2:1: "...*wise men* [**124**], from the east..."
Genesis 2:8"...*Eden* [**124**], in the east..."
Matthew 24:27: "For as the *lightning* cometh out of the east..."; "lightning" = "לפיד" (ref. 3940) = "ד+י+פ+ל" = 4+10+80+30 = **124**.

The word "magic" was negatively applied to enchantment, witchcraft, communications with the dead, divination involving serpents and corpses, etc. The "miraculous" was sometimes deemed "magic" as the two words are connected by way of *astonishment*, though they are antithetical in meaning; for example: "He [Jesus] went up the mountain and called to Him those whom He wanted, and they came to Him. And He appointed 12 [*like the Zodiac; like the Tribes of Israel*], whom He also named apostles, to be with Him, and to be sent out to proclaim the message, and to have authority to cast out demons. So He appointed the 12: Simon (to whom He gave the name Peter); James son of *Zebedee* [*Jehovah's Gift*] and *John* [*Jehovah has Graciously Given*] the brother of James (to whom He gave the names Boanerges, that is, *Sons of Thunder*); and Andrew, and Philip, and Bartholomew, and *Mathew* [*Gift of Jehovah*], and Thomas, and James son of Alphaeus, and Thaddaeus, and Simon the *Canaanite*, and Judas Iscariot {5}, who betrayed Him. Then He went home; and the crowd came together again, so that they could not eat. When His family heard it, they went out to restrain Him, for the people were saying, 'He has gone out of His mind.' And the Scribes [*who were masters of sorcery*] who came down from Jerusalem said, 'He has Beelzebul, and by the rule of demons He casts out demons.' And He called them to Him, and spoke to them in *parables* ["משל" (ref. 4911) = **370**], 'How can Satan cast out Satan? If a *kingdom* ["משל" (ref. 4915) = **370**] is divided against itself, that **house** will not be able to stand,'" (Mark 3:13-25).

"בניה" (ref. 1140) = "a structure; building" = "ב+נ+י+ה" = 5+10+50+2 = **67**

"בינה" (ref. 998) = "*knowledge; wisdom*" = "ב+י+נ+ה" = 5+50+10+2 = **67**

"גחון" (ref. 1512) = "the external abdomen; belly (**as the source of the fetus**) = "ג+ח+ו+ן" = 50+6+8+3 = **67**

"גחון" (ref. 1521) = "Gihon, a river of Paradise; also a valley (or pool) near Jerusalem" = "ג+ח+ו+ן" = 50+6+8+3 = **67**

The word "בית" (ref. 1004) = "a house," signified by the letter "ב," is rendered "daughter" in Isaiah 10:32. The word "בת" (ref. 1323) = "a daughter" is from "בנה" (ref. 1129) = "*to build,* **obtain children**." A "house" that cannot stand is a "*fallen*" house (as in Luke 11:17): "נפל" (ref. 5309) = "something *fallen*, i.e. an **abortion:- untimely birth**" = "נ+פ+ל" = 30+80+50 = **160** – this is a reason that Luke 11:17 states that "a house *divided* ["נפל" = **160**] against itself shall *fall* ["נפל" = **160**]," and this teaching was met with the exclamation, "Blessed is the *womb* which bore You..." (Luke 11:27). As the letter/number "ב" = 2 signifies a "house" in relation to *a womb*, the story of Creation in Genesis 1:1 (that thematically begins at **Virgo**, the Virgin – the first in the celestial order) begins with the letter "ב = 2" in agreement with Genesis 2:24 where two become one. Consider the Book of Job as well: "Who is this that darkens counsel by words without knowledge? Gird up your *loins* like a man, I will question you, and you will declare to Me. Where were you when I laid the *foundation* of the earth? Tell me if you have *understanding* [(ref. 998) = **67**]. Who determined its measurements – surely you know! Or who stretched a line upon it? On what were its bases sunk, or who laid its *cornerstone* when the morning stars sang together and all the sons of God shouted for Joy? Or who shut in the sea with doors when it **burst forth from the womb**?" (Job 38:2-8). Accordingly, the first letter of the New Testament's first Book is the Greek equivalent of the Hebrew "ב" (or "2") which is "B" (or "2" as well): "The book of the **generations** of Jesus Christ..." (Matthew 1:1).

The firstborn human, the event that all of creation was waiting for, the ultimate gift that God Himself gave to the first humans before they were found guilty of sin, was killed in the womb of Adam's wife after she mistakenly consumed the poison ("רוש"/"ראש" = ref. 7219) that came from the Tree of the Knowledge of Good and Evil – a substance that is described as "the venom of the serpent." The woman thought that she could become wise through artificial (and rebellious) means. The first sin resulted in a miscarriage, and the firstborn human was birthed as a corpse "...as one dead, who proceeded from the womb of OUR mother..." (Numbers 12:12). The chilling history of the murder in Eden is certainly displeasing to the ear... but, being the Holy Word of God, and being the one answer that begins to unlock the many "Why?" questions that have plagued the Church for nearly 2,000 years, this history ought never to be altered to please human ears lest it be covered over for another 2,000 years.

Humanity did not fall as the result of an arbitrary piece of fruit, but humanity fell because the fruit of Eve's womb "fell" ("נפל" = "something fallen, abortion, untimely birth") by her own ignorant, but rebellious, hand at the coaxing of the Adversary and at the foolish agreement of her husband who was to "guard" Eden but failed in doing so. Eve had no idea that her child would die as a result of her new "knowledge," as we can see that the concept behind the word "to make wise" could have been only perceived (although mistakenly) as "wisdom" by Eve, for the forbidden "tree" could, under no circumstances, have been "desirable to suffer abortion," nor was her decision wise in any way. Rather, the vaguely recollected transmission of eroded tradition was Satan's main tool that fashioned blindness.

After asking a simple question from a false premise (like reckoning the celestial "scroll" from Taurus: Genesis 3:1), Satan himself deceived Eve by providing an oral interpretation of God's Law that was (errantly) dependent on God's Word, but Satan only told a limited version of God's Word. In the same way, the Pharisees, the elite group whose main doctrine was that *the oral law was necessary to complete the Written Law* were called "vipers," (John 3:7). Consider the fact that "the woman "saw that the tree was good for food, that it was pleasant to the eyes, and that it was desirable to make one wise," (Genesis 3:6) – how could Eve have "seen" all of those things?: "Woe to those wise in their own eyes, and discerning in their own sight!" (Isaiah 5:21). How could the description of "good" be apart from evil in a tree that was named the Tree of the Knowledge of Good *and* Evil? "Woe to those who draw iniquity with an inheritance of desolating evil... Woe to those who say to evil, good; and to good, evil; who put darkness for light and light for darkness..." (Isaiah

5:18-20); "... even Satan disguises himself as an angel of light," (II Corinthians 11:14). "Woe to those... who put bitter for sweet and sweet for bitter!" (Isaiah 5:20); "Do you not know this from of old, from setting of Adam on earth? ... Even if evil is sweet in his mouth – he hides it under his tongue, he spares it, and will not leave it; yea, keeps holding it in his mouth – yet his food in his belly shall be turned; the gall of asps is within him. He swallows wealth, but vomits it; God drives it out from his belly. He shall suck the poison of asps; the viper's tongue shall slay him." (Job 20:4-16). "Either make the tree good, and its fruit good; or make the tree bad, and its fruit bad; for the tree is known by its fruit. You brood of vipers! How can you speak good things, when you are evil? For out of the abundance of the heart the mouth speaks. The good person brings good things out of a good treasure, and the evil person brings evil things out of an evil treasure. I tell you, on the day of judgment you will have to give an account of for every careless word you utter; for by your words you will be justified, and by your words you will be condemned," (Matthew 12:33-37) {6}.

[2.55] Since a new moon is considered the firstborn of the month (which then indicates the festival of the Head of the Month), a solar eclipse would darken this birth. Job 3 links the darkening of day to an abortive birth, for many ancients considered Typhon (Satan) to be the cause of solar eclipses, dark clouds, terrible storms, etc. (compare to Revelation 12). We may reflect on the cloud-cover that hung over Christ's crucifixion, for solar eclipses do not last as long as the "darkness" present at Jesus' death. Considering the link between the words "head" ("ראש" =

"ש+א+ר" = 300+1+200 = **501**) and "poison" ("ראש" = "ש+א+ר" = 300+1+200 = **501**), we might also consider these words:

"Give ear O heavens, and I will speak; let the earth hear the words of my mouth. May my teaching drop like rain... They are a nation void of sense; there is no understanding in them. If they were wise, they would understand this... Indeed their rock is not like our Rock; our enemies are fools. Their vine comes from the vinestock of Sodom, from the vineyards of Gomorrah; their grapes are grapes of poison, their clusters are bitter; their wine is the poison of serpents, the cruel venom of asps. Is not this laid up in store with me, sealed up in my treasuries?" (Deuteronomy 32:1-35).

"The years of the book [of Deuteronomy] are from the eleventh month on the first of the month unto the first month on the tenth of the month, i.e. **seventy** days, thirty of them were spent wherein they lamented and three days in which they provided food for themselves, i.e. **three and thirty**, there are left **thirty and seven** days," (*Introduction to the Ginsburg Edition of the Hebrew Old Testament*, 68). Observe how the time periods of Deuteronomy are grouped in **70**, **33** and **37**, and notice also how these numeric groupings align with the eclipse cycle called *Saros*: "...the important point is this, that if we take the prophetic reckoning of 360 days to the year, we have the following significant Biblical numbers:- In the first place, we already have the **70** +/- *Sari* divided into two portions of **33+37**. A perfect cycle is accomplished in **33** *Sari*, or 595 years, when the eclipse, by a series of unbroken *Sari*, has accomplished a passage through the year of 360 days; or, if we reckon only the whole numbers, i.e., the 18 completed years, we have for the **33** *Sari* the period of 594 years, while the remaining portion of **37** *Sari* makes 666 years (37x18); and the whole **70 +/-** *Sari* makes 1,260 years (594+666)," (*Witness of the Stars*, Bullinger; p. 181) {7}.

SECTION III

ג

A GARDEN, A VINEYARD, OR A PARADISE?

"And the Lord God planted a garden *in* Eden, in the east..." (Genesis 2:8).

"For since the creation of the world God's invisible qualities – His eternal power and divine nature – have been clearly seen, being understood from what has been made, so that men are without excuse," (Romans 1:20).

"...you drank fine wine from the blood of grapes," (Deuteronomy 32:14).

[3.1]   Let us observe a few definitions:

ג = "גמל" (ref. 1581) = from ref. 1580 (in the sense of *labor* or *burden-bearing*): a *camel*; "בכר" (ref. 1070) = "(in the sense of *youth*); *a young camel:*- dromedary"; from "בכר" (ref. 1069) = "to burst the *womb*, i.e. (caus.) bear or make early *fruit (of woman or tree)*; also to give the birthright:- make firstborn, be firstling, bring forth first child (new fruit)." As this letter "ג" is also the number "3," we can understand the fruitful union of a husband and wife that brings forth a third member into their family unit, for the "ג" is linked to the firstborn, the third member of the family, not the fourth member nor any other successive member.

"*I have spread out My hands* all the day unto a rebellious people, which walketh in a way that was not good, after their own thoughts; a people that provoketh Me to anger continually to My face; that sacrificeth in gardens and burneth incense upon altars of brick," (Isaiah 65:3). "Now there was a garden in the place where He was *crucified*, and in the garden there was a new tomb in which no one had ever been laid," (John 19:41).

"דם" (ref. 1818) = "*blood* (as that which when shed causes death) of a man or animal; by analogy, *the juice of the grape*; figuratively bloodshed (i.e. drops of blood)."

"αιμα" (ref. *129*) = "*blood* literally (of men or animals), figuratively (*the juice of grapes*) or specifically (the atoning blood of Christ); by implication bloodshed, also kindred:- blood."

[3.2] "There are several kinds of figs mentioned in the Talmudists besides these common ones; namely, figs of a better sort, which grew in gardens and paradises," (*Commentary on the New Testament from the Talmud and Hebraica*, Lightfoot; Vol. 2, p. 279).

There are distinctions between the words "garden," "vineyard," and "paradise," as these three terms apply to physical places that illustrated the grandeur of Scriptural accounts in relation to Heavenly reality. "The Greek word παραδεισος [*paradise*] occurs in the Septuagint twenty-eight times. In nine it represents the Hebrew word "Eden"; and in nineteen places the Hebrew word גן (*gan*), *garden*. In English it is rendered *Eden, Garden, Forest, Orchard*, (*How to Enjoy the Bible*, Bullinger; p. 256). English has the tendency to blend the word "paradise" with other similar but distinct terms. "Jehovah Elohim planted a garden *in* Eden, to the east, and He put the man whom He had formed there," (Genesis 2:8); that is God put the man in a specific garden within Eden. Eden housed a garden.

"And Jehovah Elohim took the man and put him in the גן [*garden* (ref. 1588)] of Eden to cultivate and to guard it," (Genesis 2:15).

"...Asaph the guardian of the of the king's פרדס [*forest* (**ref. 6508**)]..." Nehemiah 2:8.

"I made my works great – I built houses for myself; I planted כרמים [*vineyards* (ref. 3754)] for myself; I made גנות [*gardens* (ref. 1593)] and פרדסים [*paradises* (**ref. 6508**)] for myself, and I planted trees in them, of every fruit; I made pools of water for myself, to water from them the יַעַר [*forest* (ref. 3293)] shooting forth trees," (Ecclesiastes 2:4-6).

Notice how "paradise" is rendered "forest" in Nehemiah 2:8 regarding the guardian Asaph's guarded territory, but that this "forest" is a different word than what is used to describe the "forest" in Ecclesiastes 2:6 above. A paradise was "a park, a forest where wild beasts were kept for hunting; a pleasure-park, a garden of trees of various kinds..." (*The Analytical Lexicon to the Greek New Testament*, Mounce; p. 351).

A vineyard was considered a type of "garden," though a "garden" does not necessarily have to be a vineyard also. "Gardens," "vineyards," and "paradises" were guarded, as is evident in Genesis 2:15 and Nehemiah 2:8; we must discover more intricate realities regarding these three related terms in order to increase the precision of our inspection of Eden.

[3.3] Let us consider the fig-leaf* garments that Adam and Eve selected to cover their nudity. The first humans covered themselves out of shame because of the intentional and guilty actions they exacted that accidentally (from their standpoint) slew their firstborn:

*"תאנה" (ref. 8384) = "the fig (tree or fruit):- fig (tree) = "ה+נ+א+ת" = 5+50+1+400 = **456**
"תאנה" (ref. 8385) = "an opportunity; purpose; occasion" = "ה+נ+א+ת" = 5+50+1+400 = **456**

"תאן" (ref. 8384) = "fig (tree)" = "ן+א+ת" = 50+1+400 = **451**
"תאן" (ref. 8383) = "naughtiness, i.e. toil:- lie" = "ן+א+ת" = 50+1+400 = **451**

"בכורה" (ref. 1063) = "the early fig" = "ה+ר+ו+כ+ב" = 5+200+6+20+2 = **233**
"בכורה" (ref. 1062) = "the firstling of man or beast; firstborn" = "ה+ר+ו+כ+ב" = 5+200+6+20+2 = **233**

Let us reflect on the prophecy of Genesis 3:15: "I will put enmity between you and the woman, and between your offspring and hers; He will strike your head, and you will strike His heel."

"נבא" (ref. 5012) = "prophesy" = "א+ב+נ" = 50+2+1 = **53**
"גן" (ref. 1588) = "a garden (as fenced)" = "ן+ג" = 50+3 = **53**
"אבן" (ref. 70) = "a potter's wheel or a midwife's stool" = "ן+ב+א" = 50+2+1 = **53**
"אבן" (ref. 68) = "to build; a stone" = "ן+ב+א" = 50+2+1 = **53**

"The stone [**53**] which the builders rejected has become the Head [**501**] of the corner," (Psalm 118:23).

"ראש" (ref. 7217) corresponds to ref. 7218; Chaldee = "*the head;* (figuratively) the sum:- chief" = "ש+א+ר" = 300+1+200 = **501**.

"ראש" (ref. 7218) = "from an unused root apparently meaning to *shake;* the *head (as most easily shaken),* whether literally or figuratively (in many applications, of place, time, rank, etc.):- band, beginning, captain, chapter, chief, excellent, first, forefront, height, (on) high, ruler, sum, top"

= "ש+א+ר" = 300+1+200 = **501**. "ראש" or "רוש" (ref. 7219) = "a poisonous plant; poison (even of *serpents*):- gall." = "ש+א+ר" = 300+1+200 = **501**.

Many of the ancients thought that Typhon (Leviathan), by illustration at least, swallowed the sun whereby a solar eclipse was produced. Typhon was also thought to be in, or the cause of, certain storms, like the "typhonic" storm of Acts 27:14. A typhonic storm, or one like it, could darken the skies considerably in order to produce an effect similar to, but longer-lasting than, a solar eclipse. When we reflect on the darkness that hung over the crucifixion of Christ, the word "darkness" used in that account (as in Matthew 27:45) is "σκοτος" (ref. *4655*) = "darkness" = "σ+κ+ο+τ+ο+ς" = 200+20+70+300+70+6 = **666**. Solar eclipses only last for minutes and they occur at new moon (birth), and the renewing moon was celebrated as the *head* of the month. The darkness that hung over Christ lasted for hours, and Passover occurs at full moon. We can perceive why the descriptions of darkness and eclipses in Job 3 are paralleled by the "darkness' that hung over the cross of Christ; for in both apparent influences of Typhon (Leviathan), light was obscured and darkness was asserted. In a sense, the sun was "eclipsed" – if you will – by the cloud-cover that hung over Jesus' crucifixion, and as He is "Firstborn of the Dead," we can understand a link to Job 3 and Genesis 3.

[3.4]   "There is no anathema at Jerusalem... In it they do not plant trees, except gardens of roses, which were there from the days of the former prophets: they do not nourish it with peacocks, or cocks... They make no paradises in

Jerusalem... (*Commentary on the New Testament from the Talmud and Hebraica*, Lightfoot; Vol. 1, p. 48). Among the most important facts concerning gardens, vineyards, and paradises, is that all three, though beautiful in their construction and nature, were also often joined to cemeteries, or in close proximity to cemeteries, in ancient times. Despite all of their serene beauty, gardens, vineyards, and paradises (which were enclosed by hedges and walls) were also places of, or near, death.

Jesus prayed to His Father on behalf of His followers, "Now they know that everything You have given Me is from You; for the words that You gave to Me I have given to them, and they have received them and know in truth that I came from You; and they have believed that You sent Me. I am asking on their behalf; I am not asking on behalf of the world, but on behalf of those whom You gave Me, because they are Yours. All Mine are Yours, and Yours are Mine; and I have been glorified in them. And now I am no longer in the world, but they are in the world, and I am coming to You... The glory that You have given Me I have given them, so that they may be one, as We are One," (John 17:7-22). "After Jesus had spoken these words, He went out with his disciples across the *Kidron* [*Very Black; Full of Darkness; Great Obscurity; Wall; Mourner*] valley to a place where there was a garden, which He and His disciples entered," (John 18:1).

In thematic relation to the darkness present during the crucifixion of Christ, notice also how the word for "eclipse (obscuration as if from a shrinkage of light)" is "כמריר" (ref. 3650) and is from "כמר" (ref. 3648) = "כ+מ+ר" = 200+40+20 = **260**:

"כמר" (ref. 3648) = "be black; be kindled; yearn [grow warm (*Brown-Driver-Briggs Lexicon*)]" = "כ+מ+ר" = 200+40+20 = **260**; "They said to each other, 'Were not our hearts burning within us?'" (Luke 24:32).

"כרם" (ref. 3754) = "a garden or vineyard" = "כ+ר+ם" = 40+200+20 = **260**; "Now there was a garden in the place where He was crucified, and in the garden there was a new tomb in which no one had ever been laid," (Luke 19:41).

"מכר" (ref. 4376) = "to *sell* literally (as merchandise, a daughter into marriage [or] into slavery), or figuratively to *surrender*" = "מ+כ+ר" = 200+20+40 = **260**; "I feel a divine jealousy for you, for I promised you in marriage to one husband, to present you as a chaste virgin to Christ. But I am afraid that as the serpent deceived Eve by its cunning, your thoughts will be led astray from a sincere and pure devotion to Christ," (II Corinthians 11:2-3).

"מכר" (ref. 4376) = "merchandise" = "מ+כ+ר" = 200+20+40 = **260**; "When Jesus had received the wine, He said, 'Paid in full.' Then He bowed His head and died," (John 19:30).

"מרך" (ref. 4816) = "fear; faintness" = "מ+ר+ך" = 20+200+40 = **260**;
"Then He said to them, 'I am deeply grieved, even to death; remain here, and stay awake with Me,'" (Matthew 26:38).

"רמך" (ref. 7424) = "dromedary" = "ר+מ+ך" = 20+40+200 = **260**; "רכב" (ref. 1070) = "(in the sense of youth); a young camel:- *dromedary*"; from "בכר" (ref. 1069) = "to burst the womb, i.e. (caus.) bear or make early fruit (of woman or tree)."

[3.5] The word "paradise," "according to Spiegel, was derived from the Zendic pairi-daeza, a hedging round, and passed into the Hebrew in the form פרדס (Cant. 4:13; Eccl. 2:5; Neh. 2:8), a park, probably through the commercial relations which Solomon established with different countries," (*Commentary on the Old Testament: Genesis*, Keil & Delitzsch; p. 50). Παραδεισος = "a park, a forest where wild beasts were kept for hunting; a pleasure-park, a garden of trees of various kinds; used in the LXX for the Garden of Eden; in N.T. the celestial paradise, Luke 23:43; 2 Cor 12:4; Rev 2:7," (*The Analytical Lexicon to the Greek New Testament*, Mounce; p. 351).

Though the Garden of Eden is often called "Paradise," we should note the fact that gardens and paradises are two different entities, and that the garden described in Genesis 2:8 is not described as The Garden OF Eden but rather "a garden IN Eden." Eden existed prior to the garden Jehovah Elohim planted within it which is a reason why it is not written that God planted Eden, but that He planted a garden (not a paradise) in Eden (which was a paradise by definition), which is also why we read of the animals being created prior to humans in Genesis 1. The confusion arises partially because both a "paradise" and a "garden" denote an enclosure, hedging, or fortification

A Garden, A Vineyard, or A Paradise? 291

of some kind. The garden of Adam's dwelling, due to strict diction, can be understood as a smaller enclosure within the larger enclosure of Eden.

Regarding Eden, Dr. Bullinger noted: "Eden. In the cuneiform texts = the plain of Babylonia, known in the Accado-Sumerian as edin = 'the fertile plain,' called by its inhabitants Edinu," (*Companion Bible*, Bullinger; p. 5). The idea of fertility is connected to the conception of Eden and the garden within it. Let us examine the letters that constitute the word "Eden":

"עדן" (ref. 5727) = "to live voluptuously:- delight self" = "ן+ד+ע" = 50+4+70 = **124**

"עדן" (ref. 5729) = "pleasure; Eden, a place in Mesopotamia" = "ן+ד+ע" = 50+4+70 = **124**

"עדן" or "עדנה" (ref. 5730) = "delicate, delight, pleasure [used sexually as in Genesis 18:12 regarding Sarah]" = "ן+ד+ע" = 50+4+70 = **124**

"עדן" (ref. 5731) = "the region of Adam's home" = "ן+ד+ע" = 50+4+70 = **124**

"עדן" (ref. 5732) Chaldee = "a set time; technically a year:- time" = "ן+ד+ע" = 50+4+70 = **124**

[Consider some of the possible reasons why perhaps the Ramban wrote that "The structure of the Garden of Eden corresponds to the structure of the firmament," (*Ramban: Genesis*, Vol. 1, Ramban; p. 131).]

The Scriptures continually utilize aspects of nature as illustrations that accompany the principles of its accounts. Considering the connection between "Eden" and "fertility" in light of the "plain of Babylonia," it is worthwhile to note that "מערה" (ref. 4629) = "a nude place, i.e. a common:- meadows"; connect "a nude place" to the fertility of both Eden and Eve with respect to the fact that Adam was to guard these two, and we can begin to understand the shame involved when Adam and his wife recognized that they were exposed as both guilty of sin and as physically naked in an embarrassing manner. The two humans first covered their loins (fertility) with fig leaves in Genesis 3:7, and then they proceeded to hide themselves amongst the trees in Genesis 3:8 in order to escape the open exposure of "the fertile plain." *Webster's New World Dictionary* defines a "meadow" as a "low, level grassland near a stream, lake, etc." and this definition agrees with Genesis 2:6 that discusses Eden's stream that issued from a spring in connection to the creation of Adam in Genesis 2:7; as Adam was created in connection with stream (as we all are produced), so sin first entered Eden's fertility near a stream through a "nude" place to the demise of life instead of to the creation of life.

[3.6] Keil and Delitzsch wrote, "The Gihon (from גוח *to break forth*) is the Araxes, which rises in the neighborhood of the Euphrates, flows from west to east, joins the Cyrus, and falls with it into the Caspian Sea. The name corresponds to the Arabic Jaihun, a name given by the Arabians and Persians to several large rivers. The land of Cush cannot, of course, be the later Cush or Ethiopia..." (*Commentary on the Old Testament: Genesis*, Keil & Delitzsch; p. 52). "Since the four branches all split off from the same source river, it is impossible for one branch to originate in southern Africa and others in the east,"

A Garden, A Vineyard, or A Paradise?   293

(*Ramban: Genesis, Vol. 1*, Editor; p. 133). Dr. Bullinger wrote, "Gihon = the river E. of the Tigris. The modern Kerkhah, and ancient Khoaspes, rising in the mountains of the Kassi. Kas has been confused with the Heb. Cush. It is not the African Cush or Ethiopia, but the Acadian Kas," (*Companion Bible, Bullinger*, p. 6). The river Gihon is the second ramification named concerning the stream or river in Eden, and the Tree of the Knowledge of Good and Evil is the second specific tree mentioned concerning the garden God planted in Eden.

Considering the ancient recognition of initial letters and concluding letters in successive words of Scripture as a point of observation, it is interesting to note that the final letters in the words "הדעת טוב ורע" ["the Knowledge of Good and Evil"] = "תבע" = "ת+ב+ע" = 70+2+400 = **472**:

"עבת" (ref. 5686) = "to *interlace*, i.e. to pervert:- wrap up" = "ת+ב+ע" = 400+2+70 = **472**

"עבת" (ref. 5687) = "*entwined*, i.e. dense:- thick" = "ת+ב+ע" = 400+2+70 = **472** "עבת" (ref. 5688) = "something *entwined*, i.e. a string, wreath, or foliage:- band, cord, rope, thick bough (branch), wreathen (chain)" = "ת+ב+ע" = 400+2+70 = **472**. "Leviathan" is from the word "לוה" (ref. 3867) which means "*to twine*, by implication to unite, to remain, to borrow (as a form of obligation), to lend, to abide with, to cleave, and to join (self)."

"Your neck is like a tower of ivory; your eyes are like the pools in Heshbon by the gate of a princess," (Song of

Songs 8:6). "*Ḥeshbon [Reason; Device; Counting]...* the pride of *Moab [Water of a father; Seed; Progeny; Desire; Waste; Nothingness]*, was famous for its fertility, verdure of plantation, and beautiful reservoirs," (*Song of Songs*, Ginsburg; p. 179). In a parallel way, "גחון" (ref. 1521) = "Gihon, a river of Paradise" = "ג+ח+ו+ן" = 50+6+8+3 = **67**; "גחון" (ref. 1512) = "the external abdomen; belly (as the source of the fetus) = "ג+ח+ו+ן" = 50+6+8+3 = **67**; "בינה" (ref. 998) = "knowledge; wisdom" = "ב+י+נ+ה" = 5+50+10+2 = **67** (different, but related, word than that of the forbidden tree).

The word we render "Cush" (that is not Ethiopia: Genesis 2:13) concerning the river Gihon is "כוש" (ref. 3578) = "כ+ו+ש" = 300+6+20 = **326**. "Gihon" can also have the same consonantal spelling and gematria as "fetus" and "knowledge." Note that "שוך" (ref. 7753) = "*to entwine*, i.e. shut in (for formation, protection or restraint):- fence, (make a) hedge (up) [like a garden]" = "ש+ו+ך" = 20+6+300 = **326**; "שוך" (ref. 7754) = "a branch (as *interleaved*):- bough" = "ש+ו+ך" = 20+6+300 = **326**. Let us reflect (thematically) on the well in I Samuel 19:22 called *Sechu [They Hedged Up; Watchtower]* = "שכו" (ref. 7906) = "an observatory" "ש+כ+ו" = 6+20+300 = **326** in connection with Isaiah 5:1-2: "Let me sing for my beloved my love-song concerning his vineyard: My beloved had a vineyard on a very fertile hill. He dug it and cleared it of stones, and planted it with choice vines; he built a watchtower in the midst of it, and hewed out a wine vat in it; he expected it to yield grapes, but it yielded wild grapes."

A Garden, A Vineyard, or A Paradise?

Concerning the unexpected and wild productions of vines, let us also reflect on the fact that immediately following Elisha's miracle of reviving a dead child, (II Kings 4:32-37), we read that "When Elisha returned to Gilgal, there was a famine in the land. As the company of prophets was sitting before him, he said to his servant, 'Put the large pot on, and make some stew for the company of prophets.' One of them went out into the field to gather herbs; he found a wild vine and gathered from it a lapful of wild gourds, and came and cut them up into the pot of stew, not knowing what they were. They served some for the men to eat. But while they were eating the stew, they cried out, "O man of God, there is death in the pot!" (II Kings 4:38-40).

Consider the "the vine-tree" of Ezekiel: "the vine-tree" = "עץ־הגפן" = "ע+ץ+ה+ג+פ+ן" = 50+80+3+5+90+70 = **298**:

"רצח" (ref. 7523) = "to dash in pieces, i.e. kill (a human being); to murder" = "ר+צ+ח" = 8+90+200 = **298**

"צחר" (ref. 6713) = "to dazzle; sheen, whiteness, white" = "צ+ח+ר"= 200+8+90 = **298**

"צחר" (ref. 6715) = "white" = "צ+ח+ר" = 200+8+90 = **298**

"צרח" (ref. 6873) = "shrill, cry, roar" = "צ+ר+ח" = 8+200+90 = **298**

"חרץ" (ref. 2757) = "incisure, incised; a threshing-sledge (with sharp teeth)" = "ח+ר+ץ" = 90+200+8 = **298**

"חרץ" (ref. 2782) = "to point sharply, i.e. to wound; to decide, decree, determine" = "ח+ר+ץ" = 90+200+8 = **298**

"חרץ" (ref. 2783) = "the loin (as the seat of strength)" = "ח+ר+ץ" = 90+200+8 = **298**

"חרץ" (ref. 2784) = "a fetter, pain, band" = "ץ+ר+ח" = 90+200+8 = **298**
"חצר" (ref. 2690) = "to surround with a stockade" = "ר+צ+ח" = 200+90+8 = **298**
"חצר" (ref. 2691) = "a yard (as enclosed by a fence)" = "ר+צ+ח" = 200+90+8 = **298**
"רחץ" (ref. 7635) = "to attend upon, trust" = "ץ+ח+ר" = 90+8+200 = **298**

Now, let us consider Jesus' parable in Mark 12 in an abbreviated format: "A man planted a vineyard, put a fence around it, dug a pit for the wine press, and built a watchtower... he sent [his son to the tenants of the vineyard]... they seized him, killed him..."

Eastern gardens contained water sources filled by springs or rain; however, water contained in a cistern is not considered "living" as is the water that gushes forth from a spring (Genesis 2:10). Pools of water were often fed by springs and were used to irrigate land (as reservoirs were also used for similar purposes). "The Lord will guide you continually, and satisfy your needs in parched places, and make your bones strong; and you shall be like a watered garden, like a spring of water, whose waters never fail," (Isaiah 58:11). Gardens, vineyards, and paradises were irrigated, similar to the function of the stream discussed in Genesis 2:5-6: "... for the Lord God had not caused it to rain upon the earth, and there was no one to till the ground; but a stream would rise from the earth, and water the whole face of the ground." The first command given to humanity was, "Be fruitful and multiply and fill the earth..." (Genesis 1:28); "A river flows out of Eden to

A Garden, A Vineyard, or A Paradise?

water the garden, and from there it divides and becomes four branches. The name of the first is *Pishon* [*Great Diffusion*]; it is the one that flows around the whole land of *Havilah* [*Bringing Forth; Trembling with Pain; Sorrow – Especially of Pregnant Women*], where there is *gold*... The name of the second river is *Gihon* [*Great Breaking Forth*]..." (Genesis 2:10-13). "When you take a head count of the Children of Israel according to their numbers, every man shall give to Jehovah atonement-money for his soul when counting them..." (Exodus 30:12). The treasury in the second Temple was in the Court of *Women*. Our souls were ransomed by Christ. The word "ransom" is a financial term. "Shekel" (as in money) and "soul" are intimately connected: "shekel" = "שקל" (ref. 8255) = "ש+ק+ל" = 30+100+300 = **430**; "soul" = "נפש" (ref. 5315) = "נ+פ+ש" = 300+80+50 = **430**.

Fountains, natural springs that often fed gardens, vineyards, and paradises, were called the "eye" of the landscape. The word "עין" (ref. 5869) = "an eye (literal or figurative); by analogy, a fountain (as the eye of the landscape):- affliction, outward appearance" = "ע+י+ן" = 50+10+70 = **130**; "עין" (ref. 5869) = "an eye" = ע+י+ן = 50+10+70 = **130**; "כפל" (ref. 3718) = "a duplicate; double" = "כ+פ+ל" = 30+80+20 = **130**; "עלל" (ref. 5768) = "a babe, infant" "ע+ל+ל"= 30+30+70 = **130**. Similarly, "When Adam had lived **130** years, he became the father of a son in his likeness, according to his image, and named him *Seth* [*Appointed; Compensation; Substitute*]," (Genesis 5:3).

"You make the springs gush forth in the valleys; they flow between the hills, giving drink to every wild animal; the wild asses quench their thirst. By the streams the birds of the air have their habitation; they sing among the branches. From Your lofty abode You water the mountains; the earth is satisfied with the fruit of Your work," (Psalm 104:10-13).

"The water of the Pool of Siloam in Jerusalem was regarded as sacred... The question of where the Pool of Siloam was located has been examined on the basis of reports from the Bible, Josephus, ancient pilgrims and archaeological findings. There were actually two pools. The first, the 'Lower' or older 'Pool of Shiloah' (cf. Isa 8:6;22:9-11) collected water from the Gihon Spring, east of the city, via a short channel. The second, or 'Upper' Pool, also received water from the Gihon Spring, but it came through an underground tunnel that had been cut through rock by King Hezekiah around 701 B.C. Hezekiah strategically situated the Upper Pool within the city walls to serve as a secure water supply. The Lower Pool would have been located outside the city of his day," (*Archaeological Study Bible: NIV*, p. 1,739). Notice how Christ (Elohim) healed a blind man in connection with the Pool of Siloam (John 9:6) compared to how the "serpent" told the woman that, "...your eyes will be opened, and you will be like Elohim..." (Genesis 3:5).

"In I Kings 1:33,38, that which is, in the Hebrew, 'Bring ye Solomon to Gihon: and they brought him to Gihon'; is rendered by the Chaldee, 'Bring ye him to Siloam: and they brought him to Siloam.' Where Kimchi thus; 'Gihon

A Garden, A Vineyard, or A Paradise? 299

is Silom, and it is called by a double name. And David commanded, that they should anoint Solomon at Gihon for a good omen, to wit, that, as the waters of the fountain are everlasting, so might his kingdom be.' So also the Jerusalem writers; 'They do not anoint the king, but at a fountain...'" (*Commentary on the New Testament from the Talmud and Hebraica*, Lightfoot; Volume 1, p. 57). Gihon = "גחון" (ref. 1521) = "a river of Paradise; also a valley (or pool) near Jerusalem."

"Gihon" is spelled two different ways, and the spelling of "Gihon" in the I Kings 1:33 account regarding Solomon is "גחון" (ref. 1521) = "ג+ח+ו+ן" = 50+6+8+3 = **67**, and with good reason, for "בינה" (ref. 998) = "knowledge" = "ב+י+נ+ה" (ref. 998) = 5+50+10+2 = **67** – and King Solomon was the wisest man who ever lived (I Kings 3:12). We cannot help but note that "the external abdomen; belly (as the source of the fetus)" = "ג+ח+ו+ן" = 50+6+8+3 = **67** as well as "knowledge"; in a related way, as the so-called "wisdom" Eve hoped to capture caused her to unintentionally abort her fetus, so King Solomon's first display of wisdom came in I Kings 3:16-28 where King Solomon judged between the truth and a lie with an infant between the two, seemingly about to be killed. Neither Eve, nor her husband, judged properly between the two trees that were both in the midst of Eden. Solomon's prayer was not to know good and evil, but to judge "between" good and evil (I Kings 3:9).

[3.7] Since a fountain is considered "the eye of the landscape," it should be also considered again that the Tree of Life and the Tree of the Knowledge of Good and

Evil were both in the middle of the garden in Eden (Genesis 2:9) in light of the fact that the woman, "... saw that the tree was good for food, and that it was pleasant to the eyes..." (Genesis 3:6), though this text only forwards a probability and not an assertion. It is quite probable that both the Tree of Life and the Tree of the Knowledge of Good and Evil grew near a stream produced by a fountain, hence Psalm 1:1-3: "Blessed is the man who does not walk in the counsel of the wicked or stand in the way of sinners or sit in the seat of mockers. But his delight is in the law of the Lord, and on His law he meditates day and night. He is like a tree planted by streams of water, which yields fruit in season and whose leaf does not wither. Whatsoever he does prospers." Eastern gardens are irrigated, and the streams of water that irrigate them are the result of channels used to regulate the prosperity of a garden's growth. Certainly trees grow near natural streams in nature, even to the extent that they sometimes bow down into them. The point is that the descriptions of the tree, the righteous man, and the streams of water in Psalm 1:1-3 are not arbitrary, for it is quite common knowledge that the Book of Psalms consists of five segments that accord with the five books of the Torah:

Psalms 1-41 correspond to Genesis;
Psalms 42-72 correspond to Exodus;
Psalms 73-89 correspond to Leviticus;
Psalms 90-106 correspond to Numbers;
and Psalms 107-150 correspond to Deuteronomy.

As the first discussion of humanity's righteousness is explained by the first book of the Torah, so the first Psalm discusses the same. There are no arbitrary words in the Scriptures, and it can be reasonably deduced that, based on the construction of the Book of Psalms in accordance with the construction of the Torah, that righteousness was planted by such a stream, as it is also in Revelation 22:1-2: "Then the angel showed me the river of the water of life, as clear as crystal, flowing from the throne of God and of the Lamb down the middle of the great street of the city. On each side of the river stood the Tree of Life, bearing 12 kinds of fruit, yielding its fruit every month."

The concept of "living water" indicates motion. Living water, "that is, water taken from a running stream or a perennial spring, where its continual motion resembles life, in contradistinction to stale or stagnant water," (*Leviticus*, Ginsburg; p. 125); "... living waters, refers to water flowing from its natural source and not contained in a cistern, pool or utensil which prevents continuous flow. This is in contradistinction to a... mikveh, literally, gathering (see Genesis 1:10), which refers to water that has flowed or rained into a cistern or pool that does not have an outlet through which the water can flow forth," (*Baal Ha Turim*, Gold; p. 1140). Consider, "A fountain of gardens, a well of living waters..." (Song of Songs 4:15).

The concept of "living water" or "river of the water of life" has anatomical applications as well. Male emission is euphemistically called "water" in the Scriptures, similar to how private feminine anatomy is sometimes called "door" or "gate." Proverbs 5 warns the young man to refrain from visiting the "door" of the loose woman where others have also visited also so that "wealth" may not be taken from the young man. The young man is reminded to "Drink... flowing water from his own well," (Proverbs 5:15). The question is then asked, "Should your springs be scattered abroad, streams of water in the streets?" (Proverbs 5:16), alluding to forms of promiscuity. Therefore, it is better to "Let your fountain be blessed, and rejoice in the wife of your youth," (Proverbs 5:18).

As the Tree of Life in Revelation 22 stood near the river of the water of life, we can also presume that the same was true in Genesis 3 regarding the two central trees of Eden. The "river of the water of life" flows down the "middle of the great street" in Revelation 22 similar to the two trees in the "midst" of Eden in Genesis 2. The "streams of water" discussed in Psalm 1 are like those of Proverbs 21:1 which also relates to the heart of a king.

[3.8] We have no excuse to invent the geography of Eden, especially since the landscape on which Eden once stood must have been drastically altered by the flood of Noah's time as well as by nature's alterations carried out over millennia. However, we should consider that there are strict definitions attached to the diction employed in the Scriptures of which natural occurrences today allow us to deduce a picture of the possibilities of yesteryear. The Scriptures interpret themselves – so it is nearly inconceivable, regarding the descriptions of Genesis 2 in comparison with its corresponding Scriptures, that the two central trees of Eden stood in some baked climate bereft of water, especially regarding the common expression of "living water" that denoted a fountain that welled up from underground, and particularly due to the fact that gardens, vineyards, and paradises were lush places where sweet water was plentiful. Yet, it seems more than probable that Eden became parched in accordance with the curse against the ground in Genesis 3:17 and in connection with the Cherubs and the "**flaming sword**" who were stationed at the east of the Garden in Genesis 3:24. The word "flaming" = "להט" (ref. 3858) = "to blaze, to burn, to set on fire" = "ל+ה+ט" = 9+5+30 = **44**; "להט" (ref. 3858) = "a blaze (from the idea of *enwrapping*), enchantment" = "ל+ה+ט" = 9+5+30 = **44**. The word "sword" = "חרב" (ref. 2719) = "drought; cutting instrument" = "ח+ר+ב" = 2+200+8 = **210** ; "חרב" (ref. 2717) "to parch (through drought) to kill, slay, decay" = "ח+ר+ב" = 2+200+8 = **210**; "הרב" (ref. 2718) = "to demolish, destroy" = "ה+ר+ב" = 2+200+8 = **210**; "חרב" (ref. 2720)= "parched, ruined" "ח+ר+ב" = 2+200+8 = **210**; "חרב" (ref. 2721) = "drought, desolation, dry, heat, waste" "ח+ר+ב" = 2+200+8 = **210**. In other words, after the ground was cursed by God, Eden probably suffered a temporary drought that began *time's* erosion of it on earth, which is probably a reason why the Cherubs are compared to the *constellations*, for "*Cherub*" means *Celestial; as if Contending*, and likewise the word "מזלה" (ref. 4208) = "from ref. 5140 (נזל) in the sense of *raining; a constellation*, i.e. Zodiacal sign (*as affecting weather*)." "You stretch out the heavens like a tent, You set the beams of your chambers on the waters, You make the clouds Your chariot, You ride on the wings of the wind, You make the winds Your angels, a fire and flame Your ministers," (Psalm 104:2-4). "And Jehovah Elohim planted a garden in Eden, to the east; and there He put the man whom He had formed," (Genesis 2:8). The story of the Cherubs and the flaming sword that were set at the east of Eden in Genesis 3:24 is compared to the Gardener restricting water to His once irrigated garden and allowing it to become parched to death in punishment for the death that Adam sowed in its soil. "At Your rebuke they flee; at the sound of your thunder they take flight," (Psalm 104:7). The entire Torah extends from Genesis 1-3, the Prophets and the Writings extend from the Torah, and the New Testament clutches every branch of the Old Testament and allows the reader to peer backward into the mysterious root of the Scriptural accounts. The word "עַיִן" (ref. 5869) = "an eye (literal or figurative); by analogy, a fountain (as the eye of the landscape)." Adam and Eve's eyes were opened (Genesis 3:7) and they recognized their nakedness after they had sinned. Noting that the word for "eye" also means "fountain," a fountain-like eye is one that cries.

Wine is connected to water when discussing vines: "The Rabbins have a tradition. Over wine which hath not water mingled with it they do not say that blessing, 'Blessed be He that created the fruit of the vine'; but, 'Blessed be He that created the fruit of the tree,'" (*Commentary on the New Testament from the Talmud and Hebraica*, Lightfoot; Vol. 2, p. 351). Watered wine, as opposed to unwatered wine, is called the fruit of the vine, and this fact helps us to understand Habakkuk 2:15: "Alas for you who make your neighbors drink, pouring out your venom until they are drunk, in order to gaze on their nakedness!"; notice the words "venom," "drunk," and "nakedness."

The J.P.S. Tanakh renders Genesis 2:5-6 to communicate, "… the Lord God had not sent rain upon the earth and there was no man to till the soil, but a flow would *well up* from the ground…" Genesis 2:10 then says, "A river issues from Eden to water the garden, and it then divides and becomes four branches"; since a fountain (like that which sprung the water of Eden) is the eye of the landscape, it should be noted that the Hebrew word "לעינים" = "to the eyes" occurs four times in the Old Testament: (Genesis 3:6; I Samuel 16:7; Proverbs 10:26 and Ecclesiastes 11:7). "For when we were in the flesh, the motions of sins, which were by the law, did work in our members to bring forth fruit unto death," (Romans 7:5) – a description paralleled to procreation that is thematically connected with James 1:15: "…and that sin, when it is fully grown, gives birth to death," which is another description paralleled to procreation. After Adam and Eve sinned, "… the eyes of both of them were opened…" (Genesis 3:7). That is, when the eyes of Adam and Eve were opened, their eyes became as fountains; they cried.

Again, a Hebrew understanding of a "nude" place is an open meadow, and it is, most likely, in this open meadow that the two central trees of the Garden of Eden stood in Genesis 2:8-9. This "nude place" = "מערה" (ref. 4629) = "ה+ר+ע+מ" = 5+200+70+40 = **315** shares the same consonants in the same order as these words:

"מערה" (ref. 4630) = "an open spot:- army = "ה+ר+ע+מ" = 5+200+70+40 = **315**

"מערה" (ref. 4631) = "a cavern (as dark):- cave, den, hole" = "ה+ר+ע+מ" = 5+200+70+40 = **315** [pronounced "*meh-aw-raw*"]

[3.9]   Genesis 1:14-15 records, "And Elohim said, 'Let luminaries be in the expanse of the heavens, to divide between the day and the night. And let them be for signs and for seasons and for days and years. And let them be for luminaries in the expanse of the heavens, to give light on the earth.' And it was so." The word rendered "luminaries" here is "מארה" (ref. 3974) = "brightness; chandelier" – thus the creation of the sun, moon, and stars is described beautifully here as God hanging a great chandelier above the earth (Revelation 1:13-16: seven candlesticks, seven stars – "...His countenance was as the sun shining in its strength."); consider the menorah. The word "מאורה" (ref. 3975, pronounced "*meh-oo-raw*") means "something lighted, i.e. an aperture; by implication a crevice or hole of a serpent; den." Concerning the narrative of Eden in Genesis, the great chandelier of the stars (or the great lamp/tree) bears a relation to a serpent's den, and by such a description we can better understand the connection between John 3:14 and John 12:30-36; in John 3:14, Jesus compared Himself to Nehushtan (the serpent on a pole made by Moses in Numbers 21). The Gematria of "Nehushtan" and "darkness" (as in Genesis 1:2) is the same:

"Nehushtan" = "נחשתן" (ref. 5180) = "ן+ת+ש+ח+נ" = 50+400+300+8+50 = **808**

"darkness" = "חשך" (ref. 2822) = "ך+ש+ח" = 500+300+8 = **808**

In John 12:28-29, God's voice was perceived by some as thunder, as an apparent storm was brewing; "Jesus answered and said, 'This voice came not because of Me, but for your sakes. Now is the judgement of this world: now shall the prince of this world [*the serpent of Genesis 3*] be cast out. And I, if I be lifted up from the earth, will draw all men unto Me.' This He said, signifying what death He should die... Then Jesus said unto them, 'Yet a little while is the light with you. Walk while ye have the light, lest *darkness* come upon you: for he that walketh in *darkness* knoweth not whiter he goeth. While ye have the light, believe in the light, that ye may be the children of light," (John 12:30-36): "מאורה" (ref. 3975) = "something lighted, i.e. an aperture; by implication a crevice or hole of a serpent; den." When Jesus was about to be captured in a garden, He said, "... But this is your hour, and the power of darkness" (Luke 22:53), and this word "darkness" is "σκοτος" (ref. *4655*) = "σ+κ+ο+τ+ο+ς" = 200+20+70+300+70+6 = **666**; this "darkness" was discussed soon after He **sweat** drops of blood in the garden (Luke 22:44): "There are serpents... which, by their bites would occasion most bitter deaths: they are horrible pains that afflict any that are struck by them, and an issue of **sweat**, like blood, seizeth them," (*Commentary on the New Testament from the Talmud and Hebraica*, Lightfoot, Vol. 3; p. 208). Jesus is the standard. Satan is the counterfeiter. At the same time, we can understand the menorah, for it is a lamp that symbolizes a tree just like the chandelier/tree of the heavens.

[3.10] "A well is a deep reservoir fed by percolation from the soil, by a spring or by groundwater. The lower part is usually dug into impermeable rock or built with rock and then coated with a thick layer of lime plaster, which prevents seepage. It is possible either to tap into a natural spring or to dig down to the groundwater level," (*Archaeological Study Bible: NIV*, p. 1259). Water also flows naturally from rocks without having to dig for it. Caesarea Philippi (near Galilee) was a center of Baal worship and it stood in a well-watered area at the foot of Mount Hermon where natural spring-water flowed, and, at one time, water once flowed from its mouth. The ancient pagans once believed that Caesarea Philippi was the Doorway to Hell, and that the fertility gods entered into the watery cave to reside in Hades until the Spring season; as a result, sexual immorality was frequently practiced as religious worship at this "Gate of Hell," and some Biblical experts believe this to be the "rock" in which Christ declared that He would build His Church (Bride) in Matthew 16:18 – "... and on this rock I will build my Church, and the gates of Hades will not overcome it," as it is believed by some that Christ prophesied His dominance over Evil so that righteousness could burst forth as living water.

The stream that issued from Eden was, most likely, a natural spring that spouted from a rock (possibly a cave). When reflecting on "מאורה" (ref. 3975) = "something lighted, i.e. an aperture; by implication a crevice or hole of a serpent; den," consider the ancient map of the serpentine constellation Cetus as discussed in Revelation 12:13-15: "When the dragon saw that he had been hurled to the earth, he pursued the woman who had given birth to the male child. The woman was given the two wings of a great eagle, so that she might fly to the place prepared for her in the desert, where she would be taken care of for a time,

A Garden, A Vineyard, or A Paradise? 309

[two] times, and half a time, out of the serpent's reach. Then from his mouth the serpent spewed water like a river, to overtake the woman and sweep her away with the torrent." The ancient maps of the heavens depict Cetus (the sea monster) near the river Eridanus and Andromeda (the chained woman), and Cetus is opposite of Virgo (who is often depicted with wings), as it is clear why "The woman was given the two wings of a great eagle..." in Revelation 12:14. Virgo flies above the Hydra. The celestial lights discussed in Revelation 12 serve as natural illustrations in the remembrance of former times. The "time, [two] times, and half a time" is the same as the numbers 1,260, or 42, or 3.5. The "time" discussed denotes the number 360, and "time [360], times [360 x 2] and half a time [180] = 360+720+180 = 1,260 days, which is 42 months on a 360-day prophetic year. "Now the important point is this, that if we take the prophetic reckoning of 360 days to the year, we have the following significant Biblical numbers:- In the first place, we already have the 70 +/- Sari divided into two portions of 33+37. A perfect cycle is accomplished in 33 Sari, or 595 years, when the eclipse, by a series of unbroken Sari, has accomplished a passage through the year of 360 days; or, if we reckon only the whole numbers, i.e., the 18 completed years, we have for the 33 Sari the period of 594 years, while the remaining portion of 37 Sari makes 666 years (37x18); and the whole 70 +/- Sari makes 1,260 years (594+666)," (Witness of the Stars, Bullinger; p. 180-181). The number 70 = ע = "עין" (ref. 5869) = "an eye (literal or figurative); by analogy, a fountain (as the eye of he landscape), and is probably reflected by the celestial river Eridanus on the ancient star maps in order to preserve the memory of the

river that issued from Eden in Genesis 2:10, thus the four "heads," as the celestial luminaries were created on Day Fourth of Creation.

It can be reasonably deduced that the two central trees in the Garden of Eden were located together in a meadow, and that there was a cave in relatively close proximity to those trees that is paralleled to the den of a serpent and that issued a stream. It can also be reasonably considered that the constellations were so mapped as to recall the first sin in connection with the final sacrifice, as Jehovah Elohim stated, "He will bruise your head, and you will bruise His heel," (Genesis 3:15), for this prophetic declaration is remembered by the constellation we now call Hercules (who crushes the head of the Leviathan), and Hercules is reflected by Ophiuchus who wrestles with the serpent while he crushes the head of Scorpio; "then do not exalt yourself, forgetting the Lord your God, Who brought you out of the land of Egypt, out of the house of slavery, Who led you through the great and terrible wilderness, an arid wasteland with fiery serpents and scorpions. He made water flow for you from flint rock," (Deuteronomy 8:14-15). When considering that Jesus depicted Himself "spewing" out His mouth along with the fact that Satan is depicted in a similar manner by the constellation Cetus (Revelation 12:15), we can understand again that Satan desired to be like the Most High (Isaiah 14:4), for Christ is called the "Righteous Branch" in Jeremiah 23:5 and Satan is called the "loathed branch" in Isaiah 14:19, just as Christ compared Himself to a serpent in John 3:14 and Satan is compared to a serpent in Genesis 3:1. *The Exhaustive Dictionary of Bible Names* by Cornwall & Smith defines the Divine Title "Jehovah-Nissi" this way: "(Exodus 17:8-15); the Lord is a Banner; the Lord my banner; the Lord our banner; root = 'Nissi' = Banner; an ensign; a standard (Isaiah 5:26; 49:22; 62:10; compare Psalm 20:5; 60:4). A sign (Numbers 26:10); and a pole in connection with the brazen serpent (Numbers 21:9)..." The *Exhaustive Dictionary of Bible Names*, Cornwall & Smith; p. 87).

[3.11] Historically, we have deduced that Christ died on the cross, and that a "cross" is two pieces of wood crossed over each other. Yet, there is no such term to be found in the New Testament, and not all crucifixions were conducted on crosses. Some crucifixions were conducted upon mere upright poles. The Greek words that we render "cross" in English are

1) "ξυλον" (ref. *3586*) = "a stick, club, or tree," (I Peter 2:24; Revelation 2:7).

2) "σταυρος" (ref. *4716*) = "a stake, a post, a support," (used in the Gospels to indicate what Christ hung on).

The "cross" of Christ is thematically paralleled to the central "trees" of the Garden in Eden where the accursed vine coiled about the Tree of Life, as opposed to when Christ called Himself the "True Vine" in John 15:1 in opposition to the false vine, i.e. Satan by Antithetical Parallel. That is, Christ was as a vine hanging from a tree. Let us recall that the "tree" of the knowledge of Good and Evil was a "vine-tree," similar to that discussed in Ezekiel 15, as is old news to Jews. Given the information above, it is useful to remember that, "The Talmud and Midrash record a dispute regarding the species of the Tree of Knowledge. According to one view, it was a grapevine..." (*Baal Ha Turim*, Gold; p. 1397). Again, "... the tree from which Adam ate [was a grape vine, as the Midrash derives from the verse,]... their grapes are grapes of gall (Deuteronomy 32:32)," (*Baal Ha Turim*: brackets by Gold; p. 1397). "And to the passage of the [wife suspected of faithlessness], the Torah juxtaposed the passage concerning a Nazirite, because the tree from which Adam ate [was a grapevine, as the Midrash derives from...,] their grapes are grapes of gall (Deuteronomy 32:32)," (*Baal Ha Turim*; p. 1396). By recognizing the Tree of the Knowledge of Good and Evil as a "vine-tree," this tree is thematically paralleled to words like "to dash in pieces, i.e. kill (a human being); to murder, shrill, cry, roar, to point sharply, to wound; to decide, decree, determine, the loin, a yard (as enclosed by a fence)" and the like. However, it still appears that Christ died on two pieces of wood crossed over each other that were remembered in connection with a "tree" and a "steak" because a word for "anointed" is "ממשח" (ref. 4473) = "with outstretched wings; from ref. 4886," as this word is also used to describe Satan before he became Evil in Ezekiel 28 (though Christ and Satan are not equal, for Satan is only a creation). "*I have spread out My hands* all the day unto a rebellious people, which walketh in a way that was not good, after their own thoughts; a people that provoketh Me to anger continually to My face; that sacrificeth in gardens and burneth incense upon altars of brick," (Isaiah 65:3). If Christ did not die on a cross, then His hands would have been pulled straight up on an upright pole (as was commonly done); but since He had

A Garden, A Vineyard, or A Paradise? 313

"outstretched wings," He must have died on a cross. By understanding a "cross" by way of the words "tree" and "post," we can observe the connection of the cross of Christ to the midst of the garden in Eden.

Both The Tree of the Knowledge of Good and Evil and the Tree of Life stood in the midst of Eden upon the strength of the Tree of Life, for the Tree of the Knowledge of Good and Evil was a vine as such vines lack the strength to stand upright on their own. This wicked vine coiled and slithered around the trunk and branches of the Tree of Life, just as the ancient celestial maps depict the constellation we now call Hercules smashing the head of a vine-serpent. Let us recall the observation concerning the final letters in the words "הדעת טוב ורע" ["the Knowledge of Good and Evil"] = "תבע" = "ע+ב+ת" = 70+2+400 = **472**; "עבת" (ref. 5686) = "to *interlace*, i.e. to pervert:- wrap up" = "ת+ב+ע" = 400+2+70 = **472**; "עבת" (ref. 5687) = "*entwined*, i.e. dense:- thick" = "ת+ב+ע" = 400+2+70 = **472**; "עבת" (ref. 5688) = "something *entwined*, i.e. a string, wreath, or foliage:- band, cord, rope, thick bough (branch), wreathen (chain)" = "ת+ב+ע" = 400+2+70 = **472**. *Strong's Exhaustive Concordance* defines *Leviathan* as a *Wreathed Animal; Serpent*, as this name is from the word "לוה" which means "*to twine*, by implication to unite, to remain, to borrow (as a form of obligation), to lend, to abide with, to cleave, and to join (self)." The only distinction in geographical proximity between the two central trees of the garden was recognized by the fact that the those two trees had their own respective roots so that, technically speaking, the exact center of Eden was between those two trees, and perhaps this is another reason why King Solomon prayed, "Give your servant therefore an understanding mind... able to discern between good and evil..." (I Kings 3:9). The Tree of the Knowledge of Good and Evil was, most likely, only called a "tree" in the Genesis 3 account (as opposed to "vine" or "vine-tree") due to the fact that the word "tree" by itself is "עץ" (ref. 6086) = "ץ+ע" = 90+70 = **160**, just as "something fallen, abortion, untimely birth" = "נפל" (ref. 5309) = "ל+פ+נ" = 30+80+50 = **160**, in connection to the fact that Christ (The Son of *Man*) died on a "tree" as the True Vine in perfect justice and grace reflected for the Son of Adam who died on account of the false vine coiled about the Tree of Life.

[3.12] "He came a third time and said to them, 'Are you still sleeping and taking your rest? Enough! The hour has come; the Son of Man is betrayed into the hands of sinners," (Mark 14:41). Concerning the Temple during Christ's earthly days, if any watchmen was found sleeping in the Temple while he was on guard-duty, he was struck with a stick and he had his clothes taken from him which were then burned in order to shame him. Such a practice stemmed from Adam, for Adam did not say that his wife gave him of the forbidden *fruit*, but rather from the forbidden "עץ" which can mean "tree" or "stick," and as a result, Adam had his apron of fig leaves taken from him. We see similar imagery in the Garden of Gethsemane amongst Jesus' sleepy disciples in that Jesus' captors brandished "clubs," (Mark 14:43) and after His arrest, "A certain young man was following Him, wearing nothing but a linen cloth. They caught hold of him, but he left the linen cloth and ran off naked," (Mark 14:51-52). The same imagery is provided in Revelation 16:15, "Behold I come as a thief;

blessed is he that watcheth, and keepeth his garments, lest he walk naked, and they see his shame." In a similar way, let us consider the name Judas "Iscariot": "It may be inquired whether this name was given him while he was alive, or not till after his death. If while he was alive, one may not properly derive it from סקורטיא *Skortja*, which is written also as אסקורטיא *Iskortja* 'What is Iskortja?... [It is a] tanner's garment.'... A leathern apron that tanners put on over their clothes... So that Judas Iscariot may perhaps signify as much as Judas with the apron. But now in such aprons they had purses sewn, in which they were wont to carry their money... And hence, it may be, Judas had that title of the purse-bearer, as he was called Judas with the apron," (*Commentary on the New Testament from the Talmud and Hebraica*, Lightfoot; Vol. 2, p. 179). "By selecting the skins of beasts for the clothing of the first men, and therefore causing the death or slaughter of beasts for that purpose, He showed them how they might use the sovereignty they possessed over the animals for their own good, and even sacrifice animal life for the preservation of human; so that this act of God laid the foundation for the sacrifices..." (*Commentary on the Old Testament: Genesis*, Keil & Delitzsch; p. 67). In bleak despair, Judas spurned Christ's sacrifice and took his own life, as opposed to Peter who denied Christ yet accepted atonement for his sins even to the extent of professing his love for God the same number of times that he denied God.

[3.13] "The names of the north and south, denoting not only regions of the heavens, but also the winds blowing from these regions, are of the fem. gender, Isa. 43:6. The east wind [is considered] destructive and adverse [Job 27:21]... The north wind brings cold till ice is formed... and if the south wind blow, it is hot, Luke 12:55. If cold and heat, coolness and sultriness, interchange at the proper time, then growth is promoted. And if the wind blow through a garden at one time from this direction and at another from that, – not so violently as when it shakes the trees of the forest, but softly and yet as powerfully as a garden can bear it, – then all the fragrance of the garden rises in waves and it becomes like a sea of incense," (*Commentary on the Old Testament: Song of Songs*; Keil & Delitzsch; p. 561-562).

Gardens, vineyards, and paradises were originally designed to house life within a fortified environment of naturally luxuriant security. However, gardens, vineyards, and paradises later became joined to, or were located nearby, places of death; but they were also irrigated so that life could grow out of the ground, just as Jehovah Elohim made Adam out of the dust of the ground (like vegetation). These three places were often where the dead were buried, and were certainly places where new life sprang up as on Day Third of Creation, and we may recall the three days and three nights that Christ was in the tomb.

"The Rabbis taught that the spirit wandered about for three days, seeking re-admission to the body, but abandoned it on the fourth day, as corruption began then," (*Companion Bible*, Bullinger; p. 1547) which helps elucidate Martha's point when she said of the deceased Lazarus, "Lord, by this time he stinketh: for he hath been dead four days," in John 11:39. There seems to be no Scriptural evidence for the three-day wandering of the human spirit taught by the Rabbis, and it is probable that Christ waited as long as He did to raise Lazarus from the dead in order to make Lazarus' resurrection that much more potent in the minds of those who adhered to the Rabbinic teachings of the day, similar to how His body remained in the tomb for three days and three nights (which means that He could not have died on a Friday like traditions says).

[3.14] Human beings are paralleled to vegetation in the Scriptures. Consider again: "Blessed is the man who does not walk in the counsel of the wicked or stand in the way of sinners, or sit in the seat of mockers. But his delight is in the law of the Lord, and on His law he meditates day and night. He is like a tree planted by streams of water, which yields fruit in season and whose leaf does not wither..." (Psalm 1:1-3); "Blessed are those who trust in the Lord, whose trust is the Lord. They shall be like a tree planted by water, sending out its roots by the stream. It shall not fear when heat comes, and its leaves shall stay green; in the year of drought it is not anxious, and it does not cease to bear fruit," (Jeremiah 17:7-8). We know that "... a stream came up from the earth and watered the whole surface of the ground – Jehovah Elohim formed man from the dust of the ground and breathed..." (Genesis 2:5-7). "They came to *Bethsaida* [*House of Fish*], and some people brought a blind man and begged Jesus to touch him. He took the blind man... When he had spit on the man's eyes and put his hands on him, Jesus asked, 'Do you see anything?' He [the man] looked up and said, 'I see people; they look like trees walking around.' Once more, Jesus put His hands on the man's eyes. Then his eyes were opened, his sight was restored, and he saw everything clearly..." (Mark 8:22-25); "...truly it is the spirit in a mortal, the breath of the Almighty, that makes for understanding," (Job 32:8).

How ironic. How could Jesus, the Almighty Creator of the Universe (John 1:1-3; Colossians 1:16; Hebrews 1:2-3), somehow botch His first attempt at healing someone? Jesus is God, and He does not make mistakes. Jesus allowed the blind man to see spiritually before He allowed him to see physically. Since when do people ever look like trees? "At least there is hope for a tree; if it is cut down, it will sprout again, and its new shoots will not fail. Its roots may grow old in the ground and its stump die in the soil, yet at the scent of water it will bud..." (Job 14:7-9). Figures are used to heighten realistic descriptions, not to obscure reality. We can see part of the reason why irrigated gardens, vineyards, and paradises also held tombs within them (at most) or connected to/nearby them (at least), for the natural design of these three places illustrated the resurrection. It should be noted that the remainder of Job 14:10-12 says that, "...mortals die, and are laid low; humans expire, and where are they? As waters fail from a lake, and a river wastes away and dries up, so mortals lie down and do not rise again; until the heavens are no more, they will not awake or be roused out of their sleep." We know that there is no reincarnation because Hebrews 9:27-28 explicitly states, "Just as man is destined to die once, and after that to face judgment, so Christ was sacrificed once to take away the sins of many people; and He will appear a second time, not to bear sin, but to bring salvation to those who are waiting for him." "Jesus"

A Garden, A Vineyard, or A Paradise?   319

means "Jehovah is Salvation," and "*Nazareth*" means "*Branch; Preservation*" – as in the act of sprouting again continually. Jehovah Elohim is likened to a gardener in Genesis 2-3, and this is part of the significance of John 19:41: "At the place where Jesus was crucified, there was a garden, and in the garden a new tomb..." Mary Magdalene came to this garden tomb and found it empty; she saw Christ (without knowing it) first "thinking He was the gardener," (John 20:15). Mary, upon a second look, recognized Him – and we see the parallel between this account and that of the blind man who saw people as trees initially and then people as people secondarily.

[3.15] In Genesis 2:8, we are told that Jehovah Elohim planted a "garden." The English word rendered "garden" in Genesis 2:8 is the Hebrew "גן" (ref. 1588) which means "a garden (as fenced)" and is from the word "גנן" (ref. 1598) which means "to hedge about, i.e. protect, defend." In Genesis 2:15, we are told that "... Jehovah Elohim took the man and put him into the Garden of Eden to cultivate it and to guard it." The word rendered "guard" or "keep" in English is "שמר" (ref. 8104) which also means, "to hedge about" and "to guard and protect." Immediately, we ask ourselves, "What was God protecting Eden from?" Genesis 1:27 discusses that humanity was created generally, whereas Genesis 2:7 discusses how Adam, the first human, was created specifically; in other words, Genesis 1 presents the larger picture of Creation whereas Genesis 2 presents a more intricate, developmental recap – the indication is provided in Genesis 2:4a: "These are the *generations* [also rendered '*developments*'] of the earth and the heavens when they were created..." in connection with Genesis 2:4b that recounts all 6 "Days" of Creation as only one "Day."

After Adam "became a living being" (Genesis 2:7), Jehovah Elohim planted a garden (Genesis 2:8) and He placed Adam in it. Danger lurked outside of the garden planted in Eden. If there were no danger outside of the particular garden that was Adam's dwelling, Adam would not have to be hedged in at all, nor would he be paced in his home to "guard" the garden in Eden. The concept of time was a key factor in Satan's assult against the first humans, for doubt was cast upon the human mind regarding "the day" Jehovah Elohim discussed in Genesis 2:17 concerning the forbidden tree versus "the day" Satan discussed in Genesis 3:5 concerning opened eyes. Jehovah Elohim stated truthfully that "...in *the day* thou eatest thereof thou shalt surely die," (Genesis 2:17) – but which day was stated? – for "*the day* that Jehovah Elohim made the earth and the heavens," (Genesis 2:4b) encompassed the entirety of the six "days" of Genesis Chapter I, and the reader will notice that Adam did not die soon after he ate of the forbidden tree. Satan structured his deceitful argument to Adam's wife based in part by her perception (or lack thereof) of time. Genesis 1:1, 2:1 & 2:4a state creation with the word "heaven(s)" preceding the word "earth," but when the entire creation is stated as only one "day" in Genesis 2:4b, the order is reversed so that the word "earth" precedes the word "heaven" in order to show relative perspective that remains absolute and correct:

"...created the *heavens and the earth*," (Genesis 1:1)
"...the *heavens and the earth* were finished," (Genesis 2:1)

"...generations of the *heavens and the earth*..." (Genesis 2:4a)

"...in THE DAY that the Lord God made the **earth and the heavens**," (Genesis 2:4b).

In a similar way, Satan inverted the order of the words "day" and "die" in Genesis 3:4-5) compared to God's statement in Genesis 2:17:

God: "...**in the day** that you eat of it, you shall surely **die**," (Genesis 2:17).

Satan: "...You shall not surely **die**: for God doth know that **in the day** you eat of it..." (Genesis 3:4-5).

The concept of time was a key factor in Satan's assult against the first humans, for the humans did not die within a 24-hour interval following their forbidden consumption. We must then ponder whose "day" God discussed versus whose "day" Satan discussed, for "the day" of Genesis 2:4b was longer than the "days" of Genesis 1, similar to how "the day" is put for more than one 24-hour interval in Leviticus 13:14, Leviticus 14:57, Numbers 7:84, Numbers 28:26, Deuteronomy 21:16, I Samuel 20:19, II Samuel 21:12, I Kings 2:37, Psalm 18:18, Isaiah 11:16, Jeremiah 11:4,7, Ezekiel 36:33, etc. Human confusion regarding the "day" under discussion in the garden in Eden provoked faulty reasoning spurred by deceit that birthed sin. "But search your hearts *daily*, until *the day* which is called *The day*, to the end that no man among you be hardened through the deceitfulness of sin," (Hebrews 3:13).

[3.16] Again, Παραδεισος [Paradise] = "a park, a forest where wild beasts were kept for hunting; a pleasure-park, a garden of trees of various kinds; used in the LXX for the Garden of Eden; in N.T. the celestial paradise, Luke 23:43; 2 Cor 12:4; Rev 2:7," (The Analytical Lexicon to the Greek New Testament, Mounce; p. 351). The word "paradise," according to Webster's New World Dictionary, means "heaven, abode of the blessed; the Garden of Eden; the abode of the righteous after death; a place of great contentment and beauty; a place or condition of great or perfect satisfaction, happiness, or delight." However, the word "paradise" as we find it in the Scriptures is "פרדס" (ref. 6508) and "παραδεισος" (ref. 3857) which both mean "a pleasure-ground." How then did we come to understand "paradise" in such an ethereal sense when it simply means "a pleasure-ground?"– and why should we link notions of pleasure to notions of violent bloodshed regarding hunting? The first blood of animate life shed in connection to death in human history belonged to Adam's firstborn, and this blood was then commanded to be atoned for by animal sacrifice temporarily. There could not have been any killing in Eden prior to human sin, and the killing of animals became a necessary component of substitutional atonement so that the punishment fit the crime and the grace fit the punishment – which is precisely why the final sacrifice (Christ) was HUMAN, not animal, in order to match the first violent bloodshed which was also HUMAN, not animal. Christ restored the original order which was as follows: "The wolf shall live with the lamb, the leopard shall lie down with the kid, the calf and the lion and the fatling together, and a little child shall lead them. The cow and the bear shall graze, their young shall lie down together; and the lion shall eat straw like the ox. The nursing child shall play over the hole of the asp, and the weaned child shall put its hand on the adder's den. They will not hurt or destroy on all My holy mountain; for the earth will be full of the knowledge of the Lord as the waters cover the sea," (Isaiah 11:6-9). It is errant to claim that humanity progressed from hunter-gatherers to agriculturalists as Genesis 2:15 describes Adam as an agriculturalist. After Adam received his punishment (Genesis 3:17-19), agriculture became difficult for him (Genesis 3:19), and the sacrificial substitutional system of animals-for-people became practiced, thus humanity reverted to fleshly food in opposition to the initial rules of Genesis 1:29-30 where humans and animals alike were to eat but vegetation in accordance with Isaiah 11:6-9: They will not hurt or destroy on all My holy mountain; for the earth will be full of the knowledge of the Lord as the waters cover the sea." Sin brought degeneration, which is why flesh was condemned to die. If killing occurred prior to sin, there would be no need for killing on account of sin to atone for sin. Blood can be shed without death, as it is when life is born and when a marriage is consummated by a virgin male and virgin female as was the proper design from the beginning, hence, the "marriage of the Lamb" in Revelation 19:7. "For the life of the flesh is in the blood; and I have given it to you for making atonement for your lives on the altar; for, as life, it is the blood that makes atonement," (Leviticus 17:11). By shedding blood in the garden in a manner that mingled it with death (Adam's firstborn), we can also better understand the first "whoredom" of sin as specifically linked the product of a fruitful marriage. Blood can be linked to life (as it flows through veins) or to death (as it spills and becomes stagnant) similar to living water versus stagnant water. "And anyone of the people of Israel, or of the aliens who reside among them, who hunts down an animal or bird that may be eaten shall pour out its blood and cover it with earth," (Leviticus 17:13), just as the ground was cursed for the blood Adam accidentally shed (Genesis 3:17), just as Christ sweated, "...great drops of blood falling down to the ground," (Luke 22:44).

The only "bloodshed" in Eden prior to sin and death and apart from the consummation of marriage (and femininity in general) is described by *analogy* and *figure* with the word "דם" (ref. 1818) = "blood; by *analogy*, the *juice of the grape*; figuratively bloodshed (i.e. drops of blood)"; this part of the reason that Adam was placed in the garden to "guard" (Genesis 2:15) it, for the word "guard" is "שמר" (ref. 8104) = "ר+מ+ש" = 200+40+300 = **540**, and "שמר" (ref. 8105) means "something preserved, i.e. the *settlings of wine*" = "ר+מ+ש" = 200+40+300 = **540** – thus the New Covenant in Christ's "blood": "αιμα" (ref. *129*) = "blood literally (of men or animals), *figuratively (the juice of grapes)* or specifically (the atoning blood of Christ); by implication bloodshed, also kindred:- blood." Ponder the irony of the first violent bloodshed of animate life coming by way of the "blood" of a poisonous vine – a plight that was balanced and then overturned by the New Covenant in Christ's blood from the "True Vine" in order that we might be "born again."

Let us now discuss vines and vineyards.

[3.17] A Greek word for "vine" is "αμπελος" (ref. *288*) which means "a vine (as coiling about a support)" {1}. The Hebrew "vineyard" = "כרם" (ref. 3754) is also considered a "garden" as the scholars Keil and Delitzsch render this word as "vine-garden" (*Commentary on the Old Testament: Song of Songs*, Keil & Delitzsch; p. 518). Consider the Hebrew word "גפן" (ref. 1612) = "a vine (as twining), esp. the grape:- vine, tree" in comparison to the word "עכשוב" (ref. 5919) means "an asp (from *lurking coiled up*):- adder." "The fig tree puts forth its green figs, and the vines with their tender shoots give fragrance," (Song of Songs 2:13), "...the vine-blossom... fills the vineyard with an incomparably delicate fragrance," (*Commentary on the Old Testament: Song of Songs*, Keil & Delitzsch, p. 535), hence the attractive qualities of coiling nature that when kept properly produces savory aromatics and elixirs, but when neglected becomes troublesome to the delicate balance of pruned and ordered harmony.

[3.18] Again, "The Rabbins have a tradition. Over wine which hath not water mingled with it they do not say that blessing, 'Blessed be He that created the fruit of the vine'; but, 'Blessed be He that created the fruit of the tree,'" (*Commentary on the New Testament from the Talmud and Hebraica*, Lightfoot; Vol. 2, p. 351). Christ specifically said that, "I tell you, I will never again drink of this fruit of the vine until that day when I drink it new with you in My Father's Kingdom," (Matthew 26:29), but then we read that, "A jar full of sour wine was standing there. So they put a sponge full of the wine on a branch of hyssop and held it to His mouth. When Jesus had received the wine, He said, 'Paid in full.' Then He bowed his head and died," (John 19:29-30). Christ consumed the "fruit of the tree" as He hung on the "tree"– He did not receive the fruit of the vine on the cross. However, when, "... one of the soldiers pierced His side with a spear, and at once blood and water came out," (John 19:34), we may understand that the "fruit of the vine" flowed out of Christ in accordance with His New Covenant in relation to the fact that He called Himself the "True Vine" in John 15:1. Before He was crucified, Christ prayed, "Father, if you are willing, remove this cup from me..." (Luke 22:42), for as the "cup" was paralleled to His death on the cross, so He took of the cup (through a sponge) of the "fruit of the tree" – in this case, being paralleled to both His final drink and His final sacrifice through His own blood, for "I am the vine, you are the branches. Those who abide in Me and I in them bear much fruit, because apart from Me you can do nothing," (John 15:5). Christ then said, "Whoever does not abide in Me is thrown away like a branch and withers; such branches are gathered, thrown into the fire and burned," (John 15:6) as this teaching stems from Ezekiel 15:1-5: "... 'Son of man, how is the vine-tree more than any other tree, or than a branch that is among the trees of the forest? Shall wood be taken from it to do work? Or will men take from it to do work? Or will men take from it for a peg to hang every vessel on it? Behold, it is put in the fire for fuel. Both its ends the fire devours, and its middle is charred. Will it prosper for work? Behold, when it was whole it was not made for work. How much less when the fire has devoured it, and it is charred! Shall it yet be made to work?'" Notice how Ezekiel is called "Son of man" and how Christ referred to Himself as "The Son of Man." The fact that both water and blood flowed out of Christ validated His own words that He was the "True Vine," though He was treated contemptuously as a wild vine that is thrown into the fire as He entered His descent into Hades by consuming the "fruit of the tree," only to overcome the "tree" (that we call "cross") and the power of Hades in order to show Himself as the True Vine of the blood covenant that we celebrate at Holy Communion. When we take into account that Jesus' "...Father is the vine grower," (John 15:1), we can also take notice of Jesus' quotation of Psalm 22:1 when He said on the tree, "My God, My God, why have you forsaken Me?" (Matthew 27:46) as a wild vine about to be tossed into the fire.

"John said to the crowds coming out to be baptized by him, 'You brood of vipers! Who warned you to flee from the coming wrath? Produce fruit in keeping with repentance. And do not begin to say to yourselves, 'We have Abraham as our father.' For I tell you that out of these stones God can raise up children for Abraham. The ax is already at the root of the trees, and every tree that does not produce good fruit will be cut down and thrown into the fire," (Luke 3:7-9). The "tree" that John the Baptist referred to was a "vine-tree" in connection with the "vipers" that the vine-tree resembled... particularly in relation to the fact that both the vine-tree and the serpent are thrown into the fire (as in Ezekiel 15:4 & Acts 28:5). We may also observe how Satan the "serpent" (Genesis 3:1) was called a "murderer" by Jesus in John 8:44 in connection with the instance of Paul's encounter with a snake: "When the natives saw the creature hanging from his hand, they said to one another, 'This man must be a murderer; though he has escaped from the sea, justice has not allowed him to live.' He, however, shook off the creature into the fire and suffered no harm," (Acts 28:4-5). Regarding Paul's escape from the sea, we might remember that "Yonder is the sea, great and wide, creeping things innumerable are there, living things both small and great. There go the ships, and Leviathan that you formed to sport in it," (Psalm 104:25-26). There is an intimate parallel between Satan and a vine: "Who has dullness of eyes? – those who stay long at the wine; those who go to seek mixed wine. Do not look at wine when it is *red* [= אדם = א+ד+ם = **605** = '*red-faced*' = **605** = *Adam* = **605**, *as in shame, for Adam's 'eyes were opened' after he consumed the 'venom of the serpent'*], when it sparkles in the cup and goes down smoothly. At last it bites like the *serpent* [*same word for 'serpent' in Genesis 3:1*] and stings like the adder. **Your eyes will see strange things**, and your mind utter perverse things. You will be like one who lies down in the midst of the sea, like one who lies on top of a mast," (Proverbs 23:29-34); notice how the wine discussed here is red wine, for not all wine is red. A talking serpent is quite a strange thing. Consider the Hebrew word "גפן" (ref. 1612) = "a vine (as *twining*), esp. the grape:- vine, tree" in comparison to the word "עכשוב" (ref. 5919) means "an asp (from lurking *coiled up*):- adder": "At last it bites like the נחש [*serpent*] and stings like the צפעני [*adder*]," (Proverbs 23:32):

"גפן" (ref. 1612) = "a *vine* (as twining), esp. the grape:- vine, tree" = "ג+פ+ן" = 50+80+3 = **133**;

"נגף" (ref. 5062) = "to inflict (a disease):- beat, dash, hurt, plague, slay, smite, strike, stumble" = "נ+ג+ף" = 80+3+50

= **133**; "נֶגֶף" (ref. 5063) = "a trip (of the foot); (figuratively) an infliction (of disease):- stumbling, plague [used in Exodus 12:13 for the plague concerning the *death of the firstborn*: Passover]" = "ף+ג+נ" = 80+3+50 = **133**.

The Proverbs were not written in plain speech, but they were written, "to understand a proverb and a figure, the words of the wise and their riddles," (Proverbs 1:6). Vineyards were hedged in as such walls served to prevent intrusion; however, "Whoever digs a pit [*like those dug pits for wine production: Isaiah 5:2,22-24; Mark 12:1*] will fall into it; and whoever breaks through a wall will be bitten by a snake," (Ecclesiastes 10:8). Remember Adam's punishment: "...cursed is the ground because of you... thorns and thistles it shall bring forth for you," (Genesis 3:17-18); "I passed by the field of one who was lazy, by the vineyard of a stupid person; and see, it was all overgrown with thorns; the ground was covered in nettles, and its stone wall was broken down. Then I saw and considered it; I looked and received instruction. A little sleep, a little slumber, a little folding of the hands to rest, and poverty will come upon you like a robber, and want, like an armed warrior," (Proverbs 24:30-34). "The thief comes only to steal, kill, and destroy," (John 10:10). "He came a third time and said to them, 'Are you still sleeping and taking your rest? Enough! The hour has come; the Son of Man is betrayed into the hands of sinners," (Mark 14:41). "בצר" (ref. 1219) = "to clip off; to gather grapes; to be isolated (inaccessible by height or fortification, cut off, (de-) fenced" = "ר+צ+ב" = 200+90+2 = **292**; "רבץ" = (ref. 7257) = "to recline, repose, brood, lurk, fall down"

= "ר+ב+צ" = 90+2+200 = **292**; "רבץ" = (ref. 7258) = "a couch or place of repose, resting-place" = "ר+ב+צ" = 90+2+200 = **292**.

"For when it is said of generous wine, that it makes the lips of sleeper's move, a movement is meant expressing itself in the sleeper speaking. But generous wine is a figure of the love-responses of the beloved, sipped in, as it were, with pleasing satisfaction, which hover still around the sleepers in delightful dreams, and fill them with hallucinations," (*Commentary on the Old Testament: Song of Songs*, Keil & Delitzsch, p. 595). In a positive, legitimate, sober light, consider that the covenant with Abraham (Genesis 15:12), Solomon's conversation with God when he asked for a discerning mind (I Kings 3:5), and Joseph's warning (Matt 2:13), etc., all occurred during dreams – in a negative sense, consider the words of Eliphaz the Temanite's words: "Now a word came stealing to me, my ear received the whisper of it. Amid thoughts and visions of the night, when deep sleep falls on mortals, dread came upon me, and trembling, which made all my bones shake. A spirit glided past my face; the hair of my flesh bristled. I stood still, but I could not discern its appearance. A form was before my eyes; there was silence, then I heard a voice, 'Can mortals be righteous before God? Can human beings be pure before their Maker? Even in His servants He puts no trust, and His angels he charges with error; how much more those who live in houses of clay, whose foundation is in the dust...'" (Job 4:12-19). With which angels can God put no trust? – "But even if we or an angel from heaven should proclaim to you a gospel contrary to what we proclaimed to you, let that one be accursed! As we have said before, now I repeat, if anyone proclaims to you a gospel contrary to what you received, let that one be accursed!" (Galatians 1:8-9). Certainly no angel whose place remains in heaven is untrustworthy: "And war broke out in heaven; Michael and his angels fought against the dragon. The dragon and his angels fought back, but they were defeated, and there was no longer any place for them in Heaven," (Revelation 12:7-8). The only one who was personally "cursed" in Eden was Satan, not Adam or his wife. The ground was "cursed" because of Adam (Genesis 3:17), and Adam's wife received her punishment without the word "curse" (Genesis 3:16).

[3.19] Ancient Eastern vineyards were partially designed to relieve one from the scorching heat of the sun at mid-day and were constructed to elicit the tranquility of organic opulence. Archways of trained vines that snaked in and out of the constructed ceilings were erected to provide aesthetically pleasing shade to those strolling beneath them, for "To train a vine some twelve to fifteen feet straight up, engenders its rapid growth, and imparts to it a heavy, rich foliage..." (*The Vine-Dresser's Manual*, Reemelin; p. 75). "Shady arched walks, therefore, formed by vines planted in rows or avenues, and trained above a trelliswork, or airy and fragrant bowers formed by the outspread branches of trees in gardens, are retreats, the delight of which an Eastern alone can fully appreciate," (*Coheleth*, Ginsburg; p. 280). When concentrating on producing grapes other than for making wine, "The trellis, however, is better adapted to the growing of table grapes than grapes for wine," (*The Vine-Dresser's Manual*, Reemelin; p. 50). By such a magnificent design, breezes would breathe their way under the serpentine ceilings of vines and swaying leaves easily and without the extreme influence of the sun which these pathways were designed to block. Those who enjoyed the leisure of such a lovely place could recline to sip sleepy, weepy elixirs. Vineyards were used for worshipping God and entertaining friends. However, vineyards were also used for burying the dead.

[3.20] When reading Holy Scripture, it is important to account for figures of speech not found in English. The Aramaic *Peshitta* Version of the Scriptures points us to such a figure that has been commonly overlooked based on the fact that the figure does not exist in English. Let us consider the story of Sodom and Gomorrah in Genesis 19. In the account of Sodom and Gomorrah, Heavenly messengers came to lodge temporarily with Lot, who, "was sitting in the gateway of the city," (Genesis 19:1). Once the angels entered Lot's home, the Sodomites demanded intimacy with these angelic men, and, "Lot went outside to meet them and shut the door behind him," (Genesis 19:6) as he attempted to dissuade the unnatural inclinations of his neighbors. The angels saved Lot from his neighbors' wrath by blinding them, and we cannot help but notice the serpent's promise to Eve: "... your eyes will be opened..." (Genesis 3:5). The angels warned Lot that they were about to destroy Sodom and Gomorrah, and they told him, "Flee for your lives! Don't look back, and don't stop anywhere on the plain! Flee to the mountains or you will be swept away," (Genesis 3:17). "However, Lot's wife was disobedient, and when she looked back, "she became a pillar of salt," (Genesis 19:26) – an Aramaic expression "...that means that she became petrified with fear and died" (*Peshitta Version of the Holy Bible*, p. 25), a figure which is similar to the English expression "white as a ghost" as salt is also white, and also similar to the fact that tombs were beautifully whitewashed to indicate the unclean white bones within them. Why would Lot's wife have become edible?

[3.21]   Dr. Lightfoot noted the following:

"On a vineyard four years old they paint some marks out of the turf of the earth, that men may know that it is a vineyard of four years old, and eat not of it, because it is holy, as the Lord saith, Lev. xix.24; and the owners ought to eat the fruit of it at Jerusalem, as the second tithe. And an uncircumcised vineyard," [that is, which is not yet four years old; see Lev. xix. 23], "they mark with clay, that it is distinguished in fire. For the prohibition of (a vineyard) uncircumcised, is greater than the prohibition concerning that of four years old: for that of four years old is fit for eating: but that uncircumcised is not admitted to any use. Therefore, they marked not that by the turf, lest the mark might perhaps be defaced and perish; and men not seeing it might eat of it," (*Commentary on the New Testament from the Talmud and Hebraica*, Lightfoot; Vol. 2, p. 434).

Notice the use of the word "circumcise" in relation to vineyards. "*Abram*" means "*Father of Height*," and the history of Abraham parallels vine-science. Vines that occur in the wild produce a fruit for the purpose of vine-perpetuity, not for wine-making. Wild vines are engaged in a constant war with trees for height in order to obtain light and rain whereby the tallest combatant is the victor. Once the wild vine no longer feels that it is in competition with the tree it constricts, it then produces fruit with seed in it in order to drop and produce a new wild vine. *Abram* [*Father of Height*] could not produce fruit at first (Genesis 15:2). God changed Abram's name to *Abraham* [*Father of Multitudes*] (Genesis 17:5), then God's covenant with Abraham was to prune the human male's vine, and after such pruning, Abraham was able to beget offspring. Thus, God took a wild vine, humbled/reduced it, and through training and pruning, produced a fruitful and tamed vine that began the exalted family line.

[3.22] "I am the true vine, and my father is the vine grower. He removes every branch in me that bears no fruit. Every branch that bears fruit He prunes to make it bear more fruit," (John 15:1-3). When Christ described himself as a serpent in John 3:14 and as a vine in John 15, the similarity of the serpent to the vine should be noted; and to a literally smaller extent, the tendril of a vine should not be ignored, for tendrils are "a convenient appendage to the grapevine; with them they twine themselves to objects near them, maintaining thereby their fruit and branches above ground, even in a wild state – an indication which the practical vine-dressers have not failed to follow," (*The Vine-Dresser's Manual*, Reemelin; p. 12). When Jesus stated that, "I Am the true vine, and my Father is the vine grower," (John 15:1), it helpful to understand the purpose of the coiling tendrils when reading Christ's words in John 3:14: "And just as Moses lifted up the serpent in the wilderness, so must the Son of Man be lifted up…"

When wild vines battle trees for height, we must consider the fact that, as Christ hung on the tree, He must have kept His head up while He breathed alive, for concerning his death, "...Then He bowed His head and died," (John 19:30). Furthermore, the title "King of the Jews" was fastened above Christ's head, and both His Title and His head had achieved the epitome of height relative to the tree (that we render as "cross" in English), for it is certain that John must have noted the distinct bowing of Christ's head in reference to Christ paralleling Himself to a wild and a trained vine; a vine trained on a stake meant for wine-grapes has one thick and round knob with two main branches that grow out and up from it that forms a shape similar to the Hebrew letter ץ. The round knob between the two outstretched and up-stretched limbs is called "the head" of the vine. Christ wore a crown of thorns on His head as He was mocked. Concerning soil cultivation for vines, "The great point is thoroughness – that is, in turning over every part of the soil, and the most careful attention towards the destruction of all weeds, particularly around the head of the vine." (*The Vine-Dresser's Manual,* Reemelin; p.74). After Adam sinned, the ground was cursed and thorns began to be produced. Adam was to "guard" = "שמר" (ref. 8104) = "to hedge about (as with thorns); the Second Adam and the Son of Adam wore an indicator of the first sin in human history atop His holy head when He died for us on the cross – in connection with the sacrificial ram of Abraham, a ram whose head was caught in a thicket.

[3.23] Biblical accounts of vines and fig trees together often describe peace, rest, security, and guiltless tranquility. For instance, I Kings 4:25 says, "During Solomon's lifetime Judah and Israel lived in safety, from Dan even to Beer-sheba, all of them under their vines and fig trees"; Micah 4:3-4 says, "... nation shall not lift up sword against nation, neither shall they learn war anymore; but they shall all sit under their own vines and under their own fig trees, and no one shall make them afraid; for the mouth of the Lord of hosts has spoken"; Zechariah 3:9-10 says, " For on the stone I have set before Joshua, on a single stone with seven facets, I will engrave its inscription, says the Lord of hosts, and I will remove the guilt of this land in a single day. On that day, says the Lord of hosts, you shall invite each other to come under your vine and fig tree." However, "All the host of heaven shall rot away, and the skies roll up like a scroll. All their host shall wither like a leaf withering on a vine, or fruit withering on a fig tree," (Isaiah 34:4) – this description of the vine and the fig tree is of death paralleled by the stars, a fact that further explains the irony concerning the "serpent" and the man-made garments of Adam and Eve.

It is probable that the fig-tree represents the Tree of Life and that the vine-tree represents the Tree of the Knowledge of Good and Evil. Revelation 22:2 states specifically that the "leaves" of the Tree of Life are for "healing," and we find the parallel to such healing leaves in the story of King Hezekiah (II Kings 20): Hezekiah suffered from a malignant boil, and Isaiah (through God's power and provision) healed the boil with "a lump of figs," (II Kings 20:7).   After Hezekiah's blunder in II Kings 20:12-15, Isaiah told Hezekiah that, "Some of your own sons who are born to you shall be taken away," (II Kings 20:18).

Tree of Life represented by – "בכורה" *(ref. 1062)* = "the early fig" = "ב+כ+ו+ר+ה" = 5+200+6+20+2 = **233**; "בכורה" *(ref. 1063)* = "the firstling of man or beast; firstborn" = "ב+כ+ו+ר+ה" = 5+200+6+20+2 = **233**.

Tree of the Knowledge of Good and Evil represented by – "עץ־הגפן" = "vine-tree" = "ע+ץ+ה+ג+פ+ן" = 50+80+3+5+90+70 = **298**; "רצח" (ref. 7523) = "to dash in pieces, i.e. kill (a human being); to murder" = "ר+צ+ח" = 8+90+200 = **298**; "רצח" (ref. 7524) = "a crushing, a murder-cry, slaughter" = "ר+צ+ח" = 8+90+200 = **298**.

As possibly a fig-tree coiled about by a vine-tree, both the Tree of Life and the Tree of the Knowledge of Good and Evil were simply called "trees" in the Eden story:

Tree of Life – "tree" = "עץ" (ref. 6086) = "ע+ץ" = 90+70 = **160**; "to be smooth; pleasant; be sweet" = "מלץ" (ref. 4452) = "מ+ל+ץ" = 90+30+40 = **160**;

Tree of the Knowledge of Good and Evil – "a shadow, phantom, illusion, resemblance, idol, image" = "צלם" (ref. 6754) = "צ+ל+ם" = 40+30+90 = **160**; "something fallen, abortion, untimely birth" = "נפל" (ref. 5309) = "נ+פ+ל" = 30+80+50 = **160**.

[3.24] Depending on the vine, a well established tree can co-exist with a vine snaking around it as gardeners are sometimes inclined to allow a non-threatening vine-tree (that is, non-threatening to the host-tree) to coil about a tree (parasitically as they do) in order to increase the aesthetic pleasure of a garden. However, if the vine-tree is a detrimental vine (that is, detrimental to the host-tree), it is cut off and disallowed from growing with the tree. Depending on the vine and on the tree, a gardener can be willing to let a vine bond with an established tree to promote beauty, or a gardener can also safeguard a tree by prohibiting various vines from growing on it, particularly if that tree is not old enough to handle a vine. In un-pruned nature, wild vines battle trees for height (light, water) and often kill host trees in their pursuit of sustentation. Job 41:32 says that Leviathan's influence only appears to be "white-haired" or well established, though he is not. When we reflect on the concept of the serpent on the pole, we can notice the antithetical reflections of Christ via a vine on a tree (John 3:14 = Jesus on the Cross) and Satan via a vine on a tree (Genesis 3 = the "serpent"). A vine on a tree can serve as an object of beauty or an object of destruction, and as it is the case with the most intense forms of evil, the one is often mistaken for the other: "to be smooth; pleasant; be sweet" = "מלץ" (ref. 4452) = "מ+ל+ץ" = 90+30+40 = **160**; "a shadow, phantom, illusion, resemblance, idol, image" = "צלם" (ref. 6754) = "צ+ל+ם" = 40+30+90 = **160**.

Wisdom is personified as saying, "'**You that are simple, turn in here!' To those without sense she says**, 'Come, eat of my bread and drink of the wine I have mixed. Lay aside immaturity, and live and walk in the way of insight,'" (Proverbs 9:4-5)

The foolish woman says, "'**You who are simple, turn in here!' And to those without sense she says**, 'Stolen water is sweet, and bread eaten in secret is pleasant.' But they do not know that the dead are there, and that her guests are in the depths of Sheol," (Proverbs 9:16-18).

"something fallen, abortion, untimely birth" = "נֵפֶל" (ref. 5309) = "ל+פ+נ"= 30+80+50 = **160**.

[3.25] Human anatomy is often paralleled to other aspects of non-human nature: "If you will only obey the Lord your God, by diligently observing all His commandments that I am commanding you today, the Lord your God will set you high above all nations of the earth; all these blessings shall come upon you and overtake you, if you obey the Lord your God... Blessed shall be the fruit of your womb, the fruit of your ground, and the fruit of your livestock..." (Deuteronomy 28:1-4). "Then you shall again obey the Lord, observing all His commandments that I am commanding you today, and the Lord your God will make you abundantly prosperous in all your undertakings, in the fruit of your body, in the fruit of your livestock, and in the fruit of your soil..." (Deuteronomy 30:8-9). Shall I give my firstborn for my transgression, the fruit of my body for the sin of my soul?" (Micah 6:7).

The word "בכר" (ref. 1069) means "to burst the womb, i.e. make early fruit (of woman or tree); also to give the birthright:- make firstborn, be firstling, bring forth first child (new fruit)." The word "גֶפֶן" (ref. 1612) = "a vine (as twining), esp. the grape:- vine, tree," is a feminine noun; consider Malachi 3:11 where this word for vine is used: "And I will rebuke the devourer for you, and he shall not destroy the fount of your ground against you; nor shall your vine *miscarry* against you in the field, says Jehovah of hosts," just as "... the serpent was subtle above every beast of the field that the Lord God had made," (Genesis 3:1); this word "*miscarry*" is "שכל" (ref. 7921) = "ש+כ+ל"= 30+20+300 = **350**; "שכל" (ref. 7919) = "to make wise" = "ש+כ+ל"= 30+20+300 = **350** – and wine is considered Wisdom's drink in Proverbs 9:2,5, though it should be noted that the wine of Proverbs 9:2 is "mixed," and so that the Rabbis called this drink the "fruit of the vine," whereas had the wine not been mixed with water they would then call it the fruit of the tree.

[3.26] Let us reexamine Eve's conversation with the serpent regarding the reason that she did not specify which tree was under discussion in the "midst" of the garden, particularly with regard to what she "saw." Genesis 3:6 states, "So when the woman saw that

1) the tree was good for food, and
2) that it was a delight to the eyes, and
3) that the tree was to be desired to make one wise, she took of its fruit and ate..."

Consider:

1) The Tree of the Knowledge of Good and Evil was certainly not good for food.
2) The Tree of the Knowledge of Good and Evil may have been pleasant to the eyes [see Section III Notes part a].
3) The Tree of the Knowledge of Good and Evil could not "make wise," for choosing to eat from it was foolish (hence the blended wordplay of wisdom and abortion;

compare to the facts that King Solomon's reign of wisdom first became evident over the threatened life of an infant disputed over by two unsavory women in I Kings 3:16-28, and that Solomon's ultimate folly resulted in the pagan, sacrificial death of his own infant(s) in I Kings 11:5 at the hands of his own unsavory wives. The story of the wisest man to ever live begins and ends with infant death.).

Genesis 2:9 names the two central trees of the garden distinctly, but when Eve discussed the centrality of the garden, she spoke of its center only with respect to the forbidden tree and she did not mention it specifically but only referred to it as "the tree." Eve contemplated and spoke ambiguously, for both of the two specific trees were in the midst of the garden, and both of them had specific names and qualities. Eve discarded both of their names and only suggested that there was but one tree in the garden's center. In the cases of ambiguity presented in Genesis 3 regarding these two trees, outright lies did not occur, but rather half-truths that were even more deceitful than outright lies occurred as premises for arguments, and once those arguments reached full fruition, the deceitfulness of the matter took full form: "… one is tempted by one's own desire, being lured and enticed by it; then, when that desire has conceived, it gives birth to sin, and that sin, when it is fully grown, gives birth to death," (James 1:14-15).

By Eve discussing "the tree" in Genesis 3:4, two possibilities arise concerning the three qualities that she "saw" concerning "the tree": I) either what she "saw" in the wrong tree was an illusion, or 2) she described two of three characteristics of the Tree of Life, not the Tree of the Knowledge of Good and Evil. For instance,

1) Genesis 1:29 says that the fruitful seed-bearing plants and trees were fit for human consumption, but Genesis 1:30 does not restrict vegetation fit for the land animals or birds to that which bears seed in its fruit. Such a situation aligns with the fact that humanity was blessed and was commanded to be fruitful and multiply in Genesis 1:28 (as were the birds and water animals in Genesis 1:22), but the land animals were not blessed or commanded to be fruitful and multiply (Genesis 1:25).

2) Genesis 2:9 says that "Out of the ground Jehovah Elohim made to grow every tree that is pleasant to the sight and good for food," and the Tree of the Knowledge of Good and Evil only fits half of this description as it was **not good for food**.

3) Wisdom is called a "tree of life" in Proverbs 3:18. If "the tree" in the ambiguity of Eve's description was "desirable to make one wise," (as we know that it was unwise to eat from the wrong tree) and knowing that Wisdom herself is called a "tree of life," it would be inconsistent to claim that the Tree of the Knowledge of Good and Evil was desirable to make one wise when it held no such capability.

Since the Tree of Life and the Tree of the Knowledge of Good and Evil both stood in the very same location as a tree coiled about by a vine, Eve would have been forced to behold both trees simultaneously, and this may, perhaps, be why only 1/3 of her descriptions regarding "the tree" (implying the Tree of the Knowledge of Good and Evil) was accurate, as the remaining 2/3 (or .666 repeating) of her descriptions relating to "the tree" were unsuitable for the forbidden tree. As the "fruit of the vine," or watered wine, was to be proportioned with 2/3 water and 1/3 wine according to ancient practice, it is consistent with Peter's command: "Repent, and be baptized everyone of you in the name of Jesus Christ so that your sins may be forgiven; and you will receive the gift of the Holy *Spirit*," (Acts 2:38), for Paul contrasted the "Spirit" and "wine." Paul said in Ephesians 5:18-19, "Do not be *drunk* [*Hebrew:* **nooma**] with *wine*, for that is debauchery; but be filled with the *Spirit* [*Greek:* **Pnoo-ma**]." When the Holy *Spirit* rushed upon the Christians during Pentecost in Acts 2:1, "Some, however, made fun of them and said, 'They have had too much *wine*,'" (Acts 2:13). It is ironic to consider the Greek words "Pneuma Hagion" or "Holy Sprit" in light of the false accusation forwarded in Acts 2 of drunken mumbling concerning Pentecost. "Πνευμα Αγιον" or "Pneuma Hagion" is Greek and is commonly rendered "Holy Spirit":

Greek:
"Pneuma" = "Πνευμα" (ref. *4151*) = "Spirit"
"Hagion" = "Αγιον" (ref. *39*) = "Holy"

The Greek words for "Holy Spirit" sound similar to the Hebrew words for "drowsy murmuring":

Hebrew:
"noomaw" = "נומה" (ref. 5124) = "drowsiness"
"higgawyone" = "הגיון" (ref. 1902) = "murmuring sound"

Consider Adam, wine, a dead infant, and Hell in the context of this reference: "...Go and get a potter's earthen bottle, and take of the ancients of the people, and of the ancients of the priests; and go forth unto the valley of the son of *Hinnom* [*Lamentation; To Make Self Drowsy*], which is by the entry of the east gate, and proclaim there the words that I shall tell thee, and say, 'Hear ye the word of the Lord, O kings of Judah, and inhabitants of Jerusalem; Thus saith the Lord of hosts, the God of Israel; Behold, I will bring evil upon this place, the which whosoever heareth, his ears shall tingle. Because they have forsaken Me, and have estranged this place, and have burned incense in it unto other gods... and have filled this place with the blood of innocents," (Jeremiah 19:1-4).

"tree" = "עץ" (ref. 6086) = "ץ+ע" = 90+70 = **160**; "to be smooth; pleasant; be sweet" = "מלץ" (ref. 4452) = "ץ+ל+מ" = 90+30+40 = **160**; "a shadow, phantom, illusion, resemblance, idol, image" = "צלם" (ref. 6754) = "ם+ל+צ" = 40+30+90 = **160**; "something fallen, abortion, untimely birth" = "נפל" (ref. 5309) = "ל+פ+נ" = 30+80+50 = **160**.

The main point is that what seems like one thing is often another. Since the Tree of Life was coiled by the Tree of the Knowledge of Good and Evil, the woman was compelled to view the one while she beheld the other, as both trees were in the midst of the garden (Genesis 2:9). As "the fruit of the vine" was to be mixed with 2/3 water and 1/3 wine, the woman "saw" three total qualities in her ambiguous description of the "tree" in the middle of the garden: 2/3 of what she saw applied to the Tree of Life (as with water) while only 1/3 of what she saw applied to the Tree of the Knowledge of Good and Evil (as without water – called the "fruit of the tree"). As the Tree of Life is connected with the water component of the "fruit of the vine," Revelation 22:1-3 states that, "…the angel showed me the river of the water of life, bright as crystal, flowing from the throne of God and of the Lamb through the middle of the street of the city. On *either side of the river* is the Tree of Life with its 12 kinds of fruit, producing its fruit each month; and the leaves of the tree are for the healing of the nations. Nothing accursed will be found there any more…" as the only being to which the word "curse" was personally applied in Genesis 3 was the serpent (Genesis 3:14).

At this point, we must consider the earth's North Celestial Pole. The North Celestial Pole of the earth can be likened to a great, invisible column that projects upward until it intersects, or nearly intersects, a star by which all the heavens appear to rotate around for a lifetime. The North Celestial Pole of the earth gradually moves like a slowing toy-top in a motion called "Precession" that occurs once fully about every 25,800 years as the pole or column (ס) of the earth traces a circle in the night sky. The language of Genesis 3:1 orients itself (thematically) around the Age of Taurus when Leviathan (Draco) was the central point in the sky, whereas the language of Gospels is oriented around the Age of Pisces when the Lesser Winnowing Fan (called so by the Jews) or Little Bear was the central point in the sky (though the official constellation boundaries used currently differ slightly from those of yesteryear, and today's celestial maps are adorned with a greater number of constellations); in either case, one cannot view either of these two principle constellations (the *Leviathan* and the *Lesser Winnowing Fan*) without viewing the other, for the Leviathan is wrapped around the Lesser Winnowing Fan. Regarding the Solar Zodiac, as the Little Winnowing Fan is encompassed by Leviathan, we may take note that "Moreover I saw under the sun that in the place of justice, wickedness is there, and in the place of righteousness, wickedness is there also," (Ecclesiastes 3:16).

In a similar way, when the woman looked at the Tree of Life, she could not help but see the Tree of the Knowledge of Good and Evil as well, thus the 2/3 (or .666 repeating) nature of her statement. In a similar way, Psalm 19 discusses the stars by utilizing the principle of 666: Psalm 19:1-6 discusses the silent speech of the stars, while verses 7-14 discuss the celestial "scroll" on the pages of Scripture by using six titles (law, testimony, statutes, commandment, fear, judgments), six attributes (perfect, sure, right, pure, clean, true), and six effects (converting, making wise, rejoicing, enlightening, enduring, righteous) in verses 7-9. King Solomon only kept the Molten Sea filled to 2/3 its capacity, as it is written that, "it contained 2,000 baths," (I Kings 7:26) but that it, "received and held 3,000 baths," (II Chronicles 4:5); it could receive 3,000 baths, but it only contained 2,000 baths. King Solomon had to judge between one child and two mothers (2/3), as one of the mothers was deceitful (like the forbidden tree) as the life of the child was at stake in I Kings 3:16-28.

Evil is parasitic and is much weaker than righteousness. To claim that the number 666 is inherently evil is to claim that Psalm 19's discussion of God's Word is evil, that King Solomon's 666 talents of gold were evil (I Kings 10:14; II Chronicles 9:13), that the construction of King Solomon's throne of six steps with six statues on either side was evil (I Kings 10:19; II Chronicles 9:18-19), etc. The evil application of the number 666 in Revelation 13:18 is linked to the antichrist, but there cannot be an antichrist without there first being a Christ, nor can there be an "anti" anything without there first being a "thing." Regarding the number 666 in Revelation 13:18, it states that, "This calls for wisdom..." as the number 666 is linked to wisdom – which is why it is an integral component of the story of King Solomon who was the wisest man to ever live (I Kings 3:12) who specifically prayed for "an understanding mind... able to discern *between* good and evil..." (I Kings 3:9). Neither Adam nor his wife rightly discerned between good and evil; rather, the woman "saw" good and evil together when discussing the "tree" in her blended manner, which is why she named two characteristics of the Tree of Life and only one characteristic of the Tree of the Knowledge of Good and Evil: 2/3 = .666 repeating; it was the "Tree of the Knowledge of Good and Evil," not the Tree of the Knowledge of the *Difference Between* Good and Evil. Mathematically, three can be one:

.333 x 10 = 3.33 divided by the original (.333) = 3, put over 9 = 3/9 = 1/3
.666 x 10 = 6.66 divided by the original (.666) = 6, put over 9 = 6/9 = 2/3
.999 x 10 = 9.99 divided by the original (.999) = 9, put over 9 = 9/9 = 3/3 = 1

$$.999 = 3/3 = 1.$$

So we see that three are one in the last line. Furthermore, the 2/3 or .666 repeating that the woman named concerned the Tree of Life, not the Tree of the Knowledge of Good and Evil. Satan is a parasitic counterfeiter, and the antichrist is linked deceitfully to 666. As an illustration, the Tree of the Knowledge of Good and Evil was only described by one characteristic in terms of what Genesis 3:6 says that the woman "saw," and being paralleled to the 1/3, or only the unmixed "wine... the poison of dragons, and the cruel venom of asps," (Deuteronomy 32:32), the woman partook of "the fruit of the tree," not the "fruit of the vine," in a manner of speaking – just as Christ drank the "fruit of the tree" (not "the fruit of the vine") as He hung on the tree.

Though Adam and Eve were tempted by the vine-tree coiled about the Tree of Life, they were always provided with a means of overcoming the temptation, as the fruit of the correct tree hung along side the poison of the incorrect tree. Consider I Corinthians 10:9-13: "We must not put Christ to the test, as some of them did, and were destroyed by *serpents* [**365**]. And do not complain as some of them did, and were destroyed by the *destroyer* [**365**]. So if you think you are standing, watch out that you do not *fall* [consider 'נפל' (ref. 5309) = *something fallen, abortion, untimely birth*]. No testing has overtaken you that is not *common to man* [*Adam*]. God is faithful, and He will not let you be tested beyond your strength, but with the testing He will also provide the way out so that you may be able to endure it," as was the case with the first temptation concerning the two trees.

The Serpent, "*the Accuser*" = "Σατανας" (ref. *4567*) = "Σ+α+τ+α+ν+α+ς" = 6+1+300+1+50+1+6 = **365**

"destroyer" = "שׁשׁה" or "שׁסה" (ref. 8154) = "ה+ס+שׁ" = 5+60+300 = 365.

[3.27] The Tree of the Knowledge of Good and Evil was a "vine-tree" – it was the false vine of deception. Christ specifically identified Himself as the "True Vine," (John 15:1), not merely "the vine" only (John 15:5). If there is a "true" vine, there must also be a false vine, as Christ pointed us to the fact that He was preparing to hang on a tree, similar to the manner in which wild vines hang on trees. The act of hanging is also described in Ezekiel 15:3 in relation to the "vine-tree": "Is wood taken from it to make anything? Does one take a peg from it on which to hang any object?"

The wild vine hangs itself about the tree it climbs, thus: "For this reason the Father loves Me, because I lay down my life in order to take it up again. No one takes it from Me, but I lay it down of my own accord," (John 10:17-18). Evil is the parasitic opposite of Righteousness. In a related way, wild vines do not possess the strength or firmness to ascend to a viable height that offers water and light; rather, wild vines must find firm trees, use the firmness and height as a host, and climb the trees in order to achieve their goal; the righteous example of this principle can be seen in John 5:30: "I can do nothing of My own. As I hear, I judge; and My judgment is just, because I seek to do not My own will but the will of Him Who sent Me." As wine is called the blood of grapes in the Scriptures (Genesis 49:11), it should be recognized that wild vines do not produce wine-grapes, and the words of Christ show Him to parallel Himself to both trained vines and wild vines. Christ never sinned, but He "became sin" instead, for He is One with the Host (John 10:30) as He Himself is the Creator as well, and He reduced Himself to One that clings for our sakes, similar to a vine meant for wine being converted (if you will) into a wild vine – a fact that points to why the Lord's Supper (with wine-grapes) preceded His crucifixion (as He was treated as a wild vine that hung on a tree). "For our sake He made Him to be sin Who knew no sin, so that in Him we might become the righteousness of God," (II Corinthians 5:21). Christ, Who knew no sin, became sin. We, who know sin, can become the righteousness of God through Christ. "Out of his anguish he shall see light; he shall find satisfaction through his knowledge. The righteous one, my servant, shall make many righteous, and he shall bear their iniquities. Therefore I will allot him a portion with the great, and he shall divide the spoil with the strong; because he poured out himself to death, and was numbered with the transgressors; yet he bore the sin of many, and made intercession for the transgressors," (Isaiah 53:11-12).

[3.28] When reflecting on the names of the two central trees in garden, the "Knowledge of Good and Evil" is not the antithesis of "Life." At the very least, only the description of "Evil" opposes life, but this description is only half of the name of the forbidden tree; it is partially for this reason that the woman saw that the tree was desirable "to make one wise," for the wordplay between "to make one wise" (from "שכל" = **350**) and "to bereave of children" (from "שׂכל" = **350**) illustrates how death is the opposite of life, not how knowledge is opposed to life. Proverbs 3:13-18 described "Wisdom" as being a "tree of life," but this word "Wisdom" is not the same word used to describe what Eve saw in the Tree of the Knowledge of Good and Evil. The word "to make one wise" was chosen because it alludes to the word "to bereave of children," the exact opposite of the "Wisdom" that is a "tree of life" in Proverbs 3, for it was not the Tree of Wisdom, but rather it was the Tree of the Knowledge; the concept involved here is one of life versus death which is why the humans were condemned to die on account of their sins. Those saved in Christ are "born again," (John 3), and as we are to be born again, Christ told us that we are to "become like children" (Matthew 18:2) – not in immaturity, for if we were supposed to revert away from knowledge and wisdom, the Scriptures would not say: "Whom shall He teach knowledge? And whom shall He make to understand doctrine? Them that are weaned from the milk, and drawn from the breasts," (Isaiah 28:9) or "Brothers and sisters, do not be children in your thinking... but in thinking be adults," (I Corinthians 14:20). The second birth in Christ is one of innocence, not ignorance, and it was this innocence that Satan successfully stole from Adam and Eve through their ignorant slaying of their defenseless child.

Concerning Satan, "He was a murderer from the beginning and does not stand in the truth, because there is not truth in Him," (John 8:44). Consider Jesus' words: "The thief comes only to steal, kill, and destroy," (John 10:10); since when do all thieves commit murder? Thieves are thieves and murderers are murderers and therefore one criminal can commit both theft and murder and yet be guilty of but one crime. Murder does not make a criminal a thief any more than theft makes a criminal into a murderer. The "thief" discussed in John 10:10 is the Enemy who bereaved Eve of her child through her own will, for, "... one is tempted by one's own desire, being lured and enticed by it; then, when that desire has conceived, it gives birth to sin, and that sin, when it is fully grown, gives birth to death," (James 1:14-15). The evil tint placed on this "thief" is parasitic to the fact that Jesus paralleled Himself to a thief in Revelation 15:16; in other words, robbery is evil, but the suddenness by which robbery often comes is neither good nor evil, for Christ will come with such suddenness, though in righteousness and for the purposes of salvation and judgment: "Look! He comes up like clouds, His chariots like the whirlwind; His horses are swifter than eagles – woe to us, for we are ruined," (Jeremiah 4:13); "Look! He is coming with the clouds; every eye will see Him, even those who pierced Him; and on His account all the tribes of the earth will wail. So it is to be. Amen," (Revelation 1:7).

[3.29] Genesis 2:18 states that there was a garden inside of Eden, whereas Ezekiel 28:13 states that Eden was a garden. There are differences between the descriptions of "Eden" concerning Genesis and Ezekiel. Genesis discusses Jehovah Elohim's garden whereas Ezekiel discusses Elohim's garden – and this distinction is made by Satan when He first questioned Eve about Elohim's command, not Jehovah Elohim's command. Satan was cast from Elohim's garden in Ezekiel 28 whereas Adam was expelled from Jehovah Elohim's garden in Genesis 3;

this may have been the case because the Eden discussed in Ezekiel 28 describes the fall of Satan, which happened before the creation of Adam, thus the term "Eden" used between Genesis and Ezekiel describes two different places (perhaps simultaneously?), as the two distinct Titles of God named here discuss the One True God, but the separate Persons. The confusion that the woman suffered in Genesis 3:1-6 came partially on account of a confusion of God's Names and the commands that were attached to these names. Since Elohim and Jehovah are both One God, the serpent's initial question was volleyed from a singular questioning of God's commands without distinguishing the Persons specifically involved in those commands. The Names of God are of extreme importance. Both the Father and the Holy Spirit are God, but They did not die on the cross as Jesus did, even though Jesus is God and God is One.

.333 x 10 = 3.33 divided by the original (.333) = 3, put over 9 = 3/9 = 1/3
.666 x 10 = 6.66 divided by the original (.666) = 6, put over 9 = 6/9 = 2/3
.999 x 10 = 9.99 divided by the original (.999) = 9, put over 9 = 9/9 = 3/3 = 1

.999 = 3/3 = 1.

Let us now discuss "paradises."

[3.30] "Paradises (pleasure-grounds) were formed by eastern monarchs. In the British Museum may be seen the inscriptions of Gudea, the greatest of the Sumerian rulers of Chaldea (2,500 B.C.), and Tiglath-pileser I, king of Assyria (1120 B.C.) describing what could be only a botanical and zoological park. Assur-nazir-pal, king of Assyria (885 B. C.), founded such a public paradise, and describes how he stocked it; what he brought, and whence he brought the natural history collection. The British Museum contains a portion of a similar catalogue of Sennacherib," (*Companion Bible*, Bullinger, p. 908). These "... pleasure-grounds, producing all kinds of delicious fruit, and aromatics, which are most calculated to regale the sense... are so essential to Oriental luxury. The Hebrew names for different kinds of gardens denote the occupation assigned to Adam when the Lord placed him in the Garden of Eden. We are told that the Lord God took the man and put him in the garden of Eden to cultivate it... hence we find that the expressions denoting gardens signify one or the other of these two offices. ... a garden is generally cultivated by means of spades and axes (Judg. xv. 5; Job xxiv. 18), and afterwards applied especially to a vineyard. ... [concerning the word "guard," a "garden"]... is guarded and protected," (*Coheleth*, Ginsburg; p. 280-281).

A paradise was different from both a garden and a vineyard in the respect that a paradise was stocked with animate life, whereas gardens and vineyards were often designed to keep out animate life as animals (like foxes) tend to destroy the a care-taker's labors. The concept of a "paradise" is most commonly remembered from its Persian sense that denoted the beautiful and fortified pleasure-grounds of elites, and for our purposes, some of the most important Persian elites were the Magi. However, in the Persian sense of the word, *paradises* were deliberately stocked with animate life for the purposes of hunting, as one of the Persian "pleasures" involved in a paradise was the act of killing.

"Thus much I can declare of the Persians with entire certainty, from my own actual knowledge. There is another custom which is spoken of with reserve, and not openly, concerning their dead. It is said that the body of a male Persian is never buried, until it has been torn either by a dog or a bird of prey. That the Magi have this custom is beyond a doubt, for they practice it without any concealment. The dead bodies are covered with wax, and then buried in the ground.

"The Magi are a very peculiar race, different entirely from the Egyptian priests, and indeed from all other men whatsoever. The Egyptian priests make it a point of religion not to kill any live animals except those which they offer in sacrifice. The Magi, on the contrary, kill animals of all kinds with their own hands, excepting dogs and men. They even seem to take delight in the employment, and kill as readily as they do other animals, ants and snakes, and such like flying and creeping things. However, since this has always been their custom, let them keep to it. I return to my former narrative," (*Clio*, Herodotus; Section 140).

Again, the word "paradise," "according to Spiegel, was derived from the Zendic pairi-daeza, a hedging round, and passed into the Hebrew in the form פרדס (Cant. 4:13; Eccl. 2:5; Neh. 2:8), a park, probably through the commercial relations which Solomon established with different countries," (Commentary on the Old Testament: Genesis, Keil & Delitzsch; p. 50). Παραδεισος [Paradise] = "a park, a forest where wild beasts were kept for hunting; a pleasure-park, a garden of trees of various kinds..." (The Analytical Lexicon to the Greek New Testament, Mounce; p. 351). In other words, paradises were hedged in, enclosed by a wall to keep intruders out; however, in the Persian sense, paradises were enclosed by a wall to ensure that the animate life within it could not escape in order that it would be hunted down and slaughtered for "pleasure." Though the Persian sense of the word is commonly remembered, Genesis 2-3 discusses what became known later in the Persian sense but was not intended originally for any bloody purposes:

"פרדס" (ref. 6508) = "paradise" = "ס+ד+ר+פ" = 60+4+200+80 = **344**

"שמד" (ref. 8045) = "to desolate, destroy, bring to nought, overthrow, perish, pluck down" = "ד+מ+ש" = 4+40+300 = **344**

"שמד" (ref. 8046) Chaldee = "consume" = "ד+מ+ש" = 4+40+300 = **344**

Regarding the Persian sense of the word *paradise*, "The Hebrews, who had gardens at so early a period, would surely not borrow names for them from other nations. [The word "paradise"]... is a compound of... [the word] *to divide*, and [the word] *to separate, to enclose*; hence *a protected, an enclosed place, a garden*," (*Song of Songs*, Ginsburg; p. 161). The Gematria example above, regardless of the Persians, helps to relate the story of the first humans. The word "paradise" does not occur in Genesis 2-3, but

Christ makes reference to Eden (or something like it) in Luke 23:43 as He Himself was the victim of such bloody pleasure (if you will), for He was hunted down in a "garden" (paralleled to Eden) that was near graves, and He was buried in a garden (paralleled to Eden). At the same time, Christ did not employ the word "paradise" to indicate any death for the purposes of bloody sport, for He used it to describe everlasting life, as the reign of the Messiah is one where, "The wolf shall live with the lamb, the leopard shall lie down with the kid, the calf and the lion and the fatling together, and a little child shall lead them. The cow and the bear shall graze, their young shall lie down together; and the lion shall eat straw like the ox. The nursing child shall play over the hole of the asp, and the weaned child shall put its hand on the adder's den. They will not hurt or destroy on all My holy mountain; for the earth will be full of the knowledge of the Lord as the waters cover the sea," (Isaiah 11:6-9). The "holy mountain" is where Satan was expelled from in Ezekiel 28:16, and being hurled to the earth, Satan sought to turn the earthly copy of the true Paradise into the sense that the Persians cast upon "pleasure." As such, we understand in Genesis 2:15 that Adam was placed inside the fortifications of a garden inside of the larger paradise of Eden (Genesis 2:8) and was to guard against intrusion.

A garden became a paradise in the sense that a paradise was deliberately designed and cultivated (like a garden) and after these steps of progression, it was stocked with animate life, for the animate life made it a paradise by definition. The reader will notice that Adam was alone within the garden (Genesis 2:18) despite the fact that many, but not all (Genesis 2:19), of the animals existed before Adam outside of his garden home. That is, Eden was created a paradise as befits its definition by the fact that it was stocked with animate life, but Adam's garden home inside of Eden was only populated by him alone as fitting the definition of a garden (and a vineyard is also considered a type of garden).

The Magi are such a crucial element to the story of Christ because theses sorcerers who sought out the Christ Child (The Son of *Man*) mirror the sorcerer who sought out the child of Adam (the son of *Adam*). As stated previously, the title "Magi" was regarded in both a regal and a wicked sense. The readers of Matthew's Gospel in Matthew's day would have probably felt uneasiness in the beginning of his narrative regarding about the ambiguous Magi, for their true intentions were only revealed upon their discovery of the "Holy Child" (as He is called in Acts 4:27). For slightly different but related purposes, notice the alarm experienced when the Magi came to pay tribute to the new King (Jesus): "When King Herod heard this, he was frightened, and all Jerusalem with him," (Matthew 2:3), for the Magi arrived unexpectedly, and with a knowledge that Herod did not possess. Antithetically, the first and most powerful sorcerer, Satan, the "Serpent," also sought out a child, and like the Persians who eventually tinctured a paradise to be a place where both life and death were mingled with the blood of the slain, Satan sought to hunt down the rarest, most prized, and most protected inhabitant of Eden.

As the New Testament is a mirror of the Old Testament,

A Garden, A Vineyard, or A Paradise?   359

we can understand specifically why the Magi play such an important role in Christ's Kingly quest to overturn the errors wrought in Eden. The Magi are called "Wise Men," and "... the serpent was subtle above every beast of the field that Jehovah Elohim had made," (Genesis 3:1). Satan existed before Adam who existed before the *complete* creation of the animals in Genesis 2:19. Satan could not have been a mere animal, nor could Satan have been brought to Adam with the other animals of Genesis 2:19. It is significant to note that Adam gave names to all of the "cattle, and to the birds of the air, and to every animal of the field," (Genesis 2:20). Adam did not name any water-dwelling life, and Satan is also likened to a sea creature (Psalm 104:26), as some serpents are of the earth and other serpents are often found in water. However, God gave humanity (Adam: Genesis 5:2) the power to dominate (Genesis 4:7) "the fish of the sea" and "the birds of the air" and "every living thing that moves upon the earth" (Genesis 1:28) following His first command to "be fruitful and multiply," (Genesis 1:28), and it is for this reason that Satan could not merely attack the humans, but instead, Satan had to exact his will through the human mind and at human hands. Satan knew the rules, and by questioning the humans' interpretation of those rules, he coaxed humanity into breaking God's rules. Notice how Satan made no excuses for his actions during Jehovah Elohim's judgments, unlike the humans.

Adam named the animals by God's permission, and naming is an act of dominance (Isaiah 43:1); for a similar reason, God named Adam. Again, we must keep in mind that, "... out of the ground, Jehovah Elohim formed every animal... and brought them to the man to see what he would call them; and whatever the man called every living creature, that was its name," (Genesis 2: 19). If there actually was a talking snake in Eden, Adam would have named it. Furthermore, knowing that God does not tempt, God would not have "brought" Satan to Adam, which would then nullify God's designation for Adam to "guard" the garden, just as it would contradict James 1:13.

[3.31] The ancients called a certain spirit of divination the "spirit of Python," and by this name, we can understand a little more clearly why Satan is described as a "serpent," as the "serpent" concept was often linked to vines, ropes, chains, whips, and other slinky sorts of things. This "Python" is also linked to wine. "And it happened, as we went into a place of prayer, a certain slave girl having a Pythonic spirit met us, whose divining brought much gain to her lords," (Acts 16:16). Biblical accounts of serpent imagery are also accompanied by descriptions of "binding" or objects consistent with binding as in Revelation 20:1-3 which sates, "... I saw an angel coming down out of Heaven, having the key of the abyss, and a *great chain* in his hand. And he laid hold of the dragon, the old serpent who is the Devil, and Satan, and *bound* him a thousand years, and threw him into the abyss, and shut him up, and sealed over him..." The Persian wise men, the Magi, of whom many were astrologers, were familiar with the Pythonic spirit, and it is amazing how God used Jeremiah to teach heathen conquerors Who God really was.

A "familiar spirit" like Python was thought to impart to his human mediums supernatural information from a voice that sounded echoey and hollow (as if spoken out of a bottle) that projected from the armpits or chest of the human medium. Jeremiah warned the people that unless they went into the rule of their attackers, they would be killed (Jeremiah 38:1-3). Out of anger, the officials lowered Jeremiah, by ropes, into a waterless cistern (Jeremiah 38:6). "A cistern is a collection chamber that gathers runoff. Cisterns typically have a bottle or bell shape, with a narrow top to prevent evaporation. The entire interior is coated with plaster, so that every drop of water is preserved. Water was drawn from a cistern in the same fashion as from a well... DRY CISTERNS also served as detention cells," (*Archaeological Study Bible: N.I.V.*; p. 1,259). As acts 16:16 tells us that a *slave* girl who made money for her *lords* was possessed of the Pythonic spirit, we read of the antithesis of this fact in that, "...the king commanded *Ebed*[*Slave*]-*Melech*[*King*] the Cushite, 'Take 30 men with you from here, and pull the prophet Jeremiah up from the cistern before he dies,'" (Jeremiah 38:10). As is consistent with serpentine imagery (vines, ropes, etc.), Ebed-Melech took old rags [as old rags were sometimes used to fertilize vines (*A Vine-dresser's Manual,* Reemelin; p. 87)] and said, "Just put the rags and clothes between your *armpits* and the ropes," (Jeremiah 38:12). Hence, the prophet Jeremiah – the medium (if you will allow the expression) of God – was pulled from a bottle-shaped enclosure by ropes out of his empty, hollow cell (compare to the abyss of the Serpent in Revelation 20:1-3) as it was supposed that Python spoke from with his hollow voice out of the armpits as if echoed from inside a bottle. As the Scriptures often refer to human physicality in terms of pottery, clay, dust, houses, etc., the ninth letter (ט) was probably alluded to by Jesus in Luke 11:24-26: "When the **unclean spirit** has gone out of a person, it wanders through WATERLESS regions looking for a resting place, but not finding any, it says, 'I will return to my house from which I came.' When it comes, it finds it *swept* and put in order. Then it goes and brings *seven other spirits* more evil than itself, and they enter and live there; and the last state of that person is worse than the first." The eight total spirits within the one person sum to 9, and "ט" is also the number "9"; the signification of this ninth letter is "*sweeping*": "טיט" (ref. 2916) = "to be sticky, from ref. 2894, through the idea of dirt to be swept away," and also a "*leather bottle*, or a *snake*" – like the EMPTY **spirit of Python**.

The hollow sound attributed to Python's voice (as echoing in a bottle) is in stark contrast to the "filling" of the Holy Spirit. Paul said in Ephesians 5:18-19, "Do not be *drunk* [*Hebrew: nooma*] with *wine*, for that is debauchery; but be filled with the *Spirit* [*Greek: Pnoo-ma*]." That is, Python is considered to sound like the empty muttering of demonic possession whereas the Holy Spirit fills His subjects with wisdom and righteousness; this fact and imagery is made evident by Elihu in Job 32:18-21: "For I am full of words; the spirit within me constrains me. My heart is indeed like wine that has no vent; like new wineskins, it is ready to burst. I must speak, so that I may find relief; I must open my lips and answer. I will not show partiality to any person or use flattery toward anyone. For I do not know how to flatter – or my Maker would soon put an end to me!" Jesus, Who judged impartially (John 7:24) used similar imagery when He said, "Isaiah prophesied rightly about you hypocrites, as it is written, 'This people honors Me with their lips, but their hearts are far from me,'" (Mark 7:6) in connection with the fact that Christ called the Scribes and Pharisees "hypocrites" (Mark 7:6) and "vipers" (Matthew 23:33); we can better understand the force of His statement when He said, "...no one puts new wine into old wineskins; otherwise, the wine will burst the skins, and the wine is lost, and so are the skins; but one puts new wine into fresh wineskins," (Mark 2:22). Jesus compared and contrasted His disciples and John the Baptist's disciples against the Pharisees (Mark 2:18), as He alluded to the fact that the Pharisees (pythons) were empty unlike His own followers who were full. The full versus empty situation of Jesus' words was exhibited by the irony of the fast that John's disciples and the Pharisees were presently undertaking; that is, Jesus used two groups who were fasting as examples to show who was full (John's disciples) and who was empty (the Pharisees) through His own disciples who were not fasting at all. Jesus corrected the Pharisees immediately following His statement about bursting wineskins. Furthermore, as to the "new wineskins" versus "old wineskins," Elihu, "like new wineskins... [was] ready to burst," (Job 32:19) because of the Ancient Spirit within him, and Elihu criticized Job's friends who were older than Elihu himself by telling them personally, "I am young in years, and you are aged; therefore I was timid and afraid to declare my opinion to you. I said, 'Let days speak, and many years teach wisdom.' But truly it is the spirit in a mortal, the breath of the Almighty, that makes for understanding. It is not the old that are wise, nor the aged that understand what is right," (Job 32:6-9). As Elihu, being filled with the Spirit of God, was righteous in his reproof of Job and his three friends, we can see how the antithetical and wicked pythonic spirit is exhibited in the story of Judas.

Judas hung himself (Matthew 27:5) probably with a rope (like a serpent) and he was emptied as "he burst out in the middle and all his bowels gushed out," (Acts 1:18) like old wine in a new wineskin – for evil, and not for good like Elihu in Job 32:18-21; this is a reason why such an emphasis is placed on the fact that Judas "burst out" so that the reader would understand that the Pythonic spirit had entered him (John 13:27) and emptied him (Acts 1:18). The satanic spirit of Python is empty and it hollows-out those who attempt to use it, but the Holy Spirit fills His followers so that their cup overflows.

[3.32] A woman is paralleled to a paradise, a locked garden, and a sealed fountain in Song of Songs 4:12-13. The term "closed garden" became a description for a virtuous woman; the opposite terminology, a "door," applied to an unchaste woman open to seduction as in Song of Songs 8:9. "To a locked garden and spring no one has access but the rightful owner, and a sealed fountain is shut against all impurity," (*Commentary on the Old Testament: Song of Songs*, Keil & Delitzsch, p. 559). Song of Songs 4:12: "a sealed fountain" – "The scarcity of water in arid countries renders fountains very valuable. To secure them against the encroachment of strangers, the proprietors formerly fastened their fountains with some ligament, and the impression of a seal upon clay, which would quickly harden in the sun, that would soon dissolve wax. This mode of rendering pits safe is found in Dan. vi. 18; Matt xxvii. 66. A fountain sealed in this manner indicated that it was private property. Hence its metaphorical use, to represent chastity as an inaccessible fountain," (*Song of Songs*, Ginsburg; p. 160). As we will soon discover in more detail, Eden is compared to the most desirable woman of absolute purity. Regarding Adam's job to cultivate and to guard Eden in Genesis 2:15, we note "... the feminine expression to work [cultivate] it (lit. her) and to guard it (lit. her)," (*Ramban*: Genesis, Vol. 1, Ramban; p. 99).

[3.33] Christ said, "... you are *Peter* [Πετρος], on this *rock* [πετρα] I will build my church, and the gates of Hades will not prevail against her," (Matthew 16:18). The name "**Peter**" is the Greek "Πετρος" (ref. *4074*) = "Rock" (masculine). The Greek word "rock" is "**petra**" = "πετρα" (ref. *4073*) = "rock" (feminine). Christ said that the gates of Hades will not prevail against her, and a gate functions like a door. In some instances (Job 3:10; Song of Songs 8:9) Scripture compares a door or gate to human femininity, and when this concept is applied negatively, a "door" implies an unchaste woman. The word "door" = "דלת" (ref. 1817) also means "gate." The impurity of Hades (like an unchaste woman) shall not prevail against the purity of the Church (like a spotless bride). What hell births shall not prevail over what Heaven births. So when Christ declared the victory of the Church to **Peter** with respect to the rock (**petra**) of the Church's foundation, it should be noted that the Hebrew word "**peter**" = "פטר"

(ref. 6363) has the same definition as the Hebrew word "**petra**" = "פטרה" (also ref. 6363) which means, "a fissure [as in a rock]; a firstling (as opening the matrix) [i.e. *the firstborn of a womb*]." The relation of a rock to reproduction conveys the concept of a foundation, as can be observed in Job 38:4, 8: "Where were you when I laid the foundation of the earth... Or who shut in the sea with doors when it burst out from the womb?" Consider the fact that water was brought out of a rock in Numbers 20.

"אבן" (ref. 68) = "to build; a stone" = "א+ב+ן" = 50+2+1 = **53**
"אבן" (ref. 70) = "a potter's wheel or a midwife's stool = "א+ב+ן" = 50+2+1 = **53**
"גן" (ref. 1588) = "a garden (as fenced)" = "ג+ן" = 50+3 = **53**
"נבא" (ref. 5012) = "prophesy" = "נ+ב+א" = 1+2+50 = **53**

The parallel of a "rock" to a womb agrees with the parallel of a "snake" to masculinity, as can be observed in Proverbs 30:18-19 by the poetic figuration of Synonymous Parallel. Accordingly, Proverbs 30:18-19 states,

> "Three things are too wonderful
> for me;
> four I do not understand:
>
> the way of an eagle in the sky,
> the way of snake on a rock,
> the way of a ship on the high seas,
> and the way of a man with a girl."

The Synonymous Parallel shows that an eagle in the sky is reflected by a ship on the high seas. In the same way,

A Garden, A Vineyard, or A Paradise?

the Synonymous Parallel shows that the snake on a rock is reflected by the way of a man with a girl.
"snake on a rock"
"man with a girl"

God is described in the masculine, particularly in relation to His adoptive characteristics (which would be quite unsuitable if applied to femininity regarding the ancient practices of acknowledging and accepting infants). At the same time, God compared Himself to a "hen [who] gathers her brood under her wings," (Matthew 23:37); hence, "The Rock, His work is perfect, and all His ways are just. A faithful God, without deceit, just and upright is He; yet His degenerate children have dealt falsely with Him, a perverse and crooked generation... You were unmindful of the Rock That bore you; you forgot the God Who gave you birth. Indeed their rock is not like our Rock; our enemies are fools. Their vine comes from the vine stock of Sodom, and from the vineyards of Gomorrah; their grapes are grapes of poison, their clusters are bitter; their wine is the poison of serpents, the cruel venom of asps." (Deuteronomy 32:4-5...18...31-33).

Applied to God, the description of a "Rock" indicates a foundation for His creation. Applied to people, the description of a "rock" is sometimes, on a smaller level, indicative of femininity as in Job 38:4,8; Matthew 16:18; etc. Yet, Leviticus 21:21 renders "testicles" as "stones" which may help us to understand John the Baptist: "You brood of vipers! Who warned you to flee from wrath to come? Bear *fruit* [אב (ref. 3)] worthy of repentance. Do not presume to say to yourselves, 'We have Abraham as our *father* [אב (ref. 1)]; for I tell you, God is able from these *stones* to raise up children to Abraham. Even now the ax is lying at the root of the *trees* [*as in lineage*]; every tree therefore that does not bear good *fruit* [אב (ref. 3)] is cut down and thrown into the fire," (Matthew 3:7-10), as we have seen previously, the "tree" discussed here is the "vine-tree" in agreement with the "brood of vipers" and in connection with "stones" – a piercingly appropriate metaphor indicating faithlessness on the part of the Pharisees, similar to an untrustworthy and unchaste bride. As John the Baptist called the Pharisees and Sadducees "vipers" in reference to their lineage by way of their fathers' stones, let us reflect again on Proverbs 30:18-19:

the way of an eagle in the sky,
the way of snake on a rock,
the way of a ship on the high seas,
and the way of a man with a girl."

The Synonymous Parallel juxtaposes "snake on a rock" with "man with a girl" and is an elegant figure representing human marital union; the "rock" here is a figure of femininity like that figure applied to the spotless Bride, the purified Church, as indicated to Peter by Christ in Matthew 16:18. John the Baptist is described as wearing "clothing of camel's hair," (Matthew 3:4): "בכר" (ref. 1070) = "(in the sense of youth); a young *camel*- dromedary"; from "בכר" (ref. 1069) = "to burst the womb, i.e. (caus.) bear or make early fruit (of woman or TREE); also to give the birthright:- make firstborn, be firstling, bring forth first child (new fruit)."

Consider Jeremiah 3:6-9: "...she took her whoredom so lightly, she polluted the land, committing adultery with *stone and tree.*" Thus, the concept of a "stone" or a "rock" is one of "foundation" that links the sexes when employed to convey faithfulness or faithlessness. As such, it is more than fitting for the Baptist who wore the hair of a *"camel"* (to burst the womb) and indicated *"stones"* (firstborn of the womb) in connection with the impurity of the Pharisees which is why they were to "bear *fruit*" ("אב": *like a spotless bride*) worthy of repentance, despite their *lineage* ("אב").

[3.34] On account of the severity of the sun in the East, repose was sought in ancient times beneath the shade of slithering vines and sweet-smelling trees where relief could be maximized by rowed foliage that allowed breezes to sift through shady pathways. The trees planted in ancient paradises were selected for their aesthetic qualities, the fruit they produced, and the perfumes they emitted. The bark of varying aromatic trees would split and drip with liquid perfume that flowed down the trunks producing a glistening passage between the upright, teary shafts of the paradise's design.

The word "בכא" (ref. 1057) means "a weeping tree" (some gum-distilling tree) in relation." Song of Songs describes the "bag of myrrh resting in [the woman's] bosom" (Song of Songs 1:13), as the liquid perfume of weeping tree bark was bottled in tiny bags that the ancient Eastern women suspended from chains or straps that hung down the center of their chests, for the feminine body adorned as such was of the utmost practical significance concerning the often sweltering heat from which these paradises would allow one to escape. These perfumed bags "formed an article of earliest commerce... highly prized by the ancients," (*Song of Songs*, by Ginsburg; p. 138); so much was the Shulamite lover's prized that she exclaimed, "A bundle of myrrh is my beloved to me; he shall lie all night between my breasts," (Song of Songs 1:13) like a bag of perfume so grandly appreciated. Amidst this dripping, balmy, breezy environment, sweet fruits dangled in the shadows and swayed in the breeze complimented by the scent of the aromatic gusts. The sensual swirling would take place amidst the shifting, declining shadows, slinking vines, and swaying branches that dipped and bobbed until the appetite was replete and the noon-day heat was abated, as both humans and animals lounged in the leisure of organic luxury – as this description precedes the concept of a "paradise" imposed by the Persians who were in pursuit of their own distinctly destructive "pleasures."

[3.35] "Although the growth of the shrubs and sprouting of the herbs are represented here as dependent upon the rain and the cultivation of the earth by man, we must not understand the words as meaning that there was neither shrub nor herb before the rain and dew, or before the creation of man, and so draw the conclusion that the creation of the plants occurred either after or contemporaneously with the creation of man, in direct contradiction to ch. 1:11, 12. The creation of the plants is not alluded to here at all, but simply the planting of the garden in Eden. The growing of the shrubs and sprouting of the herbs is different from the creation or first production of the vegetable kingdom, and relates to the growing and sprouting of the plants and germs which were called into existence by the creation, the natural development of the plants as it had steadily proceeded ever since the creation. This was dependent upon rain and human culture; their creation was not. Moreover, the shrub and herb of the field do not embrace the whole of the vegetable productions of the earth. It is not a fact that the field is used in the second section in the same sense as the earth in the first… not 'the widespread plain of the earth, the broad expanse of the land,' but a field of arable land, soil fit for cultivation, which forms only a part of the 'earth' or 'ground.' Even the beast of the field' in v. 19 and 3:1 is not synonymous with the 'beast of the earth' in ch. 1:24, 25, but is a more restricted term, denoting only such animals as live upon the field and are supported by its produce, whereas the 'beast of the earth' denotes all wild beasts as distinguished from tame cattle and reptiles. In the same way, the 'shrub of the field' consists of such shrubs and tree-like productions of the cultivated land as man raises for the sake of their fruit, and the ' herb of the field,' all seed-producing plants… which serve as food for man an beast," (*Commentary on the Old Testament: Genesis*, Keil & Delitzsch; p. 48).

[3.36] A "paradise" is generally larger than a garden or a vineyard. As such, it makes sense that Jehovah Elohim planted a garden in Eden, for Eden was a paradise with a smaller garden within its hedge. However, since Adam was alone in the garden and knew not (for a time) of the animals outside of the boundaries of the garden (but that were within the boundaries of the paradise), it makes even more sense as to why the word "paradise" is not used in Genesis 2 or 3: Adam's garden home did not possess abundant animate life, but only abundant vegetable life. After Adam resided alone in the garden within the paradise for a time, it was then that "Jehovah Elohim formed *every* animal of the field, and *every* bird of the heavens out of the ground. And He brought them to the man to see what he would call them..." (Genesis 2:19). According to Genesis 1, animals were created prior to Adam's creation, and being contained inside the garden within the paradise (Genesis 2:8), Adam could not have had knowledge of the animate inhabitants of Eden as they lived outside the hedge of his garden home. Genesis 1 does not say that Elohim formed "every" animal prior to the creation of humanity, but Genesis 2 says that Jehovah Elohim formed "every" animal after the creation of Adam; thus the creation of the animals began before Adam and finished after Adam. When it is written, "... and He brought [the animals] to the man..." (Genesis 2:19), Jehovah Elohim must have brought them through the gates (or whatever entrance there was) of the garden, not the gates of the paradise called "Eden." "Jehovah Elohim planted a garden in Eden, to the east, and He put the man whom He had formed there," (Genesis 2:8) that is, inside the hedge of the garden, not merely inside the outlying paradise where the animals created before Adam lived.

[3.37] Eve was created from the body of Adam himself. Human femininity was the only creation made from another body prior to the termination of "Day the Sixth" and of Creation as a whole, which is the singular physical grandeur of Eve's uniqueness. Eve was the final creation and the crown of beauty, formed out of another fleshly creation, that was her counterpart – as she was to be a helper, not a subordinate, for man. As man understands the undying fervor for woman, so man can begin to understand God's undying fervor for humanity which is a reason why all saved humanity is called The Bride of Christ, for "Jesus" = "Jehovah is Salvation"; remember that it was commanded that the Christ Child be named "Jesus" in Matthew 1:21. The entire Holy Bible is the most monumental love-story ever conceived!

Men can understand the earthly Eden as the height of unimaginable sensuality in the sleekness of all its purity. Women can understand Eden as an entirely unique pulchritude that serves as the crown of natural compliments about the construction of human femininity crafted by Him Who loves women more than any mortal man ever could. By fleshly masculinity, fleshly femininity houses the most precious entity created. Thus, man is compelled rightly to prize woman righteously in all innocent humility. Woman is compelled rightly to honor man righteously in all innocent humility. Man and woman did not create each other, but both were gifted with each other by the One Who loves them more than either can love each other. There is no legitimate romance without the utmost reverence for God and His commands, as the Bible is very clear about homosexuality (Romans 1:26-27; I Corinthians 6:9; I Timothy 1:10; etc.) and is, obviously, very clear about abortion, as is evinced in the Fall of humanity in connection with the crucifixion. The Church, including both male and female members, is the "Bride" of Christ; though this concept can be difficult for men to grasp, it is good to remember that it is the Bride who is to bring forth fruit.

[3.38] Jehovah Elohim gave Adam a physical occupation that allowed him to begin to understand the nature of The Creator. At first, the notion of work seems to be far from ideal, but our concept of work is only as it is because we exist after the Fall of humanity from perfection. "The structure of the Garden of Eden corresponds to the structure of the firmament," (*Ramban*: Genesis, Vol. 1, Ramban; p. 131). Adam's occupation within the garden, his cultivation, was soft and easy, but it was turned into hard labor following his expulsion from the garden to the fulfillment of the serpent's wishes. The letters "נחש" can mean "serpent" or "brass" (or bronze or copper) depending on how they are vowelized (they have the same gematria). Considering that the "firmament" means something similar to "a beaten out sheet of of metal," we might better understand the metaphor in Leviticus 26:19: "And if in spite of this you will not obey me, I will continue to punish you sevenfold for your sins... I will make your sky like iron and your earth like brass."

Adam's original occupation allowed him to behold the Earth spring up life as it did on "Day Third" in Genesis 1 before Adam was created. Prior to sin, Adam was placed in the garden to "till" or "cultivate" it (Genesis 2:15), and this occupation was part of perfection. However, after Adam sinned, "Jehovah Elohim sent him out of the garden of Eden to till the ground out of which he was taken," (Genesis 3:23) also. Adam had to till (or cultivate) in both instances: the first in pleasure, the second in pain. "The curse pronounced on man's account upon the soil created for him, consisted in the fact, that the earth no longer yielded spontaneously the fruits requisite for his maintenance, but the man was obliged to force out the necessaries of life by labor and strenuous exertion," (*Commentary on the Old Testament*, Keil & Delitzsch; p. 65).

[3.39] The account that Adam was made from the dust of the ground describes Adam as similar to vegetation in connection with the definitions of "garden," a "vineyard," and a "paradise"; these three entities are distinct from the wilderness, and since Genesis 1 tells us that vegetation was formed prior to Genesis 2, we can understand the unpruned world of Eden's exterior as opposed to the pruned garden-vineyard-paradise of Eden's interior. Jehovah Elohim placed Adam in the garden of Eden to "guard" her in Genesis 2:15, for the garden was within Eden, and the two central trees were in the midst of the garden. It was Adam who was, at first, the only fleshly inhabitant of the garden, not the first fleshly inhabitant created altogether. Genesis 2 never claims such a contradiction, though tradition sometimes claims such a contradiction.

Remember that Elohim said to humanity, "Behold, I have given to you all herbage yielding seed that is on the surface of the earth, and every tree that has seed-yielding fruit; it shall be yours for food," (Genesis 1:29). He did not say "every tree," but rather "every tree that has seed-yielding fruit," which explains the nature of the Tree of the Knowledge of Good and Evil and Jehovah Elohim's prohibition against it Genesis 2:17: a parallel between the Tree of the Knowledge of Good and Evil to humanity is that this forbidden tree did not produce fruit with seed in it, and by consuming its peculiar fruit, it demanded the same of those who ate of it; "בכר" (ref. 1069) = "to burst the womb, i.e. (caus.) bear or make early fruit (*of woman or tree*); also to give the birthright:- make firstborn, be firstling, bring forth first child (new fruit)" = "ב+כ+ר" = 200+20+2 = **222**. Adam and Eve rebelled against Elohim's first command (Genesis 1:28) and spurned His *blessing*: "ברך" (ref. 1288) = "to bless" = "ב+ר+ך" = 20+200+2 = **222**. We can understand why the constellations of Hercules and Draco were identified in the prophesy of Genesis 3:15 regarding redemption: "He shall bruise thy head, and thou shalt bruise His heel." The constellation Hercules, "...is one of the oldest sky figures, although not known to the first Greek astronomers under that name, – for Eudoxos had Ενγουνασι; Hipparchos... *Bending on his knees*... Aratos added to these designations... *the Kneeling One*," (*Star Names*, Allen; p. 239) as the constellation we now refer to as "Hercules" was organized in its ancient map to depict a mighty warrior on bended knee (due to a wounded heel) in preparation to smash the head of a serpent and a vine held in one of his hands by a piece of wood in his other hand. In a similar way, "ברך" (ref. 1288) = "to kneel" = "ב+ר+ך" = 20+200+2 = **222**; "ברך" (ref. 1290) = "knee" = "ב+ר+ך" = 20+200+2 = **222**, as the constellations indicate time-periods similar to our present-day analog clocks, for "כבר" (ref. 3528) = "extent of time; long ago, formerly, hitherto:- already, (seeing that which), now" = "כ+ב+ר" = 200+2+20 = **222**.

[3.40] Before Eve was created, Adam found no fleshly helper that suited him, so "Jehovah Elohim caused a deep sleep to fall upon the man, and he slept; then He took one of his ribs and closed up its place with flesh. And the rib that the Lord God had taken from the man He made into a woman and brought her to the man." Jehovah Elohim made flesh from the ground except for Eve who was made from Adam. The word applied to the initial construction of the "garden" of Eden is "גַן" (ref. 1588) = "garden (as fenced)"; from "גנן" (ref. 1598) = "to hedge about; protect; defend." The chief function of the rib-cage is to guard the heart. As Adam was "hedged" into the garden in Eden by Jehovah Elohim for his protection, Adam was to "guard" the garden for his sustentation and the sustentation of his home's eventual family. The hedge of the garden was opened to other animate life besides Adam at the direction of God, and Adam's heart was exposed to his wife by the grace of God.

The creation of Eden foreshadows the creation of Eve. Eve's constitution accorded with the constitution of Eden, for the garden home of Adam was a garden "in" Eden (Genesis 2:8) but was later referred to the garden "of" Eden (Genesis 3:24). A garden and a paradise are related by cultivation and vegetation, but a paradise contains animate life; by allowing other animate life into Adam's garden home, it began to take on the characteristics of a paradise. Consider "...the feminine expression to work [cultivate] it (lit. her) and to guard it (lit. her)," (*Ramban: Genesis*, Vol. 1, Ramban; p. 99) – similarly, Eve, like Eden, became the larger that contained the smaller, as her own body eventually housed animate life in a representation of how a garden can become a paradise. Jehovah Elohim's first command to humanity was to "be fruitful and multiply," (Genesis 1:28). Fruitful multiplication is the result of cultivation for both land and humanity. As Eden was the crown of vegetation in beauty, Eve was the crown of flesh in beauty accordingly – before she became a pregnant mother, for by this pregnancy, the human infant became the most rare and exotic creation of all. As the garden in Eden was planted in the larger and preceding paradise of Eden, so Adam was commanded to plant his seed into Eve by Elohim's first command.

As Eden was a paradise and as Adam's wife was a type of paradise, Satan was the first to convert the protective enclosures of peaceful paradises (as they were intended to be) into the containing enclosures of bloody "paradises" in the sense of Luke 19:43: "Indeed, the days will come upon you, when your enemies will set up ramparts around you and surround you, and hem you in on every side." In like manner, the Magi of the Persian priesthood also came to include killing amongst the "pleasures" of a paradise, for no violent bloodshed occurred prior to sin which is of the utmost significance regarding sacrifice, the blood covenant, and atonement – for to claim that the violent shedding of any blood occurred prior to sin is to disregard the fulfillment of righteousness described in Isaiah 11:6-9 in connection with Christ's promise in Luke 23:43. The title "Magi," like the color white, can be viewed positively and negatively... and the Magi wore white. One of evil's greatest tactics is the employment of confusion. The Magi were a strange and violent order, yet those sages who paid righteous homage to Christ the King, the Creator who allowed Himself to come to earth as a Child in the redemptive stead of the stillborn son of Adam, are remembered for their regal dignity and unforgettable honesty – unlike those dark renegades who called themselves "Magi" and unlike Satan who but disguises himself as an angel of light.

When discussing paradises, the Persian priesthood can hardly be omitted from this topic, and as they are depicted in purity (although mysteriously so) in the Book of Matthew, they positively paralleled the Enemy who is compared to a renegade of their order (for there was no such order in the beginning of Adam's days).   What was meant for protection became devised for destruction. What blood was present at union and birth became a component of the sacrifice, blood covenant, and atonement. Whatever exertion was planned for pregnancy became arduous labor. Whatever ease Adam enjoyed during his cultivation prior to sin became his hard punishment. Evil is the dim reflection and exact opposite of Righteousness. The New Testament is the exact fulfillment and bright reflection of the grandeur, beauty, precision, mastery, and power of the Old Testament – both of which were so graciously, tenderly, and magnanimously given to us by God to guard us and to guide us into the design we were intended to live up to and within.

[3.41] When perfect order is reversed for antithetical purposes, that which was meant for intense beauty becomes drenched in intense hideousness to the extent that even terms of otherwise blithe grandeur can become corrupted by a tint that is against the design and dignity of pristine nature. When acts of barbarism are considered to be acts of mercy, when selfishness is painted as selflessness, when the humanity and essence of one is but regarded as the decision and "right" of another, then the chosen qualities of the life of one become converted into the unchosen suffering and death of another.

Given all of the preceding information, the reader can understand that the accidental slaying of an infant through intentional consumption sank the world into sin and death... and the reader can also understand that the intentional slaying of an infant is even worse. "Now the word of the Lord came to me saying, '**Before I formed you in the womb I knew you**, and before you were born I consecrated you; I appointed you a prophet to the nations," (Jeremiah 1:5). Arguing that an unborn human is not human defies the Holy Scriptures. The intentional slaying of an unborn human – a process that we call "abortion" – cannot be right if the unintentional slaying of an unborn human through intentional, but ignorant, actions opened the door to every evil known to humanity.

CONCLUSION
DRAWING NEAR TO THE BEGINNING

"Listen, O heavens, and I will speak; hear, O earth, the words of my mouth. Let my teaching fall like rain and my words descend like dew, like showers on new grass, like abundant rain on tender plants,"
(Deuteronomy 32:1-2).

Let us now put all of the pieces of our study together. The first sin resulted in an abortive birth, as this stillbirth was the very event that plunged the earth into a doomed state; the abortion of Adam's firstborn was carried out in this way:

Adam impregnated his wife as he was commanded in Genesis 1:28. Adam failed to guard Eden as he was designated to do so in Genesis 2:15. Satan, in the guise of something like a wise-man, deceived Adam's wife into believing she lacked a certain constructive knowledge, and Adam's wife assumed falsely that she would become wise by acquiring the knowledge she was without. Adam unintentionally allowed his wife to be deceived by the Enemy. Adam's wife partook of a destructive vine without understanding that it was poisonous prior to her consumption of it, and she also gave some to her husband. Adam vomited after being poisoned with the "poison of asps… the viper's tongue" (Job 20:15-16). A wicked tongue is also called "the venom of vipers" (Psalm 140:30). Adam's wife, who was pregnant with the first human infant, miscarried on account of the venom she consumed, but she could not have known that her forbidden consumption would kill her child prior to or during her fatal choice; God's first command to humanity (Genesis 1:28) was disobeyed, and Adam's innocent son was the first human born into death. Adam planted his infant son's corpse into the ground in accordance with his designation in Genesis 2:15. In perfect justice, God punished Eve's womb (Genesis 3:16) because she unintentionally destroyed the fruit of her womb and brought forth an abortive birth by intentionally sinning. In perfect justice, the ground became cursed (Genesis 3:17) because Adam planted death into the soil. However, before God punished humanity, He prophesied the Savior (Genesis 3:15). Jesus came to earth and lived in pure innocence as The Son of *Man (Adam)* and Jesus fulfilled the whole Torah so that all who follow Him will be saved and brought to the eternal paradise: "Therefore we are **buried** with Him by baptism into death: that like as Christ was raised up from the dead by the glory of the Father, even so we also should walk in the newness of life. For if we have been **planted** together in the likeness of His death, we shall be also in the likeness of His resurrection," (Romans 6:4-5). The story of the sin in Eden was considered "indecent" by the ancient Scribes who deliberately altered and limited the Eden narrative of Genesis 2-3 and, accordingly, these deceitful Scribes (like the "serpents" of Matthew 23:33) did their best to stifle the elucidation of Christ in order to cover their own errors, hence these Scriptures: "How can you say, 'We are wise, and the law of the Lord is with us,' when, in fact, the false pen of the Scribes has made it into a lie?" (Jeremiah 8:8); "Woe to you, scribes! For you have taken away the keys of knowledge; you did not enter, and those who were entering you hindered," (Luke 11:52). Likewise, "Our sages submit, 'All the verses wherein are written indecent expressions, decent expressions are read in their stead,'" (*Introduction to the Rabbinic Bible*, Jacob Ben Chajim Ibn Adonijah; p. 51). However, what people consider indecent does not always reflect proper consideration, for "Every word of God is pure; He is a shield to those who put their trust in Him. Do not add to His words; lest He reprove you, and you be found a liar," (Proverbs 30:5-6).

Satan desired to be like God (Isaiah 14), and as such, we may recall that Jesus described Himself as a serpent in John 3:14, and Satan is referred to as a "serpent" in Genesis 3:1. Jesus described Himself as, "the bright Morning Star" in Revelation 22:1; Satan is referred to as "morning star" in Isaiah 14:12. Jesus said, "Behold, I come like a thief..." in Revelation 16:15; Jesus said of Satan, "The thief comes only to steal and kill and destroy" in John 10:10. Jesus is described as a "lion" in Revelation 5:5; Satan is described as a "lion" in I Peter 5:8.

God is entirely righteous, but Satan is entirely evil. The ancients linked violent storms, like the "typhonic" storm of Acts 27:14, to the Devil (Typhon/Leviathan/Satan), and we may observe that *Strong's Exhaustive Concordance* tells us that the word "Torah" (the first five Books of Scripture) comes from the word "ירא" or "ירה" (ref. 3384) = "to flow as water (i.e. to rain), to lay or throw (i.e. to shoot an arrow); figuratively, to point (the finger), hence, to teach"; the idea of rainwater and arrows points us to something like a storm. "Then the Lord will appear over them; His arrow will flash like lightning... He will march out in the storms of the south," (Zechariah 9:14). "The clouds overflowed with water; the atmosphere resounded; Thine arrows also issued forth; the voice of Thy thunder was in the skies; the lightnings enlightened the world; the earth trembled and shook," (Psalm 78:18-19). "The Lord also thundered in the heavens, and the Most High uttered His voice. And He sent out His arrows, and scattered them; He flashed forth lightnings, and routed them," (Psalm 18:13-14). "The Lord also shall thunder from Zion, and from Jerusalem will He utter His voice; and the heavens and the earth shall shake," (Joel 3:16). As the word "Torah" relates to a finger pointing, we should remember that the first set of 10 Commandments were written, "When all the people witnessed the thunder and lightning..." (Exodus 20:18) and "When God finished speaking with Moses on Mount Sinai, He gave him the two tablets of stone, written with the finger of God," (Exodus 31:18). Jesus said, "...'Father, glorify Your Name.' Then a voice came from Heaven, 'I have glorified it, and I will glorify it again.' The crowd that was there and heard it said it had thundered; others said an angel had spoken to Him," (John 12:24-29). "The voice of the Lord strikes with flashes of lightning," (Psalm 29:7); "Our God comes and does not keep silence, before Him is a devouring fire, and a mighty tempest all around Him," (Psalm 50:3).

In light of the sin in Eden, we may consider the *origin* of the imagery found in this passage of Scripture: "Then your covenant with death shall be annulled, and your agreement with Sheol will not stand; when the overwhelming storm passes through you will be beaten down by it. As often as it passes through, it will take you; for morning by morning it will pass through, by day and by night; and it will be sheer terror to understand the message," (Isaiah 28:18-19).

"דם" (ref. 1818) = "blood (as that which when shed causes death) of a man or animal; by analogy, the juice of the grape; figuratively bloodshed (i.e. drops of blood). Bloodshed defined sin, and in perfect justice bloodshed defined victory over sin. Consider: "one yielding purple grapes, the richest variety:- choice (-est, noble) wine =

"שרקה" (ref. 8321) = "ה+ק+ר+ש" = 5+100+200+300 = **605**; "derision, hissing" = "שרקה" (ref. 8322) = "ה+ק+ר+ש" = 5+100+200+300 = **605**; "Adam" = "אדם" (ref. 121) = "ם+ד+א" = 600+4+1 = **605**; "wealth" = "הם" (ref. 1991) = "ם+ה" = 600+5 = **605**; as man was created on Day the Sixth, "give the sixth part" = "ששה" (ref. 8341) = "ה+ש+ש" = 5+300+300 = **605**; "destroyer" = "ששה" (ref. 8154) = "ה+ש+ש" = 5+300+300 = **605**.

"Do you not know this from of old, from setting of Adam on earth? For the exultation of the wicked is but recent; the happiness of the hypocrite lasts but a moment. Though his eminence ascends to heaven and his head touches the clouds, he will perish forever like his own dung; those who had seen him will ask, 'Where is he?' He will fly away like a dream and they will not find him; he will be hustled away like a nighttime vision. The eye that beheld him will not [see him] again; [the people of] his place will not observe him again. His children must appease the poor, and his hands must make restitution for his robbery. His power filled his youth, but it will all lie with him in the dust. Even if evil is sweet in his mouth – he hides it under his tongue, he spares it, and will not leave it; yea, keeps holding it in his mouth – yet his food in his belly shall be turned; the gall of asps is within him. He swallows wealth, but vomits it; God drives it out from his belly. He shall suck the poison of asps; the viper's tongue shall slay him," (Job 20:4-16).

NOTES

THE KNOWLEDGE OF GOOD & EVIL

THE HISTORICAL COVER-UP OF THE WORD "ABORTION" IN THE BIBLE

OPENING WORDS NOTES

{1} *The Analytical Lexicon to the Greek New Testament*, Mounce; p. 303.

{2} *Strong's Exhaustive Concordance of the Bible,* Strong; p. 45; *A Greek-English Lexicon of the New Testament and other Early Christian Literature,* Danker & Bauer; p. 600.

{3} The best book I have read on Biblical numbering is *Number in Scripture* by E.W. Bullinger.

●

The Introduction to the Lamsa translation of the Peshitta version of the Holy Bible argues that Jesus and His disciples "never heard [Greek] spoken," (p. ix). Though this argument is not universally accepted, the Peshitta is certainly a treasure, and Lamsa's fluid translation and astounding scholarship are marvelous.

SECTION I
NOTES

Some considerations possibly worth examining:

a) Consider the Torah, the Law, the Books of "Moses" in light of the word "dough":

"Moses" = "מֹשֶׁה" (ref. 4872) = "ה+שׁ+מ" = 5+300+40 = **345**

"dough" = "עֲרִיסָה" (ref. 6182) = "ה+ס+י+ר+ע" = 5+60+10+200+70 = **345**

"Moses" means *"Taken out of the water."* Moses was set upon the water as a child, was raised an Egyptian, but then returned to the Hebrew people, and it may be that this facet of the number "345" formed part of Coheleth's impetus for writing, "Cast thy bread [*dough* = **345**] upon the waters [*Moses* = **345**]: for thou shalt find it after many days [*as Moses returned*]," (Ecclesiastes 11:1).

b) "Jesus" = "Ιησους" = "Ι+η+σ+ο+υ+ς" = 10+8+200+70+400+200 = 888; Genesis 2:4: "Jehovah Elohim made" = "עשות יהוה אלהים" = "ם+י+ה+ל+א+ה+ו+ה+י+ת+ו+שׁ+ע" = 40+10+5+30+1+5+6+5+10+400+6+300+70 = 888.

Consider, "חפף" (ref. 2653) = "to cover (in protection)" = "ף+פ+ח" = 800+80+8 = 888 along with this passage: "Then Moses, the servant of the Lord, died there in the land of Moab [Seed; Progeny of a Father], at the Lord's command. He was buried in a valley in the land of Moab, opposite Bethpeor [House of the Hiatus], but no one knows his burial place to this day," (Deuteronomy 34:5-6).

c) Upon one's first exposure to Gematria, one may be inclined initially to argue that Gematria shows but the symmetry of Hebrew and Greek. However, one of the major points of this book is to display how the accounts of the Bible are framed by Gematria in order to show the unity of the Text Itself. In other words, Gematria is not some entity unto itself, which is precisely why each example of Gematria displayed in this book shows parallel STORIES in Scripture, not mere parallel words. Showing parallel words can be accomplished artificially in any alphabetic system where the rules of Gematria are imposed for the purposes of Numerology and the like. The congruence of Biblical words frames Biblical stories so that history itself is understood to be constructed by the Word. If it is thought mistakenly that the words of Scripture are no different than any other system of written communication, that they have no absolute value, and that they are subject to "evolution," then there is no reason to adhere to anything said from antiquity, and a (false) concession can be made that antiquity itself has the power of erasing the accuracy of God's message – a line of thinking which was part of the temptation in Genesis 3.

d) Aeschylus (525-456 B.C.) preserved portions of the Eden story in his play *The Suppliant Maidens*. Furthermore, the myth of Io discusses the alteration concerning the indentification of the first constellation in the celestial "scroll" (Zodiac/Mazzaroth), i.e. the false change from Virgo to Taurus regarding the beginning of the Zodiac.

b) Both Adam and his son Cain were workers of the soil (Adam – Genesis 2:15; Cain – Genesis 4:2). When Cain deliberately killed his brother Able in full knowledge of his own deeds, Cain was personally cursed and told by God, "When you till the ground, it shall no more yield to you its strength..." (Genesis 4:12) and "...Cain went out from the presence of the Lord, and dwelt in the land of *Nod* [*Wandering*], on the **east** of Eden," (Genesis 4:16). When Adam deliberately sinned regarding his ignorance, he was not personally cursed, but the ground was cursed instead, and the ground continued to yield its strength to Adam, though Adam had to exert a punishing strain to obtain the fruits of his labors; Adam was also driven away from Eden, and guardians were placed "...at the **east** of the Garden of Eden..." (Genesis 3:24). It is important to note that both Adam and Cain (*tillers of the earth*) were condemned to endure punishments regarding earth's *soil*, and both were driven in the direction of the **rising sun**. "Therefore we are *buried* with Him by baptism into death: that like as Christ was **raised up** from the dead by the glory of the Father, even so we also should walk in the newness of life. For if we have been *planted* together in the likeness of His *death*, we shall be also in the likeness of His **resurrection**," (Romans 6:4-5).

SECTION II
NOTES

{1} Dr. Bullinger wrote that, "Whatever the modern meanings of such symbols as I.H.S. may be given, the fact remains that it was part of the name of Bacchus: and, the letters I.N.R.I., which were changed by Rome into Iesus Nazarenus Rex Judaeorum (Jesus of Nazareth King of the Jews), originally formed the pagan symbol that by fire nature will be renewed in its entirety (*Igne Natura Renovetut Integra*). See *The Rosicrucians: their Rites and Mysteries*, by Hargrave Jennings (Vol. ii. 1887), quoted by the authors of *The Computation of 666* (p. 70, published by James Nisbet)," in his book *Commentary on Revelation* (Bullinger; p. 396).

{2} "Wisdom" is personified in the Proverbs, and she says, "Come, eat of my bread and drink of the wine I have mixed," (Proverbs 9:5). On the other hand, folly's grasp on fools presents a seemingly impossible situation: "Do not answer fools according to their folly, or you will be a fool yourself. Answer fools according to their folly, or they will be wise in their own eyes," (Proverbs 26:4-5); in a parallel way, Jesus presented a ludicrous situation when He said, "For John came neither *eating nor drinking*, and they say, 'He has a demon'; the Son of Man came *eating and drinking*, and they say, 'Look, a glutton and a drunkard, a friend of tax collectors and sinners!' Yet *wisdom* is vindicated by Her deeds," (Matthew 11:18-19).

By using examples of literal consumption, a point about wisdom and folly was made.

{3} "Now the only entrance into Egypt is by this desert: the country from Phoenicia to the borders of the city Cadytis belongs to the people called the Palestine Syrians; from Cadytis, which it appears to me is a city almost as large as Sardis, the marts upon the coast till you reach Jenysus are the Arabian king's; after Jenysus the Syrians again come in, and extend to Lake Serbonis, near the place where Mount Casius juts out into the sea. At Lake Serbonis, where the tale goes that Typhon hid himself, Egypt begins. Now the whole tract between Jenysus on the one side, and Lake Serbonis and Mount Casius on the other, and this is no small space, being as much as three days' journey, is a dry desert without a drop of water," (*Thalia*, Herodotus; Section 5).

{4} "We have already observed elsewhere, that there stood by the reader of Law and the Prophets in the synagogues an interpreter, that was wont to render what was read to the people in the Hebrew into their own language, and that it was a very usual thing for those interpreters to expatiate, and, by way of comment, to preach upon the words that had been read... a thing also observable in the Chaldee paraphrasts," (*Commentary on the New Testament from the Talmud and Hebraica*, Lightfoot, Vol. 4; p. 155).

According to Dr. Lightfoot, the leadership of the Synagogue was structured as follows:

1) The Magistracy or "The Bench of Three" (referred to as The Rulers of the Synagogue) who judged financial matters, moral actions, the admission of proselytes, etc.
2) The *Angel* of Ecclesia [*Messenger* of the Church], who prayed publicly and managed the Scripture reading of the Synagogue by appointing readers.
3) The Deacons, who regarded the poor and collected alms.
4) The Interpreter, skilled in tongues, who stood by the reader of the Hebrew Scriptures and orally rendered the Hebrew Scriptures into the tongue of the attendees, passage by passage.
5) (Assumedly) the Master of the Divinity School and his interpreter.

Compare these designations to the Spiritual Gifts of I Corinthians 12:

"To one is given, through the Spirit, the utterance of wisdom," (v. 8) – like The Magistracy; "and to another the utterance of knowledge," (v. 9) – like the Master of the Divinity School; "...to another various kinds of tongues, to another the interpretation of tongues," (v. 11) – like a selected reader in the Synagogue who read the divine Hebrew Scriptures, and his Interpreter who interpreted and translated the divine Hebrew into the common language of the congregation when listening to these divine Words – all under the direction of the Angel of Ecclesia.

{5}   "It was not unusual for a master to kiss his disciple; but for a disciple kiss his master was more rare.

Whether or not [Judas] did this under pretence of respect, or out of open contempt and derision, let it be inquired," (*Commentary on the New Testament from the Talmud and Hebraica,* Lightfoot. Vol. 2, p. 357).

{6}   Can anyone possibly believe that the Jews of Jesus' earthly days were taught in the Synagogue by talking snakes that crawled on the floor, slithered on scales, and hissed with actual FORKED tongues? – for many of the elites of Jesus' earthly days were called "vipers" and if such a description is taken without respect to the context in which it was given, then we can conclude that these men were actually talking snakes... "Either make the TREE good, and its fruit good; or make the tree bad, and its fruit bad; for the tree is known by its fruit. You brood of vipers! How can you speak good things, when you are evil? For out of the abundance of the heart the mouth speaks. The good person brings good things out of a good treasure, and the evil person brings evil things out of an evil treasure. I tell you, on the day of judgment you will have to give an account of for every careless *word* you utter; for by your words you will be justified, and by your words you will be condemned," (Matthew 12:33-37). The Hebrew letter "צ" (which is also "ץ") signifies a "FORK" and a "TREE": "Deacons likewise must be serious, not DOUBLE-TONGUED..." (I Timothy 3:8): consider one who is FORK-TONUGED as in ץ. In the same way, can it be possible that Eve actually had converse with a talking snake? It is beneficial to note that Joseph was renamed "Zaphnath-paaneah" by Pharaoh in Genesis 41:45 which means "of food for the living" or "abundance of life"; "The thief comes only to steal and kill and destroy. I came that they may have life, and have it abundantly," (John 10:10).

{7} "The relations between 595 years and 1,262 years 36 days, are the same as the relations between 594 years and 1,260 years. The difference of the 2 years 36 days is due to the excess of the 10.96 days over the 18 completed years in each *Saros*," (*Witness of the Stars*, Bullinger; p. 181).

●

Some considerations possibly worth examining:

    b)   "The Massorah points out that the word Ariel occurs thee times, in [2 Sam. xxiii.20] and Isa. xxix. 1. In Isa. the word is twice transliterated as a proper name, while in 2 Sam. xxiii. 20, margin, it is translated *lions of God*: the first part of the word ירא (*aree*) *a lion*, and the second part אל (*el*) *God*. But if we keep it uniformly and consistently as a proper name we have with the *Ellipsis* of the nominative (*sons*) the following sense: "He slew the two *sons* of Ariel of Moab," (*Figures of Speech Used in the Bible*, Bullinger; p. 5).

SECTION III
NOTES

{1}   "'If a man plants one row of five vines,' the school of Shammai saith, 'That is a vineyard,'" (*Commentary on the New Testament from the Talmud and Hebraica*, Lightfoot; Vol. 2, p. 433).

"Misled by tradition and the ignorance of mediaeval painters, it is the general belief that only two were crucified with the Lord. But Scripture does not say so. It states that there were two 'thieves' (Gr. *lestai* = robbers, Matt. 27:38. Mark 15:27); and that there were two malefactors' (Gr. *kakourgoi,* Luke 23:32).

"It is also recorded that both the robbers reviled Him (Matt. 27:44, Mark 15:32); while in Luke 23:39 only one the malefactors 'railed on Him,' and 'the other rebuked him' for so doing (v. 40). If there were only two, this is a real discrepancy; and there is another, for the two malefactors were 'led with Him to be put to death' (Luke 23:32), and when they were come to Calvary, 'they' then and there 'crucified Him and the malefactors, one on the right hand and the other on the left' (v. 33).

"But the other discrepancy is, according to Matthew, that after the parting of the garments, and after 'sitting down they watched Him there,' that 'THEN were there two robbers crucified with Him, one on the right hand and the other on the left,' (Matt. 27:38. Mark 15:27). The two malefactors had already been 'led with Him' and were therefore crucified 'with Him,' before the dividing of the garments, and before the two robbers were brought.

"The first two (malefactors) who were 'led with Him' were placed on either side. When the other two (robbers) were brought, much later, they were also similarly placed; so that there were two (one of each) on either side, and the Lord in the midst. The malefactors were therefore nearer, and being on the inside they could speak to each other better, and the one with the Lord, as recorded (Luke 23:39-43).

"John's record confirms this for he speaks only of place, and not of time. He speaks, generally of the fact: 'where they crucified Him, and with Him others, two on this side, and that side, and Jesus in the midst,' (John 19:8). In Rev. 22:2 we have the same expression in the Greek (*enteuthen kai enteuthen*), which is accurately rendered, 'on either side.' So it should be rendered here: 'and with Him others, on either side.'

"But John further states (19:32,33): 'then came the soldiers to brake the legs of the first, and of the other which was crucified with Him. But when they came (Gr. = having come) to Jesus, and saw that He was dead already, they brake not His legs.' Had there been only two (on either side) the soldiers would not have come to the Lord, but would have passed Him, and then turned back again. But they came to Him after they had broken the legs of the first two. There are two words used of the 'other' and 'others' in John 19:32 and Luke 23:32... In the former passage we read, 'they brake the legs of the first and of the other.' Here the Greek is also, which is the other (the second) of the two when there are more (see Matt. 10:23; 25:16,17,20; 27:61; 28:1. John 18:15,16; 20:2,4,8, and Rev. 17:10

"In the latter passage (Luke 23:32) the word is *heteros* = different... 'and others also, two, were being led with Him.' These were different from Him with Whom they were led, not different from one another; for they were 'in the same condemnation,' and 'justly,' while He had 'done nothing amiss' (vv. 40,41).

"From this evidence, therefore, it is clear that there were four 'others' crucified with the Lord; and thus, on the one hand, there are no 'discrepancies,' as alleged; while, on the other hand, every word and every expression, in the Greek, gets (and gives) its own exact value, and its full significance.

"To show that we are not without evidence, even from tradition, we may state that there is a 'Calvary' to be seen at Ploubezere near Lannion, in the Cotes-du-Nord, Brittany, know as *Les Cinq Croix* ('The Five Crosses'). There is a high cross in the center, with four lower ones, two on either side. There may be other instances which we have not heard," (*Companion Bible*, Bullinger; Appendix 164).

As Abram had the letter/number "5" added to his name (Abra-H-am), we have also read how his personal history parallels a vine. The number 5 is often used to signify "Divine Grace" in the Scriptures, a fact that is most befitting in the crucifixion account. However, Christ completed the mission of redemption, and it may be that the crucifixion account is told respectively in a manner that at first glance appears to indicate three people, probably because the letter/number "3" indicates "completeness" (as a number) and "firstborn" (as a letter). As Christ was the "True Vine" in light of the five crosses of the crucifixion, "If a man plants one row of five vines,' the school of Shammai saith, 'That is a vineyard,'" (*Commentary on the New Testament from the Talmud and Hebraica,* Lightfoot; Vol. 2, p. 433). Regardless of how the crucifixion took place as to the arrangement of the crosses specifically, it is interesting to consider the constitutions of ancient vineyards in relation to the story of Salvation.

•

Some considerations possibly worth examining:

a) "And out of the ground made the Jehovah Elohim to grow every tree that is *pleasant* [נחמד] to the sight, and good for food; the Tree of Life also in the midst of the garden, and the Tree of the Knowledge of Good and Evil," (Genesis 2:9). It cannot be that God planted the Tree of the Knowledge of Good and Evil, for He made "every tree that was pleasant to the sight **and good for food**," but the Tree of the Knowledge of Good and Evil was certainly **not good for food**. Furthermore, Genesis 2:9 states that every tree that God made was *pleasant* [נחמד (ref. **2530**)] to the sight, but the forbidden "tree" described in Genesis

3:6 was *pleasant* [תאוה (ref. **8378**)] to the eyes – and the reader will notice that the two words rendered *"pleasant"* are NOT THE SAME. When Genesis 3:6 states that the ambiguous "tree" was "desireable to make one wise," the word *desireable* is the same as the word *pleasant* in Genesis 2:9. Since Proverbs 3:18 describes Wisdom as a "tree of life" that gives "long life," we can understand why God prohibited the humans from eating of the Tree of Life after they had sinned (Genesis 3:22); the forbidden tree shortened life. In Genesis 3:6, first and third description of "the tree" describes the Tree of Life, and knowing that the vine coiled around it was the Tree of the Knowledge of Good and Evil, the second description of "the tree" applies to that which was forbidden.

These facts can seen by knowing that every tree God made was good for food (therefore the forbidden tree could not have been planted by God), every tree that God made was

"pleasant [נחמד (ref. **2530**)] to the SIGHT," (Genesis 2:9),

but the tree that Satan planted was

"pleasant [תאוה (ref. **8378**)] to the EYES," (Genesis 3:6).

Knowing that sin brings death and that righteousness brings life, we may grasp the fact that every tree God made was "pleasant [נחמד (ref. 2530)] to the SIGHT," (Genesis 2:9) and that the Tree of Life was "pleasant [נחמד (ref. 2530)] to make one wise," (Genesis 3:6) – thus, "The wise man's eyes are in his head…" (Ecclesiastes 2:4). The mirrored deception of Satan is evident in the fact that the Tree of Life was "desireable להשכיל to make one wise [ref. 7919]," (Genesis 3:6) but the Tree of the Knowledge of Good and Evil ["להשכיל" (ref. 7921)] bereaved the woman of her child (Genesis 3:6), hence the word-play – for despite shifting mirrored perspectives from good to evil, the 2/3 (.666 repeating) ultimately remains consistent with both, as only the Tree of Life was "good for food." Such a truth is exhibited in Jesus' parable in Matthew 13:24-30 concerning the plants that "an enemy" planted. Since only the Creator can create, seedless plants can be made by a manipulation of nature. In other words, Satan cannot "create," but he can fashion. We cannot "create," but we can construct. Satan could have manipulated nature and produced a seedless, poisonous vine through scientific means motivated by unwholesome purposes with methods similar to the production of seedless fruit today. Anyone who has eaten a seedless watermelon understands how simple such a manipulation of nature is.

b) A non-viable infant (an "abortion" or an "untimely birth") was called a "נפל" = "**nay-fel**" in Hebrew. Eve "saw that the tree was... desirable to make one wise..." (Genesis 3:6), and this word "to make one wise" is from "שכל" = "**circumspect**, intelligent" which was then written without vowels, as these same letters also spell "שכל" = "*to suffer abortion.*" It is interesting to note that Adam's **nay-fel** (Hebrew) was killed accidentally by his parents amidst their desire to become *circumspect* in light of the fact that the word νηφαλεος (Greek) means "sober, i.e. **circumspect**" and is pronounced "**nay-fal**-eh-os." Perhaps we may gain insight as to why the ancient Scribes read the words "to make wise" exclusively with regard to Genesis 3:6 in order to forward their euphemized traditions – for eating of the forbidden tree was not wise at all. The mandate of sobriety in spirituality was advanced in like manner regarding the similarity of sounds between Hebrew and Greek when Paul said in Ephesians 5:18-19, "Do not be *drunk* [*Hebrew:* **nooma**] with *wine*, for that is debauchery; but be filled with the *Spirit* [*Greek:* **Pnoo-ma**]."

The Knowledge of Good and Evil

All credit, glory, and honor belong to God Almighty, and I thank Him for allowing me to research this topic and to write this book.

Printed in the United States
209141BV00005B/14/P